126853

D1492478

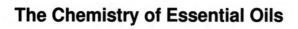

The Chemistry of Essential Oils

The Chemistry of Essential Oils

An Introduction for Aromatherapists, Beauticians,
Retailers and Students

David G. Williams

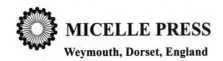

MICELLE PRESS
Weymouth, Dorset, England

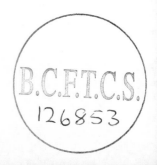

First published 1996. Reprinted with corrections 1997

A catalogue record for this book is available from the British Library

ISBN: 1-870228-12-X

Published by
Micelle Press, 10-12 Ullswater Crescent, Weymouth, Dorset DT3 5HE, England

http://www.wdi.co.uk/micelle

Cover design by Slade Design & Marketing

Printed and bound in Great Britain by Redwood Books, Trowbridge, Wiltshire

To my Wife

Contents

Acknowledgements

Thanks to:

R.C Treatt Limited for the supply of the chromatograms of essential oils and for identifying the named constituents.

Norfolk Lavender Limited for the use of the photograph of lavender on the cover.

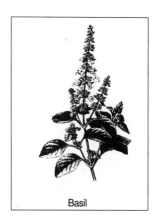

Basil

Foreword

The practice of aromatherapy as a generally available form of health care is of comparatively recent emergence in Britain. Involving, as it does, the use of essential oils from plant sources as therapeutic agents, aromatherapy demands of practitioners sound knowledge of human anatomy and physiology, and of the composition and properties of essential oils.

The purpose of this book is to bring to students of aromatherapy and beauty therapy a foundation of knowledge of the composition and physicochemical properties of essential oils which may be used as a basis for further study.

Aromatherapy shares common ground with perfumery in the use of essential oils, albeit for different purposes and, more closely, in the practice of aromachology. It was these relationships which prompted the inclusion of the chapters on perfumery, which it is hoped will also encourage readers to explore the pathways of the subject in greater depth.

The book is addressed also to practising aromatherapists and beauticians and to retailers of essential oils seeking to extend their knowledge into the areas of essential oil composition and perfumery, to students in the sixth forms of schools and in college and university, to life-long students whose thirst for knowledge can never be wholly satisfied, and to those who find hope for the future and solace in the study of subjects of unlimited interest and practical value.

David G. Williams
Eltham, London (June, 1996)

Safety Note

It is recommended that when working with aromatic materials and chemicals of all kinds, both appropriate eye protection and skin protection (i.e. suitable protective gloves) should be worn.

Chapter 1

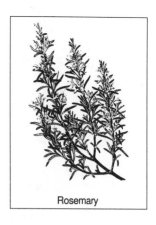

Rosemary

Some Basic Chemistry

1.1 The Nature and Purpose of Chemistry

Chemistry is the study of the composition and properties of matter, which comprises the solids, liquids and gases of the physical world, and of the changes of composition that matter can undergo.

Everyday living brings us into contact with many different varieties of matter: the air we breathe, with its vital 20% of oxygen, water and other foodstuffs, garden soil, the materials of buildings, forms of transport, living things, medicinal, personal-care and household products of almost endless variety. Some of these materials are apparently of uniform composition; water, for example, looks much the same from whatever domestic tap it is drawn, and filtered seawater appears little different, whereas even a casual glance at garden soil reveals the presence of several, individual materials which are seemingly of different composition.

But appearances can be deceptive, and on closer examination similar materials may turn out to be quite different from one another. Tap waters in different parts of the country do not have the same taste, while sea-water is intensely salty, and rather bitter as well. By simply allowing saucers of tap water and seawater to evaporate in a warm place, further and very clear evidence of their difference soon becomes apparent, as colourless crystals slowly form and grow in the seawater, but not in water from a domestic supply. If the two waters are allowed to evaporate completely, a hand lens will reveal a slight, chalky deposit in the tap water saucer if the water was 'hard', but not if it was 'soft', whereas the seawater saucer will contain a residue of colourless, glittering crystals. Quite evidently, seawater contains very much more dissolved matter than tap water.

Without some use of chemistry, this is about as far as we could hope to go with a comparative investigation of tap and seawaters.

Using chemistry, however, very much more becomes possible. We could, for example, take small samples of the seawater, also of the crystals deposited from it at different stages during evaporation, and by observing the results of simple tests deduce important facts as, for example, the presence of sodium, magnesium and calcium as their sulphates, chlorides and bromides; a fascinating and instructive series of experiments.

Information of this kind is known as *qualitative* information; it states *what* is present in a material but not *how much* there is of whatever is present, which is called *quantitative* information: the difference between saying that a cake contains sugar and that it contains 15% of sugar. Quantitative information on the composition of a material can be obtained also by the use of chemical techniques.

The investigation of the composition of seawater is an example of *analysis*, meaning 'taking apart'. The opposite of analysis is *synthesis* — 'putting together'. Chemical synthesis is any process in which more complex molecules are formed from simpler ones. Analysis and synthesis are the two main practical aspects of chemical science.

1.2 Photosynthesis and Respiration in Green Plants

Chemical synthesis occurs naturally in the leaves of green plants as the process of *photosynthesis*, i.e. synthesis mediated by light. It is the process by which green plants manufacture the food they need for growth and reproduction. When the plant is illuminated, carbon dioxide, diffusing naturally from the surrounding air into the leaf tissue via minute pores, or stomata, interacts with water, absorbed by the root system of the plant from the soil in which it rests, to form the sugar *glucose*. Like all other synthetic processes, photosynthesis can occur only under certain conditions, which are in this case as follows:

a) a supply of energy, in the form of light in the red region of the solar spectrum (leaves reflect the other colours of the spectrum, and so are green);

b) the presence, in structures known as *chloroplasts* (Greek: *chloros*: green) of the green, magnesium-containing pigment chlorophyll, which acts as a catalyst for the reaction;

c) a cool temperature, maintained by the evaporation of water from the leaves through the stomata — the process of *transpiration*.

During photosynthesis, the hydrogen and oxygen atoms of six molecules of water and the carbon and oxygen atoms of six molecules of carbon dioxide become rearranged to form a single molecule of glucose and six molecules of oxygen. Biochemists, who study the chemistry of living cells, represent photosynthesis in the form of an equation, as follows:

$$6\,CO_2\ (g)\ +\ 6\,H_2O\ (l)\ +\ \text{energy from} \longrightarrow\ C_6H_{12}O_6\ (aq)\ +\ 6\,O_2\ (g)$$
$$\text{sunlight}$$

6 mols	6 mols		1 mol	6 mols
Carbon dioxide	Water		Glucose	Oxygen

Glucose dissolves in water, and as it forms in the leaves most of it is distributed, in solution, to all other living parts of the plant through conducting vessels. In the leaves and elsewhere in the plant glucose is used for many purposes, among which is the process of *respiration*. Respiration amounts to almost the reverse of photosynthesis, in that glucose is oxidized by oxygen to form carbon dioxide and water:

$$C_6H_{12}O_6\ (aq)\ +\ 6\,O_2\ (g) \longrightarrow\ 6\,CO_2\ (g)\ +\ 6\,H_2O\ (l)\ +\ \text{energy}$$

The letters enclosed in brackets following formulae for the reacting substances or reaction products are state symbols, expressing their physical state or condition:

(l) = liquid; (g) = gas; (aq) = dissolved in water

The energy produced by this reaction, which is a form of low-temperature combustion, takes the form not of light, but of *chemical potential energy* — energy which is *available* when required, provided the conditions for its release are right. An analogy, here, though a very much more violent one, is the potential energy contained in an explosive, which is released when the material experiences detonation. Until released, the energy of an explosive is locked up in its molecules, as energy is locked up in a structure such as an old chimney stack before it crashes to the ground.

The chemical energy of respiration is used to synthesize complex molecules (organic phosphates) which hold the energy used for their construction until it is required, whereupon it is released for the building of other molecules necessary to the growth and development of the plant. Thus glucose, synthesized with the energy of sunlight, transmits the chemical energy it contains to organic phosphates, which yield it wherever needed to sustain the life processes of the plant.

Glucose not used for respiration takes part in the formation of the proteins of protoplasm. This requires a supply of nitrogen, contained in the nitrates present in absorbed soil water. It is used also for a process of polymerization, the joining together of smaller molecules of the same kind to form larger molecules, yielding starch in the form of water-insoluble grains which lodge wherever they are formed. Starch, familiar in cereals and potatoes, acts as a reserve of food for the plant, as, when necessary, it is depolymerized to re-form glucose.

The leaves of green plants perform the vital function of maintaining the content of oxygen in the earth's atmosphere, since during the hours of daylight most of it produced by photosynthesis diffuses out of the leaves into the air, in the opposite direction to the inward diffusion of carbon dioxide. At night, when photosynthesis cannot take place except under artificial light, the energy requirements of the plant are met by the oxidation of glucose produced by the depolymerization of starch, with the formation of carbon dioxide as a waste product.

1.3 Essential Oils from Plant Sources

Parts of many plants are odorous as a result of their content of essential oils. Because, once produced, an essential oil is either released, as from a fragrant flower, or is stored by a plant until it eventually evaporates or deteriorates when the plant dies, it is regarded as an end-product of the metabolism of the plant.

The essential oil of an aromatic plant is stored in oil cells, glands or vessels and is in most instances of extremely complex composition, consisting of hundreds of different constituents. The fragrance of a scented flower is given by the vapour of an essential oil, released from specialized oil glands, the purpose of which is not to delight our senses, but to attract pollinating insects. Essential oils produced by plants which give fragrance when stroked, such as the mints, may in this way use the oil to deter hungry herbivorous animals, whose noses will give warning of the proximity of inedible leaves.

Essential oils stored in the heartwood of oil-bearing trees, such as those of Cedarwood, Rosewood and Sandalwood, may act to preserve the integrity of the trunk against the ravages of microorganisms and insects, so maintaining the leaves at a height sufficient to receive maximum sunlight; those present in aromatic plant exudates may function to kill pathogenic micro-organisms. Examples, here, are the exudates known as Gum Benzoin (really an oleoresin), Myrrh and Olibanum (Frankincense). These are produced at a very slow rate naturally, but in very much larger amounts if the bark is wounded, to seal off the living, girth-increasing and conducting tissues beneath, which perform functions vital to the continued life of the plant.

Aromatic plants and the essential oils that they contain have long found extensive use in medicine and pharmacy, perfumery and flavouring, and are the subject of continuing and increasingly penetrating research to elucidate their composition, with particular interest being centred upon the discovery of novel constituents. The essential oils of aromatherapy are those of proven value for the relief of stress-related and certain other conditions amenable to this form of alternative and supportive, holistic medicine, and which are harmless as recommended for use by professionally trained and fully experienced aromatherapists. In aromachology, certain essential oils are smelled for the purpose of transforming negative mood states, such as depression, into positive mood states, such as happiness and normal physical appetite.

Essential oils in regular use in the perfume and flavour industries, which are the main consumers of these products, number no more than about two hundred, with perhaps a further one hundred well-known but 'rare' or 'unusual' oils available when required.

Essential oils are the subject of continuing research for analytical purposes, and yield valuable information to scientists working in this field. Most of them remain of academic, rather than commercial, value, since to be of commercial interest an essential oil must offer properties of importance to end-users for their novel odour, flavour or medicinal properties, to the extent that demand will support the growing and processing of crops.

Users of essential oils demand guarantees of unfailing supplies within reasonable limits of certainty. An essential oil of outstandingly novel fragrance or flavour interest cannot be used to boost the competitive position of a manufacturer if supplies of the oil are likely to fail, as it is likely to be an irreplaceable ingredient of those formulations in which it appears. The wanton destruction of earth's natural resources renders the gathering and investigation of plants unknown to science an urgent necessity, before constituents of possibly great value are lost for the foreseeable future. The development of genetic engineering into a technology capable of regenerating lost species no doubt lies far in the future.

1.4 Atoms, Molecules and Ions

For many years the evidence has been overwhelming that the different forms, or states, of matter, solids, liquids and gases, are 'grainy'; that is, that they consist of minute particles, separated by empty space. The Greek philosopher Democritus, who lived from about 460 to 370 B.C., put forward the suggestion that matter is composed of individual particles, but this idea was rejected by Aristotle who, with Plato, held that substances consisted of different proportions of the four, ancient elements: earth, air, fire and water. Those Greeks who believed in the ideas of Democritus referred to the supposed particles of matter as *atomos*, meaning *indivisible*, a term from which the modern word *atom* is derived. Plato and Aristotle, however, would not accept the hypothesis of Democritus, and since Greek scientists of this era were devout followers of the doctrine of Aristotle, the notion of the existence of atoms fell by the wayside. Even if the possibility of the existence of atoms had at that time been given serious consideration, any hope of settling the issue of their reality was quite beyond possibility in those ancient times.

The atomic hypothesis was revived at the turn of the nineteenth century, by the famous British chemist John Dalton, who wrote a book of two volumes entitled *A New System of Chemical Philosophy*.

By this time, chemists had abandoned the four 'elements' of the ancients, and had established that there were certain substances, such as oxygen, hydrogen, sulphur, phosphorus, iron and copper, which could not be decomposed into simpler substances by any chemical process. These substances were, therefore, true elements, which could combine with one another to form compounds. In Part 2 of Dalton's book, published in 1810, the author set forth his views in a series of statements which we can summarize as follows:

Dalton's atomic theory

Matter is composed of minute particles (atoms) which can neither be created from nor divided into smaller particles. All atoms of any given element are identical in weight and properties, but are different from the atoms of other elements. When elements combine to form compounds, small whole numbers of atoms of the elements involved combine to form 'compound atoms' (molecules). All molecules of a given compound are identical.

It was to be nearly a century before firm evidence of the existence of atoms began to accumulate.

One of the many forms of experimental proof that matter consists of particles is the behaviour of X-rays, discovered by Wilhelm Röntgen in November 1895, when directed onto a crystalline substance, such as ordinary salt. The rays are reflected, forming a pattern which can be photographed using special film. It can be shown that such a pattern could be formed only by the scattering, or diffraction, of the rays from minute particles, arranged in the case of common salt in a cubic pattern. The fact that a strong solution of salt deposits cubic crystals if allowed to evaporate gives visible evidence of the arrangement of the particles of which it is composed. Supporting proof of the minute structure of crystals is provided by X-ray diffraction and crystallization experiments on other crystalline substances.

An atom

An *atom* is defined as *the smallest particle of an element which can exist*.

Some idea of the size of an atom can be gained from the fact that an ordinary metal milk bottle top is composed of about three thousand five hundred million million million (3·5 sextillion, or $3·5 \times 10^{21}$) atoms of the element aluminium.

An element

An *element* may be defined as *a substance consisting of chemically identical atoms*.

The number of known elements stands currently at 107, of which some 30 are commonly encountered either as the elements or as compounds with other elements.

A molecule

A *molecule* is *the smallest particle of an element or compound which can exist alone.*

Most metals are capable of existing as single atoms, although in any quantity of a solid metal the atoms of which it is composed are bonded together by strong attractive forces, balanced by repulsive forces, between adjacent atoms. Something of the great strength of these interatomic forces may be demonstrated by trying to pull apart or compress an iron nail — the former experiment difficult, though not impossible given the right equipment, the latter impossible by normal means.

A compound

A *compound* is a substance consisting of elements combined together in fixed and definite proportions by weight.

Some, but by no means all, compounds exist as molecules. A familiar example is carbon dioxide, commonly called by its chemical formula 'CO_2', a form of shorthand expressing the composition of molecules of the gas, as one atom of carbon combined with two of oxygen. We have met the molecular compound glucose when discussing photosynthesis and respiration.

Water is a poor conductor of electricity. If glucose is dissolved in water the solution is about as poor a conductor of electricity as pure water. If, however, common salt is dissolved in water, the conductivity of the water is greatly improved, for the reason that salt, unlike glucose, consists not of molecules, but of electrically charged atoms of sodium and chlorine called *ions*.

An ion

An *ion* is *an electrically charged atom, or group of atoms.*

Common salt, sodium chloride, is a typical ionic compound, formula Na^+Cl^-. A crystal of salt is composed of aggregates of equal numbers of sodium and chloride ions. When salt is dissolved in water, the ions disperse in the water freely, and because they are mobile are able to carry currents of electricity. Since in any quantity of sodium chloride the numbers of positive and negative charges are equal, and since the strength of the positive charge on a sodium ion is equal and opposite to the charge on a chloride ion, the compound is electrically neutral and we can handle it without fear of electric shock.

1.5 Chemical Symbols and Formulae

In English and many other languages, letters or other symbols are used to express the consonants and vowels which are the elements of speech; letters written together, or combined, produce words having meaning ascribed to them by general agreement. In a similar way, letters are used in chemistry as symbols representing atoms of the chemical elements. Symbols for elements (each consisting of one or two, or in a few cases three, letters) when written close together, express the formulae of compounds. Table 1.1 gives the names of some common elements, together with their symbols, each of which stands for one atom of the respective element.

There are several things to notice about the table:

1. The symbols for copper, iron and sodium are derived from the old Latin names for these elements.
2. The names and symbols in heavy type refer to those elements which are of particular importance to our studies of the chemistry of essential oils.
3. Most nonmetallic elements do not occur naturally as single atoms, but exist normally as molecules consisting of two or more atoms combined (polyatomic molecules). However, the atoms of these elements can exist singly in the molecules of compounds.

Table 1.1 — Symbols and formulae of common elements

Name of element	Symbol representing one atom	Symbol or formula for one molecule of the element*
Calcium	Ca	Ca
Carbon	**C**	**C**
Chlorine	Cl	Cl_2
Copper (*Cuprum*)	Cu	Cu
Hydrogen	**H**	$\mathbf{H_2}$
Iodine	I	I_2
Iron (*Ferrum*)	Fe	Fe
Nitrogen	**N**	$\mathbf{N_2}$
Oxygen	**O**	$\mathbf{O_2}$
Phosphorus	P	P_4
Sodium (Natrium)	Na	Na
Sulphur	**S**	$\mathbf{S_8}$

*N.B. The molecules of metals and of the ordinary forms of carbon consist of single atoms, which are the smallest particles of these elements that can exist alone, as further explained in paragraph 4, below.

4. Single atoms of carbon can exist, but any quantity of carbon, in the form of a single mass of either diamond or graphite, consists of carbon atoms bonded together. A faultless diamond of one carat, weighing 0·2 gram, is a single molecule consist-

ing approximately of ten sextillion (10^{22}, or 10,000,000,000,000,000,000,000) atoms of carbon.

5. The letters of symbols consisting of two or three letters are inseparable, as the letters of multi-letter words are inseparable. Thus Ca represents one atom of calcium. Notice that the second letter of a two-letter symbol is always lower case.

The formula for one compound, water, is widely known as H_2O. This formula represents one molecule of water (hydrogen monoxide, or di-hydrogen oxide) consisting of two atoms of hydrogen and one of oxygen bonded together. Chemical symbols written close together always mean that the atoms of the elements represented are bonded together to form molecules, or ion-aggregates, of a compound. It is very important to note that the elements present in the combined state in a compound, though not losing their identity, do not possess the properties they had in the uncombined state.

In this book we are concerned mainly with molecules, not ion-aggregates, and so it will be helpful if we now make a statement about the properties of molecules.

Properties of molecules

The properties of a molecule depend on the nature, number and arrangement of the atoms of the elements of which it is composed; and taking a further step, *the properties of a molecular compound depend on the nature, number, arrangement and positions in space of the atoms in its molecules.*

Notice, in the formula H_2O, the absence of a numerical suffix to the symbol 'O'. The formula for water could be written H_2O_1, but it never is, because a symbol lacking a numerical suffix is understood to represent one atom only of the corresponding element.

The formula H_2O represents the composition of *all* water molecules, an example of the general principle that *all molecules of the same, pure compound are chemically identical.*

Most samples of compounds, including water, are not chemically pure, but are purified to conform to specifications of purity which ensure their suitability and safety for the purposes for which they are to be used. For example, the richly fragrant Dark Muscovado Sugar, used for making irresistible fruit cakes and succulent Christmas puddings, contains about 89·3% of sucrose, whereas Pure Cane Sugar is stated to be 100·0% pure, meaning that its content of impurities is so low as to be negligible — it is almost chemically pure, i.e. within the very low levels of permissible impurities, it consists of identical molecules of sucrose. Demerara Sugar contains about 95·4% sucrose.

All of these products, as packed by the manufacturers, are completely acceptable grades of sugar, the brown varieties of which contain natural and necessary flavour substances which are absent from white sugar. All are purified to strict standards of purity, so that it is true to say that they are *pure food products*, but it is equally true that of these products only Pure Cane Sugar is *chemically* pure. An essential oil, consisting, as all essential oils do, of many different constituents, cannot possibly be *chemically* pure; it can, however, be of high *odour* purity, *in reference to the odour of a sample of the same essential oil kept as an odour standard.* We shall return to the subject of the purity of essential oils later in this book.

Table 1.2 includes molecular compounds which we have already mentioned, together with some further examples. We have, with limonene and linalöl, introduced here two very common constituents of essential oils, representative of the two main classes of constituents of essential oils: i) terpenes, and ii) oxygenates, respectively, to which we shall return in Chapters 2 and 3.

Table 1.2 — Symbols and formulae of some molecular compounds

Name of compound	Formula for one molecule	Notes
Carbon dioxide	CO_2	Colourless, odourless, nonflammable gas.
Water	H_2O	Colourless, odourless liquid, blue in deep layers.
Ammonia	NH_3	Extremely pungent-smelling, colourless, alkali-forming gas.
Hydrogen sulphide	H_2S	Colourless, toxic gas, with an odour of rotten eggs.
Sulphur dioxide	SO_2	Colourless, asphyxiating, acid-forming gas. Partly responsible for 'acid rain'.
Nitrogen dioxide	NO_2	Brown, acid-forming gas. Common atmospheric pollutant from motor vehicle exhaust fumes.
Methane	CH_4	Forms the bulk of North Sea gas.
Alcohol (Ethanol)	C_2H_6O	The alcohol of alcoholic beverages. Widely used as a solvent for perfumes.
Glucose	$C_6H_{12}O_6$	A sugar: organic product of photosynthesis.
Sucrose	$C_{12}H_{22}O_{11}$	The sugar obtained from sugar cane or sugar beet.
Limonene	$C_{10}H_{16}$	A member of the chemical family of monoterpenes; occurs as a constituent of citrus oils. Colourless liquid.
Linalöl	$C_{10}H_{18}O$	A member of the chemical class of terpenoid alcohols; a chief constituent of Rosewood, Lavender and Bergamot oils. Colourless liquid.

1.6 Atomic Structure

An atom consists of a minute, dense, central body — the nucleus — around which one or more larger, and much lighter, particles, called *electrons*, move at high speed. The electrons occupy regions of space known as *orbitals*. Unlike the orbit of a planet moving around a star, an atomic orbital is three-dimensional. The simplest orbitals are spherical in shape, with the nucleus of the atom placed centrally.

An atomic nucleus consists of one or more *protons*: dense particles, each carrying a unit positive charge of electricity. Each electron weighs about 1/2000 of the weight of a proton and carries a unit negative charge. The electrical charges on a proton and on an electron are therefore equal and opposite.

Particles of similar electrical charge repel one another, and so an atomic nucleus containing two or more protons alone could not exist. Such a nucleus is, however, stabilized by the presence of two or more electrically neutral particles called *neutrons*, the presence of which generates powerful forces, binding the protons together.

Particles of opposite electrical charge attract one another; hence an electron, moving in its orbital around an atomic nucleus, tends to be pulled into the nucleus. The reason why this does not happen is that the electron obeys one of the sets of physical laws which govern the existence of matter, to which there are no satisfactory analogies on the infinitely larger scale of our everyday experience. However, some appreciation of the balance of forces involved may be experienced by whirling a ball attached to a length of string around in the air, when it is found necessary to exert a pulling force on the string to prevent the centrifugal force, which is easily felt, from hurling the ball away at a tangent, which will happen if the string is released.

Hydrogen and helium atoms

The simplest atom is that of ordinary hydrogen, the nucleus of which consists of a single proton, around which a single electron moves in a spherical orbital. This may be represented in two dimensions thus:

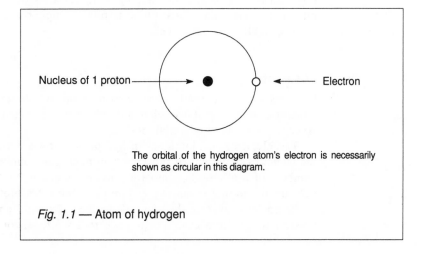

Nucleus of 1 proton ⟶ • ○ ⟵ Electron

The orbital of the hydrogen atom's electron is necessarily shown as circular in this diagram.

Fig. 1.1 — Atom of hydrogen

In the discussion which follows, we can conveniently omit further consideration of neutrons because, as we shall see, their presence does not affect the number of electrons in an atom, and hence does not affect the chemical properties of an atom.

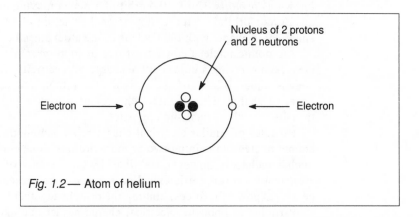

Fig. 1.2 — Atom of helium

The atom of next greater complexity, following hydrogen, is that of the element helium. The nucleus contains two protons and two stabilizing neutrons. The two electrons of the helium atom occupy the same orbital, which can hold no more than two electrons. The paired electrons of helium form a spherical layer of negative electrical charge around the nucleus. This layer is known as an *electron shell.*

[If the reader has found these notes on atomic structure so far somewhat heavy going, it would be best to take a break from studies of about an hour, then return to this section, to read it carefully over again before continuing.]

Summarizing, the helium atom consists of a nucleus of two protons and two neutrons, surrounding which is a single, spherical orbital of two electrons. This orbital is fully occupied, and it forms an electron shell around the nucleus.

1.7 The First Ten Elements

In this section, we shall continue to develop the subject of atomic structure, to include those elements which are of particular importance to the study of essential oils.

The elements, beginning with hydrogen, form a series in which the nuclei of the atoms of those beyond hydrogen contain increasing numbers of protons. Remembering that the electron shell of helium can contain no more than two electrons, if one more proton is added to the nucleus, to form the atom of the next element, the electron to balance its positive charge will have to go into an outer electron shell. This next element in the series is the reactive metal lithium, and later on we shall represent its atom by a diagram.

For the present, it will be sufficient simply to represent the number and arrangement of electrons in the two shells of the lithium atom as 2.1, and to adopt the same notation for the next seven elements (table 1.3). Since the electron shell of helium is filled with two electrons, the third electron of lithium cannot be accommodated in this shell, and occupies an outer shell, as we have noted.

Passing down the list to carbon, the four electrons of the outer electron shell of the carbon atom occupy three orbitals: one containing a pair of electrons, and the other two containing single, unpaired electrons. However, in diamond and in most compounds of carbon, the two paired electrons separate, and all four unpaired electrons form pairs with unpaired electrons of other carbon atoms or with atoms of other elements, such as hydrogen, oxygen, nitrogen or sulphur.

The outer shell of a nitrogen atom consists of one orbital containing a pair of electrons (called a 'lone pair') and three orbitals containing unpaired electrons. In all the nitrogen-containing compounds with which we shall be concerned, the unpaired electrons of the nitrogen atom form pairs with electrons of other atoms.

The outer shell of an oxygen atom consists of two orbitals, each containing a pair of electrons (i.e., two 'lone pairs') and two orbitals each containing an unpaired electron. In all the oxygen compounds with which we shall be concerned, the unpaired electrons of the oxygen atom form pairs with unpaired electrons of other atoms.

Table 1.3 — The first ten elements, formed by filling the first two electron shells

Element	Description	Symbol	Protons in nucleus	Electron arrangement
Hydrogen	Colourless, flammable gas	**H**	1	1
Helium	Colourless, inert gas	He	2	2
Lithium	Soft, very reactive white metal	Li	3	2.1
Beryllium	Light, white, lustrous metal	Be	4	2.2
Boron	Hard, black, lustrous nonmetal	B	5	2.3
Carbon	As diamond, very hard, lustrous nonmetal	**C**	6	2.4
Nitrogen	Colourless, unreactive gas	**N**	7	2.5
Oxygen	Colourless gas, supporter of combustion	**O**	8	2.6
Fluorine	Greenish-yellow, highly reactive gas	F	9	2.7
Neon	Colourless, inert gas	Ne	10	2.8

This leaves us with sulphur which, though not of importance regarding essential oils used in aromatherapy, is nevertheless present, as sulphur-containing compounds, in several important essential oils. Grapefruit Oil, for example, contains the barest traces of a sulphur compound of enormous odour power, which forms an essential feature of the natural odour profile of this essential oil. Of interest to flavourists, too, are the very highly odorous sulphur compounds found in the essential oils of Onion, Leek, Garlic and Asafoetida. Sulphur appears in the following abridged extension of the previous table of elements, beginning with sodium, in the atom of which the eleventh electron occupies a third electron shell, the second having been completely filled with eight electrons in neon (table 1.4).

Table 1.4 — Elements formed by filling the third electron shell

Element	Symbol	Protons in nucleus	Electron arrangement
Sodium (*Natrium*)	Na	11	2.8.1
Magnesium	Mg	12	2.8.2
Aluminium	Al	13	2.8.3
Silicon	Si	14	2.8.4
Phosphorus	P	15	2.8.5
Sulphur	**S**	16	2.8.6
Chlorine	Cl	17	2.8.7
Argon	Ar	18	2.8.8

The third electron shell is completely filled in the Argon atom.

We shall complete this section of Chapter 1 with two important statements:

1. As in the examples of helium, with two electrons, and neon and argon, having eight electrons in an outermost electron shell, *the electrons of a completely filled shell form a very stable arrangement, which atoms of other elements tend to assume, by the loss, gain or sharing of electrons.* We shall exemplify this statement in the following two sections of this chapter.

2. *The number of unpaired electrons in an atom determines the structures and shapes of the molecules that it can form in combination with other atoms.*

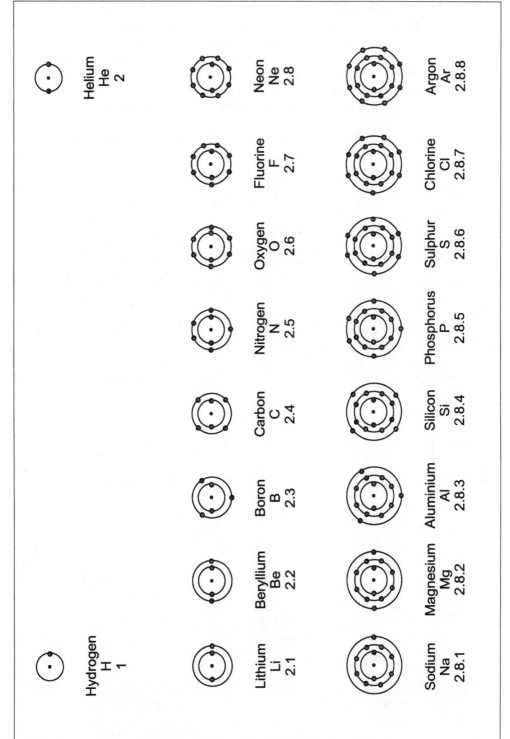

Fig.1.3— Electron arrangement of the elements from hydrogen to argon

1.8 Electrovalent or Ionic Combination

In this section and in section 1.9, we shall consider two different ways in which elements combine to form compounds. It will be helpful to both discussions if we first represent the structures of the elements we have listed diagrammatically (fig. 1.3), and according to the arrangement of the periodic table of elements to be found in any textbook of general chemistry written to GCSE level or above.

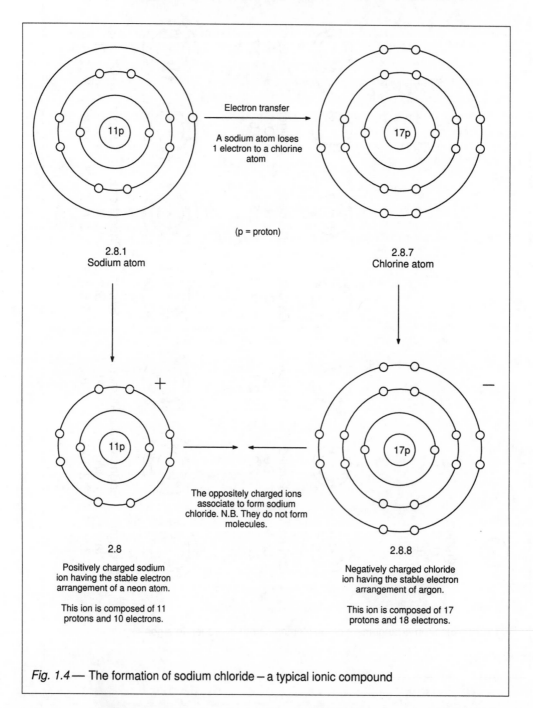

Electron transfer

A sodium atom loses 1 electron to a chlorine atom

(p = proton)

2.8.1
Sodium atom

2.8.7
Chlorine atom

+

The oppositely charged ions associate to form sodium chloride. N.B. They do not form molecules.

−

2.8

Positively charged sodium ion having the stable electron arrangement of a neon atom.

This ion is composed of 11 protons and 10 electrons.

2.8.8

Negatively charged chloride ion having the stable electron arrangement of argon.

This ion is composed of 17 protons and 18 electrons.

Fig. 1.4— The formation of sodium chloride – a typical ionic compound

When a typical metal, such as sodium, combines with a typical nonmetal, such as chlorine, electrons from the metal are transferred to atoms of the nonmetal. *In general, the number of electrons lost by the metal atom is the number required to give that atom the very stable number of two or eight electrons in its outermost shell. The number of electrons gained by the nonmetal atom is the number required to give that atom the very stable number of two or eight electrons in its outermost shell.* This is illustrated in figure 1.4.

The products of this reaction are oppositely charged atoms, called *ions.* Because of their opposite charges, the sodium and chloride ions attract one another, forming an ion-aggregate of sodium chloride. Many such ion-aggregates form a crystal of sodium chloride — common salt. The formation of sodium chloride may be represented more simply, in the form of equations, where *e* stands for an electron:

$$Na - e \longrightarrow Na^+$$

$$Cl + e \longrightarrow Cl^-$$

$$Na^+ + Cl^- \longrightarrow Na^+Cl^-$$

Taking into account the fact that chlorine exists as molecules, each consisting of two chlorine atoms, we can summarize the reaction between sodium and chlorine thus:

$$2\,Na + Cl_2 \longrightarrow 2\,Na^+Cl^-$$

Sodium chloride is a typical electrovalent or ionic compound. It consists of aggregates of sodium chloride ions, not molecules.

1.9 Covalent Compounds

Covalent compounds consist of true molecules, in which the constituent atoms are bonded together by shared pairs of electrons.

A typical essential oil consists of a mixture of some two or three hundred individual chemical substances, all of which are covalent compounds. They are, moreover, all based on carbon, meaning that each of their molecules has a skeleton of carbon atoms bonded together by covalent bonds — shared pairs of electrons.

This kind of molecular structure is made possible by the unique character of the carbon atom, in that it can bond with other carbon atoms to form chains, branched chains, ring structures, multiple-ring structures, chains bonded to rings, and so on, in virtually limitless variety. Resulting from this property of the carbon atom, which is not possessed to anything like the same, vast extent by atoms of other elements, the total number of carbon compounds by far exceeds the total number of compounds of all the other elements added together.

Purely for convenience of study, therefore, chemistry is divided into organic chemistry, the study of carbon compounds, and inorganic chemistry, the study of compounds of elements other than carbon.

These two great branches of chemistry are not separated by an impregnable wall, but are closely related and interwoven to form the magnificent edifice of chemistry, which rests upon a massive foundation of a third branch of the subject — physical chemistry, a body of knowledge concerned with explanations of how chemical reactions work, measurements of the energy changes which always accompany chemical reactions and the scientific laws which govern the behaviour of substances of all kinds.

Some of the most fundamental discoveries in physical chemistry have resulted in explanations of how atoms are bonded together in organic compounds; that is, of the nature of the chemical bond. We have noted that hydrogen gas does not normally exist as single atoms of hydrogen, but as molecules consisting of two hydrogen atoms bonded together. This is represented in figure 1.5.

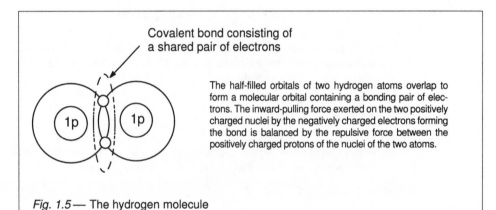

Covalent bond consisting of a shared pair of electrons

The half-filled orbitals of two hydrogen atoms overlap to form a molecular orbital containing a bonding pair of electrons. The inward-pulling force exerted on the two positively charged nuclei by the negatively charged electrons forming the bond is balanced by the repulsive force between the positively charged protons of the nuclei of the two atoms.

Fig. 1.5— The hydrogen molecule

Here, we have a shared pair of electrons, one from each of the two hydrogen atoms, forming the bond between the atoms. The electrons are negatively charged, and they hold together the positively charged nuclei of the hydrogen atoms by the force of attraction which exists between opposite charges; they form a bonding pair. This kind of bond is typical of all organic compounds, which is remarkable in view of the fact that, being of like charge, electrons repel one another. When joining atoms, however, two electrons form a stable bonding pair and usually a strong bond.

The simplest organic compound is the gas methane, the molecule of which consists of one carbon atom bonded to four hydrogen atoms (fig. 1.6).

We shall return to the subject of organic compounds in section 1.11.

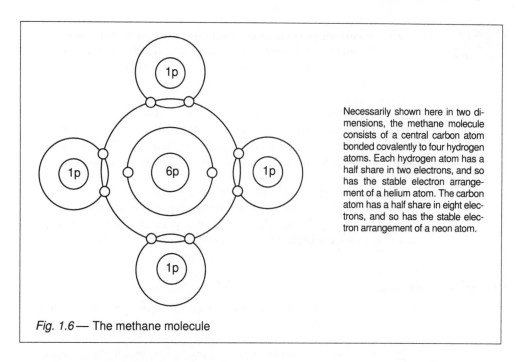

Necessarily shown here in two dimensions, the methane molecule consists of a central carbon atom bonded covalently to four hydrogen atoms. Each hydrogen atom has a half share in two electrons, and so has the stable electron arrangement of a helium atom. The carbon atom has a half share in eight electrons, and so has the stable electron arrangement of a neon atom.

Fig. 1.6 — The methane molecule

1.10 The Combining Power of Atoms

In figure 1.3, notice the numbers of *un*paired electrons in the atoms represented, particularly those of hydrogen, carbon, nitrogen and sulphur. They are as follows:

Table 1.5 — Unpaired electrons in some atoms

Element	No. of unpaired electrons
Hydrogen	1
Carbon	4
Nitrogen	3
Oxygen	2
Sulphur	2

Because, in covalent compounds, bonds are formed by the sharing of pairs of electrons which were, before bonding took place, the unpaired electrons of the atoms bonded together, *the above numbers are the numbers of covalent bonds which the respective atoms can form with other atoms.*

Valency — the combining power of an atom

The combining power, or valency, of an atom is the number of single bonds which that atom can form with atoms of other elements; it is equal to the number of unpaired electrons in the outermost electron shell of the atom.

In general, when atoms combine to form molecules all available unpaired electrons are involved in the formation of bonds. Thus in organic compounds, carbon atoms form four bonds with other carbon atoms or atoms of other elements, nitrogen forms three, oxygen and sulphur two and hydrogen one.

It should be mentioned here that carbon atoms and atoms of certain other elements can form double or triple bonds, of which the double bond only is of relevance to our present studies. We shall discuss the double bond a little later on, when the need arises.

1.11 Organic Compounds

Until the mid-nineteenth century it was assumed that carbon compounds such as the alcohol of wine, the nitrogen-containing urea excreted by man and some other mammals, and the acid of vinegar, acetic acid, could be made only by living cells, under the influence of a mysterious 'vital force' which did not exist in nonliving things, such as the chemicals and apparatus of the laboratory. Then, in 1845, the German chemist, Hermann Kolbe, succeeded in synthesizing acetic acid from its elements — carbon, hydrogen and oxygen — so providing powerful evidence that the so-called 'vital force' did not in fact exist, and encouraging attempts at the synthesis of other organic compounds. Arising from such beginnings, the name 'organic chemistry' has persisted in reference to the chemistry of carbon compounds.

1.12 Inorganic Compounds

Inorganic compounds are, with certain exceptions, those of elements other than carbon. They include such chemicals as sodium chloride (common salt), water, sulphuric acid, calcium sulphate (plaster of Paris), copper sulphate, ammonia, caustic soda, calcium oxide (builders' lime) and, among the carbon-containing inorganic compounds, sodium carbonate (washing soda), calcium carbonate (occurring as chalk, limestone, Iceland spar, etc.) and sodium bicarbonate (bicarbonate of soda). Many inorganic compounds exist as ion-aggregates, others as true molecules.

1.13 The Law of Constant Composition

The law of constant composition is a fundamental law of chemical science concerning the composition of chemical compounds, which states that:

Law of constant composition

All pure samples of the same compound, however prepared, consist of the same elements combined together in the same proportions by weight.

The idea of the constant composition of a compound came eventually to be accepted as the result of the analysis of samples of any given pure compound which had been prepared by different methods, when within the limits of experimental error no difference was found in the proportions by weight of the different elements of which it was composed.

The law of constant composition does, in fact, generalize the results of the precise analysis of countless pure compounds over many years. This law, together with other laws and principles discovered by experiment, played a major role in establishing the concept that any pure compound consists of molecules, or aggregates of ions, in which the atoms or ions of the elements present are united always in the same proportions by number.

1.14 Atomic and Molecular Weights

The fascinating story of how inspired ideas and principles, discovered as the result of deduction from the results of innumerable experiments, gave rise to the determination of atomic and molecular weights is beyond the scope of this book. However, consideration of the weights of atoms and molecules is very helpful in explaining the behaviour of an essential oil when it is allowed to evaporate.

Since it is impossible to weigh individual atoms by any ordinary means, the weights of different atoms are expressed comparatively, by reference to a unit of weight. The original unit for atomic weights was adopted, quite arbitrarily, as the weight of the atom of the lightest element, hydrogen, taken as 1·000. This will suffice for our purposes (though we should note that for accurate work the unit adopted is one-twelfth of the weight of an atom of the isotope — see below — carbon-12, taken as 12·0000).

Since by far the greatest contribution to the weight of an atom is made by its nucleus, the weight of the electrons it contains can for most purposes be ignored. On this basis, the weight of the nucleus, relative to the weight of an atom of ordinary hydrogen, consisting of a single proton, is the sum of the weights of the protons and neutrons present in its nucleus. Since the weight of a neutron is the same as that of a proton, the weight of an atom is, numerically, for all but the most accurate work, the sum of the number of protons and neutrons in its nucleus.

If the atomic weights of other elements are determined relative to the weight of a hydrogen atom (i.e. H = 1), it is found that they are not whole numbers. The reason is that although all atoms of the same element are identical with respect to the numbers of protons and electrons they contain, any quantity of a given element consists of

Isotopes

certain proportions of atoms containing different numbers of neutrons in their nuclei. These atoms are known as *isotopes* of the element. However, *the chemical properties of an atom depend only on the number and arrangement of its electrons* and this is, in turn, dictated by the *number of protons* in its nucleus. So although the presence of isotopes gives rise to atomic weights which are not whole numbers, *the presence of isotopes does not affect the chemical properties of an element.*

The reason for the adoption of the isotope carbon-12 (C = 12, precisely) as the standard for atomic weights ($\frac{1}{12}$ of 12 = 1, precisely) was the existence of isotopes. On the carbon-12 standard, the atomic weight of hydrogen is slightly greater than 1, because ordinary hydrogen, though consisting mainly of atoms with a single proton in their nuclei, contains a very small proportion of an isotope (called *deuterium*) of twice the weight, owing to the presence of a neutron in addition to a proton in its nucleus, also an even heavier isotope (*tritium*), in minute proportion, with one proton and two neutrons.

For many purposes, as we noted, H = 1 serves very well, and using this standard the atomic weights of elements occurring in the constituents of essential oils may be given, and used, as whole numbers (table 1.6).

Atomic weight

We can now define, for the purposes of this book, the *atomic weight of an element* as *the number of times that one atom of the element is heavier than one atom of hydrogen taken as 1.*

Table 1.6 — Atomic weights of some elements

Element	Atomic weight
Hydrogen	1
Carbon	12
Nitrogen	14
Oxygen	16
Sulphur	32

Molecular weight

The *molecular weight of a compound* is *the number of times that one molecule of the compound is heavier than one atom of hydrogen taken as 1.*

Using the above values for atomic weights, we can easily calculate the molecular weights of compounds (table 1.7). It is now a simple matter to relate the results of these calculations to the law of constant composition, taking any one of them as an example:

a) If, by experiment, carbon dioxide is found always to consist only of the elements carbon and oxygen in the proportions of 12 to 32 by weight, then carbon dioxide is of constant composition, or, conversely,

b) If carbon dioxide is of constant composition, then the gas will always consist of the elements carbon and oxygen only, in the same proportions by weight, however it may be prepared. Since these proportions are always in the ratio of 12 to 32, then the law is upheld. Similar reasoning can be applied to any other compound.

Table 1.7 — Molecular weights of some compounds

Compound	Formula	Calculation	Molecular weight
Carbon dioxide	CO_2	$1 \times 12 + 2 \times 16 =$	44
Water	H_2O	$2 \times 1 + 1 \times 16 =$	18
Methane	CH_4	$1 \times 12 + 4 \times 1 =$	16
Ethanol	C_2H_6O	$2 \times 12 + 6 \times 1 + 1 \times 16 =$	46
Glucose	$C_6H_{12}O_6$	$6 \times 12 + 12 \times 1 + 6 \times 16 =$	180
Sucrose	$C_{12}H_{22}O_{11}$	$12 \times 12 + 22 \times 1 + 11 \times 16 =$	342
Limonene	$C_{10}H_{16}$	$10 \times 12 + 16 \times 1 =$	136
Linalöl	$C_{10}H_{18}O$	$10 \times 12 + 18 \times 1 + 1 \times 16 =$	154

When a typical essential oil is allowed to evaporate from a smelling strip, the odour of the oil is observed to change. This is readily shown using Geranium Oil or one of the citrus oils, by taking a ½ cm dip of the oil, allowing it to evaporate for, say, 20 minutes, then comparing the odour with that of a fresh dip. The difference in odour is caused by the evaporation of constituents of the oil of lower molecular weight, leaving behind others of higher molecular weight. Since different constituents have different odours, the odour of the sample changes.

1.15 Mixtures

The important difference between a compound and a mixture is that whereas a compound, if pure, is of invariable composition, the composition of a mixture is variable. We define a mixture as follows:

Mixtures

A mixture is composed of elements, compounds, or both elements and compounds, brought together in any proportions by weight.

We can, for example, mix common salt and white sugar, or water and alcohol, together in any proportions we may choose, but the proportions of the elements present in any of the compounds named in table 1.7 or, for that matter, in any other compound, are always the same. An essential oil is a mixture par excellence, as we have noted. The molecules of all constituents of essential oils contain atoms of carbon and hydrogen; many of them contain atoms of oxygen as well, and a few contain atoms of nitrogen or sulphur, bonded together in a great variety of different arrangements.

In an essential oil-bearing plant the production of the oil takes place in living cells, by a series of reactions, known as reaction pathways, under the influence of enzymes, which are biochemical catalysts. The precise nature of the reaction pathways by which the constituents of an essential oil are synthesized by the plant is, like all other reactions which take place in living cells, genetically determined, and so, provided these processes of cell chemistry are unaffected by other influences, the composition of the essential oil also will be genetically determined.

On this basis it is to be expected that, provided the genetic information is faultlessly passed on from one generation of the plant to the next, the composition of its essential oil will be constant within the limitations of natural genetic variability; i.e. as human offspring of the same parents vary in their form and body chemistry, so do offspring of the same parent plants vary in their form and chemistry for the same reason. The limits of variability in plants are, however, narrower than they are in the human species because plants, being relatively simpler organisms, carry less genetic information for their reproduction. Such constancy of composition is, however, never found among different samples of an essential oil produced from plants of the same species and variety, even if the processing conditions have been identical for all samples.

The reasons for variations in the composition of an essential oil will be discussed in Chapter 4; for the moment, a mental picture of the situation will suffice. The leaves of a plant, such as those of *Pelargonium graveolens,* the Geranium plant of perfumery, which can easily be grown in the home, all have the same general shape, showing that the prescribing template for the chemical reactions by which the leaves are formed is the same for all leaves of the same species — it is genetically determined. However, no two leaves of the plant are ever identical, showing that the dictates of genetic inheritance must be modified by other influences. The composition of an essential oil from a plant of a single species and variety always follows the same *general* pattern of constituents and their proportions, but differs in detail from sample to sample.

1.16 Odour Properties of Essential Oils

Using the technique of gas–liquid chromatography, to which we shall make further reference in Chapter 7, a minute, vaporized sample of an essential oil may be separated almost completely into its individual, pure constituents. This analytical process can be adapted to permit smelling of the vapours of the constituents after separation, when it is observed that the odours of no two of the constituents are identical in character. Some of the constituents of a given essential oil, such as Lavender, Rosemary or Citronella, are in most cases to be found also in other oils, but wherever a particular constituent may occur its odour is always the same. The odours of identical molecules are identical; the odour of a chemically pure substance is determined by the geometry of its molecules and the nature of its constituent atoms.

The property of odour

Odour is a property of certain gases and vapours only. A liquid or solid is odorous only if

a) it is capable of evaporating to form a vapour; that is, only if, on exposure to air, molecules of the substance can become detached from it and mix with the molecules of gases of air. Such substances are said to be *volatile*;

b) the molecules of the vapour are able to stimulate the odour-sensitive receptors of the olfactory organ of the nose.

Olfactory receptors take the form of extremely minute, hair-like extensions of the nerve fibres of the olfactory organ, lying submerged in the extremely thin layer of mucus by which the twin membranes of this organ are covered.

Occupying a surface area of about 2·5 square centimetres on each side of the nasal septum, the human olfactory organ supports some 50 million receptor hairs, called olfactory hairs, each of which, it is believed, is capable of responding to either a single kind of odour stimulus or to several kinds of such stimuli. From experimental evidence, the theory has been developed that each olfactory hair carries a number of sites, of molecular dimensions, into which odorous molecules, but not those which are inodorous, can fit, as a key fits into the lock for which it is made. Perhaps only part of an odorous molecule can make a good fit, perhaps all of it does so; whichever may be true, the 'site-fitting' theory of odour stimuli, first advanced by J.E. Amoore in 1962, states that when this occurs the nerve ending responds by initiating nervous impulses which travel via a succession of olfactory nerve fibres to the brain. The recently advanced theory of Luca Turin suggests that odour-sensitive sites on the olfactory hairs are stimulated by the vibrations of odorous molecules. The question of just how we and other mammals are able to detect odours is as yet far from settled.

We shall consider the odour properties of essential oils and their constituents in Chapter 5. For the present, we should remember that when an essential oil is allowed to evaporate, its odour changes as time passes, and note that the various features of its total odour profile are expressions of the combined odours of those of its constituents which are in the process of evaporating at any given instant. Hence the total odour profile of an essential oil is a reflection of its composition which, in turn, determines the quality of the oil.

Careful sensory evaluation can therefore yield valuable information on the quality of an essential oil, within the limitations that small differences in the proportions of weakly odorous constituents are difficult or impossible to detect by smelling alone, as are odourless or weakly odorous adulterants. It is also usually impossible positively to detect, by smelling alone, the presence of any synthetic chemicals, added to make up deficiencies of the same chemicals occurring as normal constituents of an unadulterated essential oil; the incidence of such practice needs instrumental analysis for its detection.

Chapter 2

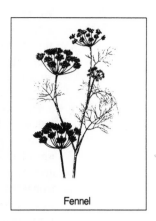

Fennel

Hydrocarbons

2.1 Saturated Hydrocarbons

A hydrocarbon is a compound of hydrogen and carbon only. The simplest hydrocarbon, methane, is a colourless, odourless gas, familiar, as we have noted, as the main constituent of North Sea gas for domestic use. Since the gas is highly flammable, forming explosive mixtures with air, it is 'marked' with a trace of the vapour of a highly malodorous organic sulphur compound to render any leakage quickly detectable by smell.

The methane molecule (*see* p. 21) may be represented on paper in two convenient ways:

$$\begin{array}{c} H \\ | \\ H-C-H \\ | \\ H \end{array} \qquad\qquad CH_4$$

Methane
(structural formula)

Methane
(molecular formula)

Fig. 2.1 — Representations of the methane molecule

A more accurate impression of a methane molecule, and of the molecules of other organic compounds mentioned in this book, may be gained by making a model of the molecule, using drilled, plastic spheres, colour-coded to represent the atoms of different elements, and bonding-pieces representing the bonds joining them together.[1]

---

1. A suitable set of models, the Molymod 003 Organic Set, is available from Spiring Enterprises Ltd., Beke Hall, Marringdean Road, Billingshurst, West Sussex RH14 9HF.

We have mentioned the ability of carbon atoms to bond to one another to form an almost infinite variety of molecular structures. This ability may usefully be explored on paper or by using models, or preferably both, with respect to the different molecules we encounter, remembering the valencies of carbon and of the atoms of hydrogen, oxygen, nitrogen and sulphur. In a set of molecular models, the valencies of the different atoms are represented by the numbers of holes drilled in the plastic spheres, so there can be no mistake once the colour code has been memorized, provided the rule 'all valencies must be satisfied' is obeyed. In terms of the electrons of which bonds are composed, this means that to form a molecule the unpaired electrons of the outermost electron shell of an atom always form bonding pairs with unpaired electrons of other atoms. Thus the following formulae are *wrong*:

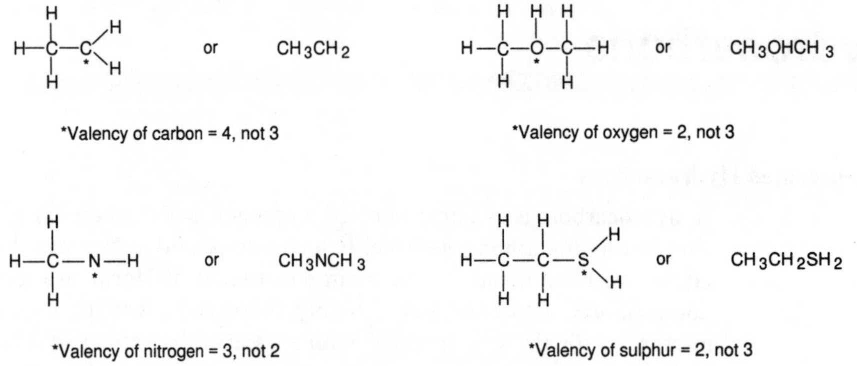

*Valency of carbon = 4, not 3   *Valency of oxygen = 2, not 3

*Valency of nitrogen = 3, not 2   *Valency of sulphur = 2, not 3

Fig. 2.2 — Incorrect structural formulae

The following are the correct formulae:

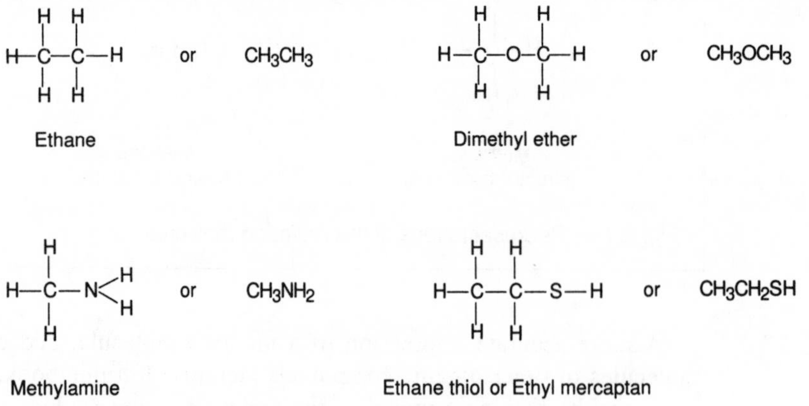

Ethane   Dimethyl ether

Methylamine   Ethane thiol or Ethyl mercaptan

Fig. 2.3 — Correct structural formulae

N.B. Oxygen-, nitrogen- and sulphur-containing organic compounds will be discussed in Chapter 3.

When studying the bonding together of carbon atoms to form different molecular structures, it is best to join the carbons together first, to give the 'carbon skeleton' of a molecule, and then to bond the carbon atoms to whatever other atoms are involved. If atoms other than carbon are part of the skeleton, these must of course be included, as shown (fig. 2.4).

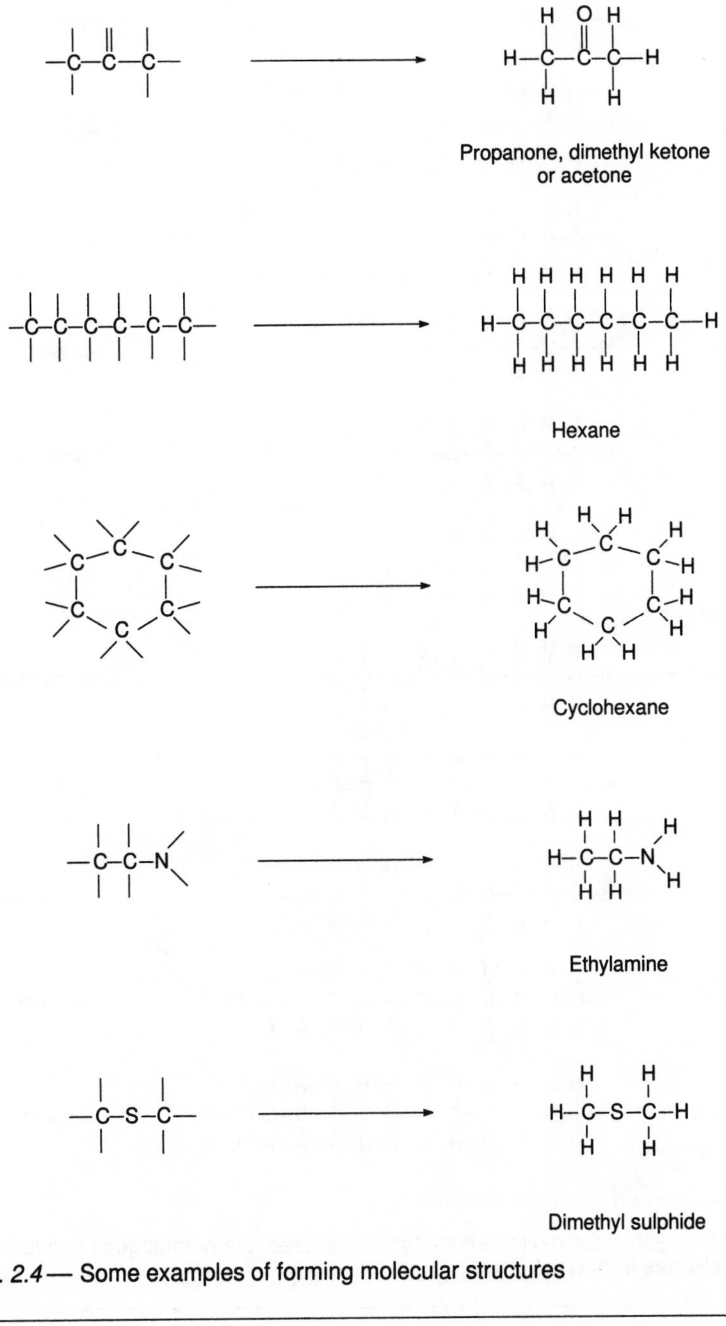

Propanone, dimethyl ketone or acetone

Hexane

Cyclohexane

Ethylamine

Dimethyl sulphide

Fig. 2.4 — Some examples of forming molecular structures

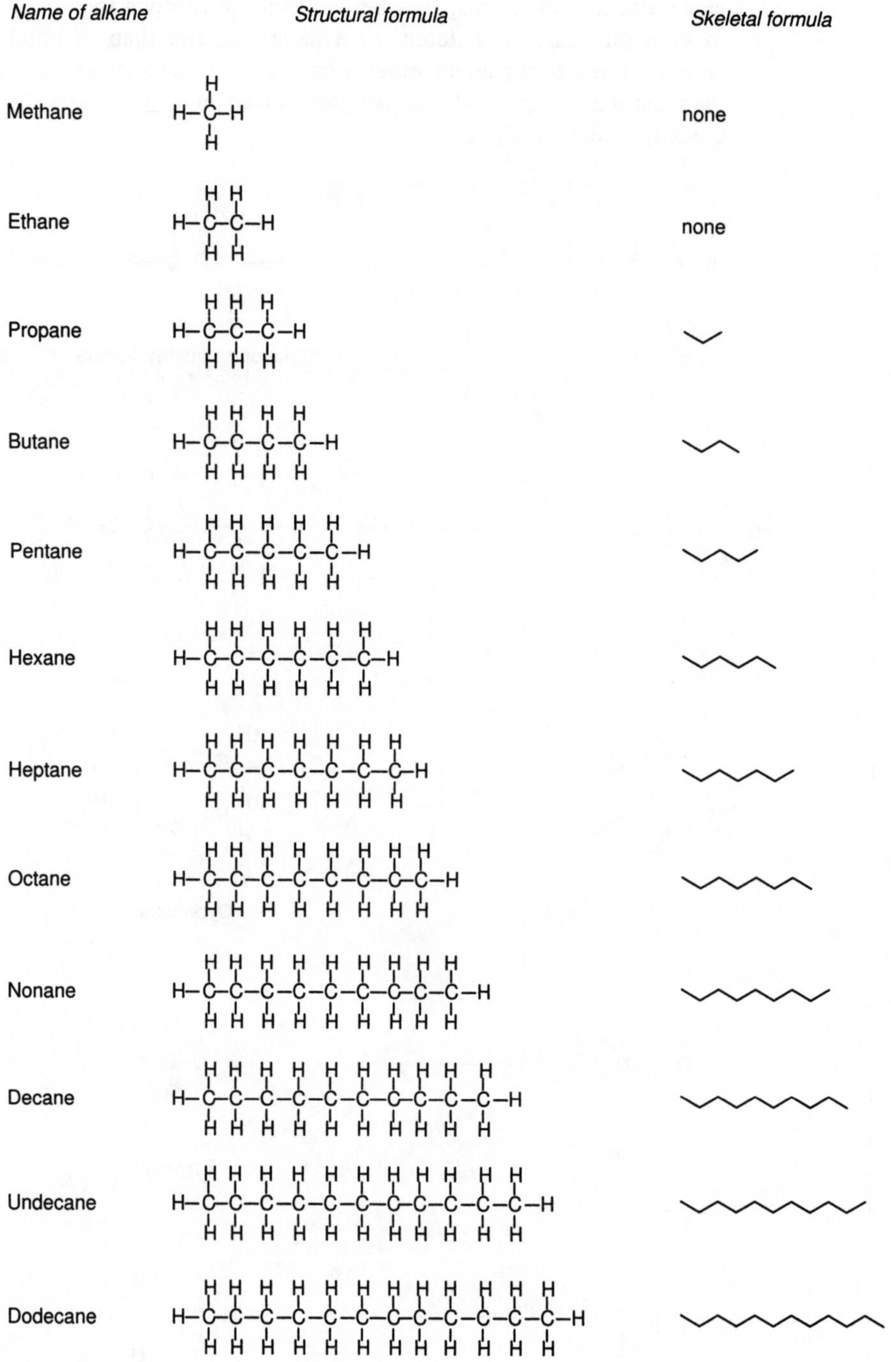
Name of alkane
Structural formula
Skeletal formula
Methane
none
Ethane
none
Propane
Butane
Pentane
Hexane
Heptane
Octane
Nonane
Decane
Undecane
Dodecane

Fig. 2.5 — Saturated hydrocarbon chain structures; the homologous series of straight-chain alkanes from C_1 to C_{12}.

The useful exercises of writing structural formulae for, and making models of, hydrocarbon molecules may be continued to form longer and longer chains, whereupon it soon becomes clear that in so doing we are representing the members of a series, each of which differs from those immediately adjacent to it by one carbon atom and two hydrogen atoms. Such a series is called a *homologous* series, and it will be helpful if we now list the members of the homologous series of straight-chain, saturated hydrocarbons from methane (which we can call C_1) to dodecane, C_{12}. The skeletal formulae included in figure 2.5 will be explained in section 2.2. Hydrocarbon chain structures extending to more than a hundred carbon atoms represent compounds which either exist in nature (in crude oil, for example) or which could be made in the laboratory. Such compounds are known as straight-chain, saturated hydrocarbons, or straight-chain alkanes (fig. 2.5).

If a model is made of a straight-chain alkane of three or more carbon atoms, it is immediately noticed that the chain is far from straight, taking a zig-zag form. The model is, in fact, a better representation of the molecule than the corresponding structural formula, because in the model the plastic spheres representing the atoms occupy positions in space relative to one another which are similar to the relative positions of the atoms in the actual molecule. This can be shown in a structural formula to only a limited extent, for the reason that the four bonds of a carbon atom are spaced equally around the atom in three dimensions. Taking the example of methane, we can attempt a perspective diagram of the molecule by using wedge-shaped lines to represent three of the bonds. If we then join the ends of the bonds, a regular tetrahedron is formed:

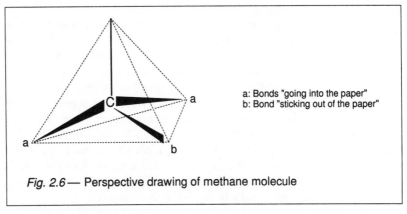

a: Bonds "going into the paper"
b: Bond "sticking out of the paper"

Fig. 2.6 — Perspective drawing of methane molecule

The point of this discussion is that the four bonds formed by a carbon atom in an alkane are *uniformly directional in three dimensions*, and that the molecule is therefore a three-dimensional structure. The angle formed at a carbon atom by any two of the bonds is the *bond angle*, which in an alkane has normally the value of 109° 28′.

2.2 Skeletal Structural Formulae

In television advertisements intended to depict the wonders of science, efforts always seem to be made to portray the laboratory as a place of incomprehensible complication, and chemists as people who revel in matters too difficult for anyone else to understand. In fact, chemists constantly strive towards simplification but would never, of course, admit that they have to do this in order to understand chemistry themselves!

An outstanding example of simplification in chemistry is the adoption of skeletal formulae to represent the molecular structures of organic compounds. This is easily appreciated by comparing the full structural formula for, say, hexane with the skeletal formula for the same compound. The following formulae for hexane show how the skeletal formula is derived:

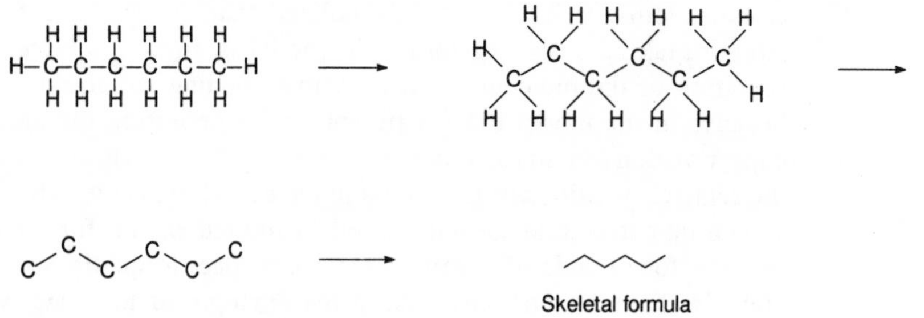

Fig. 2.7— Deriving a skeletal structural formula for hexane

In the skeletal formula a carbon atom is assumed to be present at each end of the zig-zag line, and at each of the angles in between. Thus the lines making up the zig-zag represent the bonds joining the carbon atoms of the molecule. The hydrogen atoms of the molecule are not represented unless specifically required, being assumed to be present. Skeletal formulae may seem strange at first, requiring much to be assumed for their interpretation. This is counterbalanced by their clarity and simplicity, and by their rather better representation of molecular geometry. Models representing skeletal formulae may be made by joining black 'carbon atom' spheres with short bonding-pieces; then, if desired, hydrogen and any other atoms present in the molecules may be joined to the carbons.

2.3 Saturation and Unsaturation

If we look for a moment at either of the full structural formulae for hexane, above, we notice that this molecule, like the molecules of all other alkanes, contains the maximum number of hydrogen atoms which it could possibly contain (remembering that a carbon atom forms four bonds only). Alternatively, we can say that all of the carbon atoms of hexane (or of any other alkane) are bonded to the maximum number of other atoms. Such molecules are said to be *saturated*.

There is a different way in which two carbon atoms can bond together, which is by sharing *two* bonding pairs of electrons, so forming a *double bond* between them. Compare the bonding of the carbon atoms in the following formulae for eth*ane* and eth*ene:*

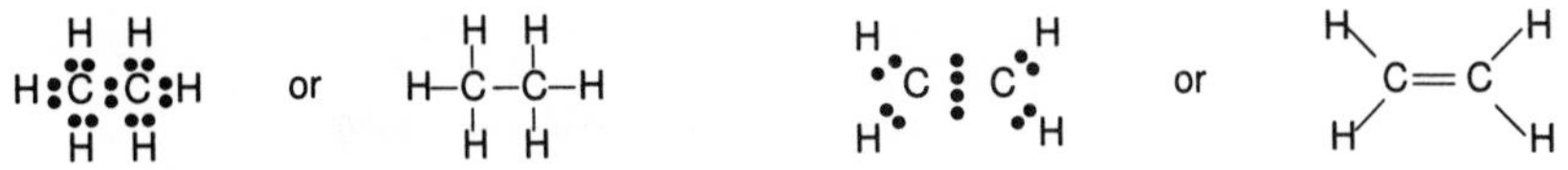

Ethane   Ethene

Fig. 2.8— Comparison of structures of eth*ane* and eth*ene*

Clearly, in ethene, the two carbon atoms are not bonded to the maximum number of other atoms to which they could be bonded, and so ethene is an *unsaturated* hydrocarbon; it is a member of the family of alk*enes*.

Alkanes

To summarize, the molecule of an alk*ane* contains single bonds only. Alkanes are *saturated* hydrocarbons; their names end in '-ane'.

Alkenes

The molecule of an alk*ene* contains a double bond between two of its carbon atoms. Alkenes are *unsaturated* hydrocarbons; their names end in '-ene'. The carbon-carbon double bond has special properties, which we shall now discuss.

The attractive bonding force between the positively charged nuclei of two carbon atoms joined by a double bond and the *four*, negatively charged electrons of the bond is, as might be expected, greater than that between two carbon atoms joined by a single bond and the *two* electrons of the bond. Evidence for this reasonable assumption comes from measurement of the distance between the respective carbon atoms, which is found to be shorter in the case of a double bond than it is with a single bond. Atoms joined by a bond can be pulled together by the electrons of the bond to only a certain, minimum distance from one another before the repulsive force between their nuclei prevents their further approach. Thus a double bond is stronger than a single bond.

There is, however, a further consideration, which is that in a double bond we have two pairs of negatively charged electrons situated very close to one another: a powerful repulsive force exists between

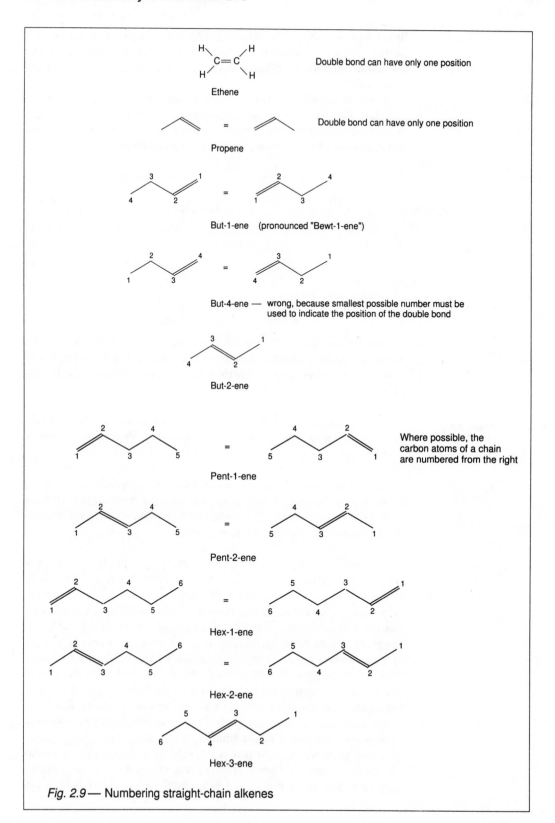

Fig. 2.9 — Numbering straight-chain alkenes

these pairs of electrons, tending to break the bond, or allowing it to be broken if the molecule containing it is attacked by another molecule, or ion, capable of doing this. Unsaturated compounds are for this reason less stable in the presence of certain other substances (oxygen, for example) than saturated compounds.

The names of alkenes are derived from those of the corresponding alkanes, but in the case of alkenes containing more than three carbon atoms in their molecules the position of the double bond has to be taken into account.

2.4 Nomenclature of the Straight-Chain Alkanes and Alkenes

The naming of organic molecules was the subject of recommendations made by the International Union of Pure and Applied Chemistry (IUPAC) in 1957. Since then, organic nomenclature has been systematic and very much simpler than beforehand.

The straight-chain alkanes are named by adding the suffix '-ane' to prefixes derived mainly from Greek roots, e.g. *penta:* five, hence *pentane*, is the name of the straight-chain alkane having five carbon atoms in its molecule. The one exception, *nona:* nine, hence *nonane*, comes from Latin, as an alternative to the Greek *ennea:* nine, hence 'enneane', which was perhaps too indefinite a proposition to be acceptable.

With the straight-chain alkenes the position of the double bond has to be indicated for all members of the family beyond propene. This is accomplished by numbering the carbon atoms of a chain, so that the position of the double bond is indicated by the *smaller* of the two possible numbers. A few examples will make this clear (fig. 2.9).

Hence to name an alkene the same prefix root is used, as for the corresponding alkane (that having the same number of carbon atoms in its molecule) together with a number giving the position of the double bond and the suffix '-ene'.

2.5 Isomerism

Isomerism is the existence of two or more molecules containing the same numbers of atoms of the same elements, but in which the atoms are bonded together, or arranged, in different ways.

Thus the two straight-chain butenes are isomers, because the position of the double bond in but-1-ene is different from what it is in but-2-ene. The same applies to the pentenes and the hexenes and to the molecules of any other alkenes in which the only difference is the position of the double bond; all exhibit *position isomerism*.

There is a further kind of isomerism concerning the double bond, which arises from the fact that two carbon atoms joined by this bond are unable to rotate with respect to one another. Let us take, for example, a model of the molecule of eth*ene*. It is impossible to twist the two carbon atoms through any more than a very small angle with respect to one another without breaking the bond, whereas such a rotation is easy in a model of eth*ane*. Studies show that the same restriction of relative rotation exists for all pairs of carbon atoms joined by double bonds in the molecules of the actual compounds, compared with rotational freedom for those joined by single bonds.

In the following structural formulae for but-2-ene we have shown the hydrogen atoms bonded to carbon atoms numbers 2 and 3 on opposite sides, and on the same side, of the double bond.

trans-But-2-ene   *cis*-But-2-ene

Fig. 2.10 — Structural formulae for the two but-2-enes

These are the molecules of two different substances, as is shown by differences in their physical properties. Their chemical properties are very similar, but not identical. This is an example of *geometrical isomerism*, otherwise known as *cis-trans* isomerism, as implied by the names of the but-2-enes. In modern textbooks and recent litera-ture the bracketed letter *(Z)*- stands for *cis*-, and *(E)*- for *trans*-; these letters refer to the German words *zusammen* and *entgegen*, respec-tively. A little thought will reveal that there cannot be *(Z)*- and *(E)*-isomers of but-1-ene, and this is always so where the double bond of an alkene occurs at one end of a molecule.

In figure 2.9 the formulae for four of the compounds all represent *trans*-geometrical isomers, but have not been so named. Can you find them?

2.6 Branched-Chain Alkanes and Alkenes

There is only one way in which three carbon atoms can be joined together by either single or double bonds to form a chain, and that is in the form of a 'straight' chain. With four carbon atoms, however,

n-Butane   iso-Butane, or methyl propane

Fig. 2.11 — Two different butane molecules

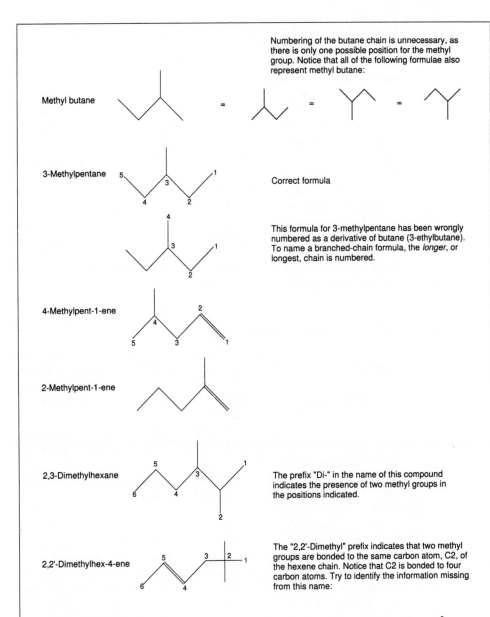

Numbering of the butane chain is unnecessary, as there is only one possible position for the methyl group. Notice that all of the following formulae also represent methyl butane:

Methyl butane

3-Methylpentane

Correct formula

This formula for 3-methylpentane has been wrongly numbered as a derivative of butane (3-ethylbutane). To name a branched-chain formula, the *longer*, or longest, chain is numbered.

4-Methylpent-1-ene

2-Methylpent-1-ene

2,3-Dimethylhexane

The prefix "Di-" in the name of this compound indicates the presence of two methyl groups in the positions indicated.

2,2'-Dimethylhex-4-ene

The "2,2'-Dimethyl" prefix indicates that two methyl groups are bonded to the same carbon atom, C2, of the hexene chain. Notice that C2 is bonded to four carbon atoms. Try to identify the information missing from this name:

The two molecular structures to the right are of particular importance to our discussion of constituents of essential oils.

Methylbuta-1,3-diene, or isoprene

trans-3,7-Dimethylocta-2,6-diene

Fig. 2.12 — Numbering branched-chain alkanes and alkenes

two chain structures are possible, one straight, the other branched (fig. 2.11). Containing four carbon atoms, these structures are molecules of different butanes, and in older nomenclature they were named normal, or *n*-butane, and iso-butane, respectively. The prefixes *n*- for 'normal', and *iso*- are still in use, but where branching of chains occurs in hydrocarbons having more than four carbon atoms further prefixes, such as *neo*-, have to be used, leading to complicated nomenclature. In the IUPAC system, the carbon atoms of a molecule are numbered, and the position of a branch in a chain indicated by the smallest possible number, as in the case of denoting the position of a double bond. Where there is a choice, the longer, or longest, chain is the chain to be numbered, and this chain gives the root of the name. A few examples are shown (fig. 2.12) in which a methyl group, the smallest possible branch, is used. This consists of a single carbon atom bonded to three hydrogen atoms, and is derived from methane. It is called a methyl group or methyl radical. We shall discuss the subject of radicals in the next section of this chapter.

2.7 Monoterpenes Having Chain Structures

Methylbuta-1,3-diene (*see* fig. 2.12), known also as isoprene, is the molecular structural unit from which all members of a large and very important family of naturally occurring, unsaturated hydrocarbons are derived. This is the family of *terpenes*, members of which are constituents of almost all essential oils.

The terpenes of essential oils are formed in living, oil-producing plant cells by complex, natural chemical processes. They are classified according to the number of isoprene units that their molecules contain, the *mono*terpenes, containing two such units, being the simplest. Isoprene is therefore classified as a hemiterpene (Greek *hemi*: half).

We can approach an understanding of the molecular structures of terpenes by means of outline diagrams of isoprene molecules. It must, however, be clearly understood that *outline diagrams of molecules are not formulae*. They are merely helpful stepping-stones on the way to an appreciation of the actual formulae of chemical compounds (fig. 2.13).

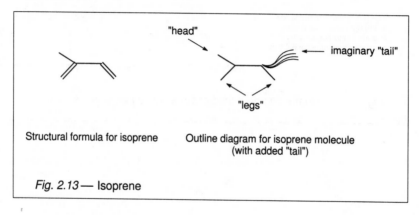

Structural formula for isoprene

Outline diagram for isoprene molecule (with added "tail")

Fig. 2.13 — Isoprene

Organic chemists do have a sense of humour (of sometimes quite unmentionable character) which gave rise long ago to the description 'the running horse' for the isoprene molecule. If two isoprene structures are linked together 'front legs to back legs', we have the outline of the molecular structure of one kind of monoterpene, taking the form of a branched chain (fig. 2.14).

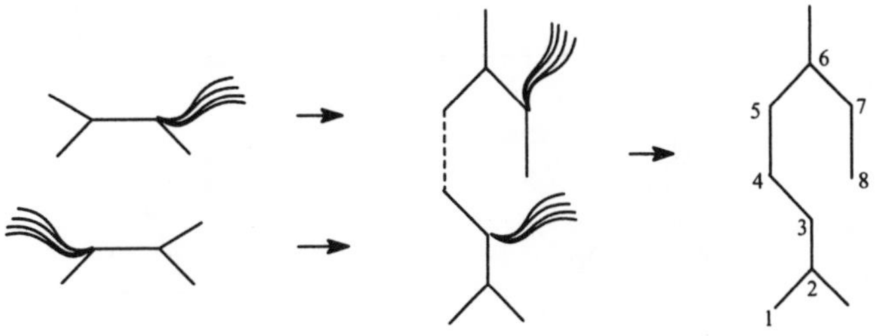

Fig. 2.14 — Outline diagrams to show how the molecular structure of an acyclic monoterpene may be regarded as being formed from two isoprene units

This outline diagram is easily seen to represent the saturated hydrocarbon 2,6-dimethyloctane, which can be regarded as the 'parent hydrocarbon' structure of the chain-type monoterpenes.

The question may arise, What happens to the double bonds?, to which the answer is that nothing happens to them, because the above series of diagrams does not represent how terpenes are formed in living cells, but merely attempts to show how the molecular structure of a chain-type monoterpene can be regarded as consisting of two isoprene units bonded together. Scientifically, chain-type monoterpenes are termed 'acyclic', meaning 'not in the form of a ring'.

Different acyclic monoterpenes are distinguished by the positions of the double bonds in their molecules; these are three in number, as shown by the structural formulae of two important examples:

Myrcene
(occurs, e.g., in Bay Leaf Oil)

Ocimene
(occurs, e.g., in Basil Oil)

Fig. 2.15 — Structural formulae of myrcene and ocimene

2.8 Monoterpenes Having Ring Structures

Very many organic compounds are known in which all or part of the molecular skeleton takes the form of a ring of carbon atoms. These are called *cyclic* compounds, hence the name 'cyclic monoterpenes' for monoterpenes having this kind of molecular structure. Before we discuss cyclic monoterpenes, note the examples of some simple, saturated, non-terpenic cyclic compounds in figure 2.16.

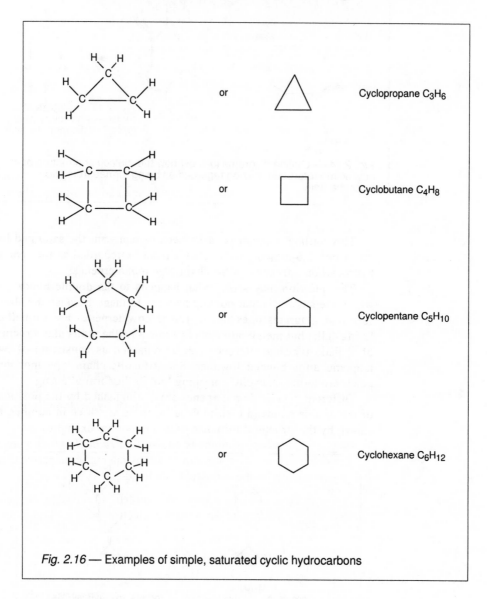

Fig. 2.16 — Examples of simple, saturated cyclic hydrocarbons

If the carbon atoms C3 and C8 of the acyclic monoterpene outline diagram shown in figure 2.14 are linked, we have the *outline* of a typical cyclic monoterpene molecular structure, based on a cyclohexane ring (fig. 2.17).

Notice the numbering of the carbon atoms in the diagram, which is the same for all monocyclic terpenes of this form. Notice also the two 'side chains', of one carbon atom (at C1) and three (at C4), bonded to the ring. Branches or side chains of various kinds are found in the molecules of countless organic compounds. Most of them are bonded to a carbon atom of a main chain or ring by a single bond, consisting of a shared pair of electrons, one from a carbon atom of the main chain and the other from a carbon atom of the side chain (fig. 2.18).

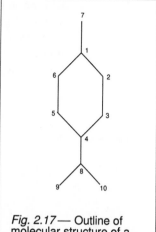

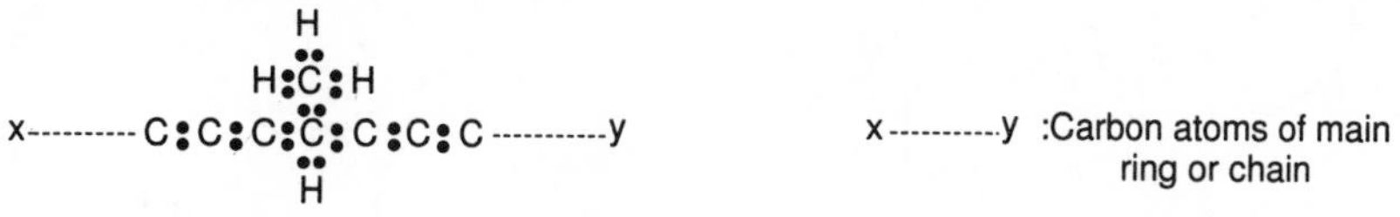

Fig. 2.17— Outline of molecular structure of a typical cyclic monoterpene

All electrons are of course identical, and so the question of identifying either of the electrons of a single bond, or any of those of a double bond, with either of the atoms joined by the bond does not arise.

Radicals

The methyl group of atoms is known as a *radical*, which may be defined as an atom or a group of atoms having an unpaired electron available for the formation of a bond.

Thus the methyl side chain may be regarded, structurally, as being formed by the pairing of an unpaired electron of a methyl radical

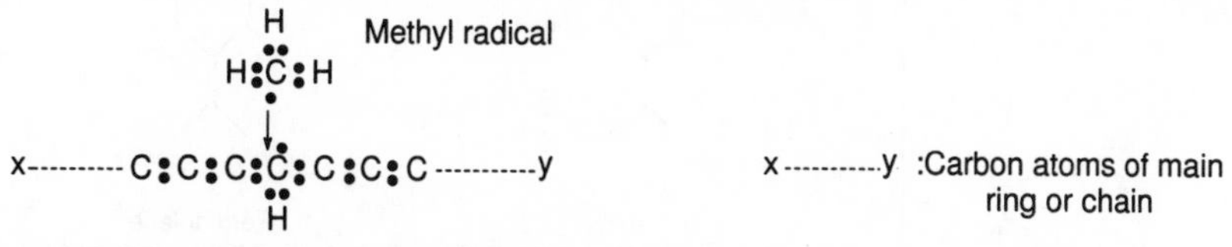

Fig. 2.18 — Sharing of electrons by side chain and main chain or ring

x---------y :Carbon atoms of main ring or chain

Methyl radical

Fig. 2.19— Pairing of unpaired electron of methyl radical with unpaired electron of carbon in main chain or ring

x---------y :Carbon atoms of main ring or chain

with an unpaired electron of a carbon atom of a main chain or ring system (fig. 2.19).

Some further examples of simple hydrocarbon radicals, frequently found in the molecules of constituents of essential oils are shown in figure 2.20.

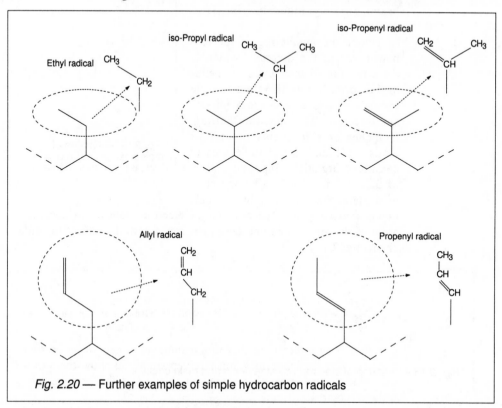

Fig. 2.20 — Further examples of simple hydrocarbon radicals

The outline diagram shown in figure 2.17, which may be considered as the 'parent hydrocarbon' structure of the cyclic monoterpenes, is 1-methyl-4-isopropyl-cyclo-hexane, otherwise known, for reasons which we shall later explain, as *para*-menthane.

Two important examples of cyclic monoterpenes are shown in figure 2.21. Note that each has two double bonds.

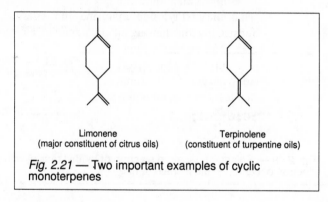

Limonene
(major constituent of citrus oils)

Terpinolene
(constituent of turpentine oils)

Fig. 2.21 — Two important examples of cyclic monoterpenes

There are many cyclic monoterpenes in which the molecules take the form of 'bridged' structures. This may be readily understood by first considering the molecular structure of *para*-menthane, and then rotating the isopropyl group into the cyclohexane ring (fig. 2.22).

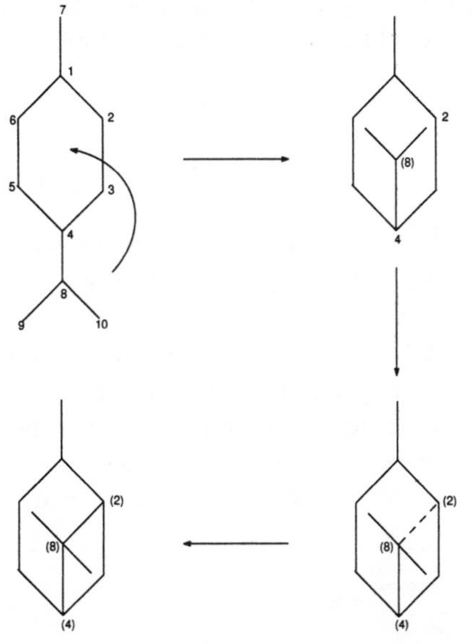

Fig. 2.22 — Rotating the iso-propyl side chain of *para*-menthane into the cyclohexane ring

It should be understood that this manipulation cannot be carried out directly in the laboratory, but is given simply to show the structural relationship between the *para*-menthane and the bridged molecular structures of figure 2.23.

Two very important cyclic monoterpenes having bridged molecular structures are shown in figure 2.23. Both of these pinenes are major constituents of Turpentine Oil, from which they are isolated to be used as feedstocks for the large-scale synthesis of a range of some of the most widely used of all aroma chemicals — the monoterpenoids.

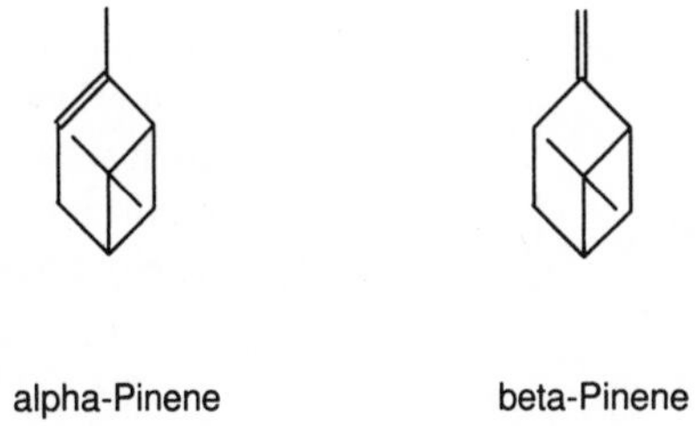

alpha-Pinene   beta-Pinene

Fig. 2.23 — The "bridged" structures of two pinenes

2.9 Sesquiterpenes

The prefix *sesqui-* means 'half as much again', which in reference to terpenes denotes a class of unsaturated hydrocarbons of molecular formula $C_{15}H_{24}$ — one-and-a-half times the molecular formula for a monoterpene $C_{10}H_{16}$. It is worth comparing the molecular weights of monoterpenes and sesquiterpenes:

$$C_{10}H_{16} = (12 \times 10) + (1 \times 16) = 136$$

$$C_{15}H_{24} = (12 \times 15) + (1 \times 24) = 204$$

The difference in molecular weight explains why sesquiterpenes evaporate more slowly than monoterpenes under the same conditions — their heavier molecules need more energy to pass into the vapour state than the lighter molecules of monoterpenes.

Sesquiterpenes are of very common occurrence in essential oils, to the odours of some of which they make significant contributions. We can again use outline diagrams to show how the molecular structure of a typical sesquiterpene is derived from three isoprene units:

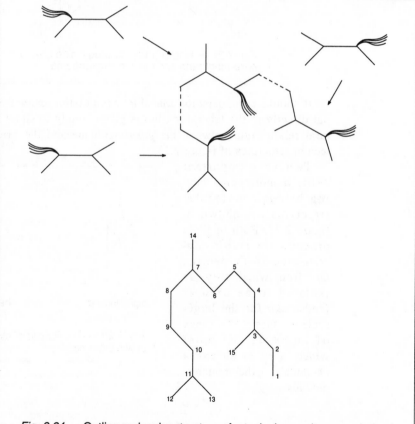

Fig. 2.24 — Outline molecular structure of a typical sesquiterpene derived from three isoprene units

Two important sesquiterpenes are the branched-chain farnesene, and bisabolene, the latter having a cyclohexene ring as part of its molecule:

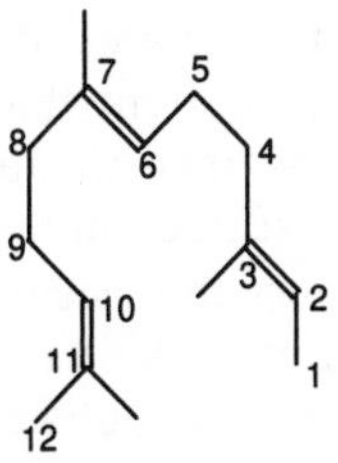

Farnesene
(occurs in Cassie Absolute)

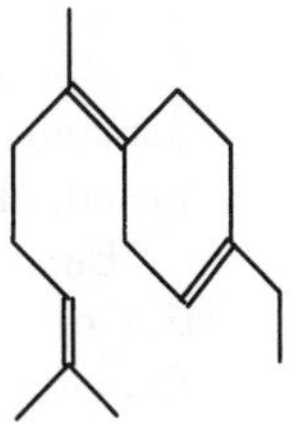

Bisabolene
(occurs in Myrrh Oil)

Fig. 2.25 — Branched-chain farnesene and bisabolene

By inspection of the structural formula for farnesene it can be seen that *cis-trans* isomerism is possible at the double bonds between C_2 and C_3 and between C_6 and C_7, but not between C_{10} and C_{11} because, here, two identical radicals (methyl groups) are bonded to C_{11}.

2.10 Benzene

Benzene is a colourless, highly flammable liquid hydrocarbon, discovered in 1825 by the eminent British scientist Michael Faraday as a constituent of an illuminating gas obtained from Whale Oil. Analysis of benzene showed its molecular formula to be C_6H_6, but it was not until 1865 that the famous German chemist Friedrich August Kekulé von Stradonitz (known as Kekulé) deduced its structural formula as a ring of six carbon atoms, each bonded to a hydrogen atom, and to one another by alternating single and double bonds (fig. 2.26).

However, experiments with benzene clearly showed that it did not undergo the chemical reactions typical of an unsaturated compound, but that the hydrocarbon possessed peculiar chemical properties of its own. From the results of further research, coupled with the development of bonding theory, it was later concluded that the electrons forming the bonds between the carbon atoms of the benzene molecule must be distributed evenly round the ring, with just one bonding pair (i.e. single bonds) between all adjacent carbon atoms and the remaining electrons forming doughnut-like clouds above and below the ring. This is sometimes indicated by writing the structural formula for benzene, as shown in figure 2.27.

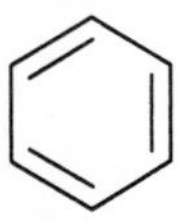

Fig. 2.26 — Benzene (Kekulé structure)

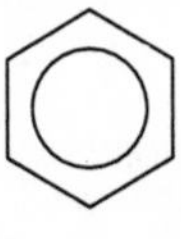

Fig. 2.27 — Benzene. Diagrammatic formula to represent later ideas on molecular structure

Many modern textbooks of organic chemistry use the original ring formula for benzene, possibly because in recent years some doubt has been cast upon a completely even distribution of electrons in the ring. This situation is typical of a science such as chemistry, the established laws and principles of which hold fast until someone finds a weakness — an exception which, far from 'proving the rule', demands that the rule be investigated and thereafter possibly adjusted, altered, or even discarded in the light of new knowledge.

Benzene itself is of very rare occurrence as a constituent of essential oils. Oxygen-containing derivatives of benzene are, however, found in many oils, and are exemplified in Chapter 3.

2.11 The Phenyl and Benzyl Radicals

If a hydrogen atom is removed from a benzene molecule, C_6H_6, the radical C_6H_5- is formed This is the *phenyl-*, not benzyl-, radical, which can bond with other radicals to form benzene derivatives. The *benzyl-* radical is in fact derived from methyl benzene, or toluene, by removal of an electron from the methyl group (fig. 2.28).

Substituents   A radical, such as a methyl group, substituting for hydrogen in benzene or another molecule is known as a *substituent*.

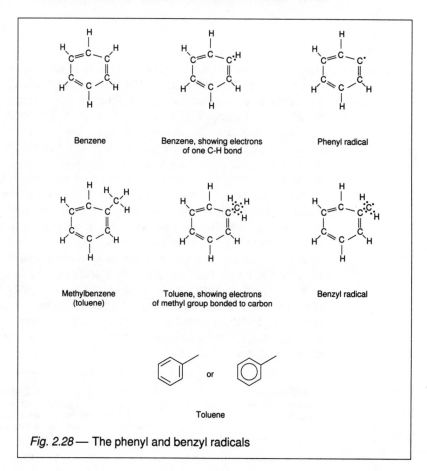

Fig. 2.28 — The phenyl and benzyl radicals

2.12 Disubstitution in Benzene

Many derivatives of benzene are known in which two or more of the hydrogen atoms of the ring are substituted by other atoms or groups of atoms. There are three relative positions which two substituents, such as methyl groups, can occupy around the ring; these are denoted as shown (fig. 2.29). Further substitution in benzene is denoted numerically.

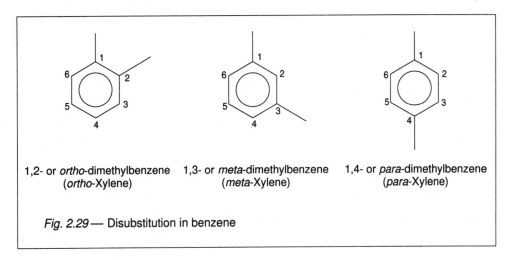

1,2- or *ortho*-dimethylbenzene   1,3- or *meta*-dimethylbenzene   1,4- or *para*-dimethylbenzene
    (*ortho*-Xylene)   (*meta*-Xylene)   (*para*-Xylene)

Fig. 2.29 — Disubstitution in benzene

2.13 Functional Groups

A molecule, such as a molecule of a terpene, which has as part of its structure one or more pairs of carbon atoms joined by double bonds, is found to be more chemically reactive than one in which all of the carbon atoms are joined by single bonds. Furthermore, if the molecule undergoes interaction with another molecule, atom or ion, the reaction usually involves a rearrangement of atoms in the region of the double bond(s). For this reason, the group of atoms $>C=C<$ is known as a *functional group*.

A functional group may be defined as a group of atoms in a molecule which is the part of the molecule most likely to undergo chemical reaction; it is that part of a molecule which tends to determine the chemical behaviour of the molecule. We should note that there are exceptions to this general rule, in that certain reactions can take place in parts of molecules other than functional groups that may be present, but this need not concern us here.

Terpenes, particularly monoterpenes, are unsaturated hydrocarbons which are vulnerable to oxidation by oxygen in the air. The attack occurs in the region of the $C=C$ double bonds of terpene molecules and is a main cause of the onset of spoilage in essential oils, such as the citrus oils, which are rich in monoterpenes. Monoterpenes can also undergo polymerization, a further cause of deterioration. Oxidation and polymerization reactions in relation to essential oils are discussed in Chapters 3 and 8 of this book.

In the following chapter we shall consider examples of functional groups containing oxygen, nitrogen and sulphur atoms.

Chapter 3

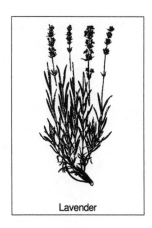

Lavender

Functional Groups
Containing Oxygen, Nitrogen and Sulphur

3.1 Oxygen-Containing Functional Groups

In Chapter 1 we noted that the valency, or combining power, of an oxygen atom is two, in reference to the fact that the atom of oxygen has two unpaired electrons in its outer electron shell which can form bonding pairs with unpaired electrons of other atoms.

Figure 1.3 of Chapter 1 shows the arrangement of electrons in the atoms of elements from hydrogen to argon, and Chapter 2 (fig. 2.28) includes a structural formula for the benzenoid hydrocarbon toluene. This shows dots representing the electrons bonding the three hydrogen atoms to the carbon atom of the methyl group (consisting of one carbon and three hydrogen atoms), and the pair of electrons bonding this carbon atom to a carbon atom of the 'benzene ring'. 'Electron dot' diagrams will be useful in this chapter to show how oxygen is involved in the structures of a number of important functional groups; they can then be translated into the relevant parts of conventional structural formulae.

In organic chemistry, the letter R is used when we wish to denote any hydrocarbon radical rather than a particular radical; R' and R" are also used where there is more than one radical in a formula which is either the same as, or different from, R. The symbols R, R' and R" can be used also to have the meaning 'a hydrogen atom or a radical', but in this case there is always an explanatory footnote to that effect. We shall use these convenient symbols as we discuss the families of organic compounds arising from the different functional groups.

3.2 Alcohols and Phenols: Functional Group -OH

Molecules of both alcohols and phenols contain the -O-H, or hydroxy functional group, but for reasons to be explained the chemical behaviour of members of the two families is distinctively different.

Alcohols

The oxygen atom of a hydroxy- group is joined to a hydrogen atom and to a carbon atom of a radical *except phenyl-* (*see* p. 53) by single bonds:

Now, in using this kind of diagram, we need to be crystal clear as to its meaning. Suppose R to represent the simplest of all hydrocarbon radicals — a methyl group; then we have the full 'electron dot' formula:

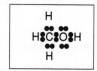

In this formula the individual atoms are represented as follows:

| H | C | O |

H represents the hydrogen atom nucleus — a proton;
C represents the carbon atom nucleus *and the two inner electrons* of the carbon atom; and
O represents the oxygen atom nucleus *and the two inner electrons* of the oxygen atom.

Thus we have taken the quite permissible step of changing the meaning of C and O, which otherwise refer to *whole atoms* of the respective elements, in order to indicate the electrons involved in bonding. The inner electrons of carbon and oxygen are omitted from consideration because they are *never* involved in bonding or in chemical reactions involving these elements.

The formula A, then, of figure 3.1 represents a hydroxy- func-

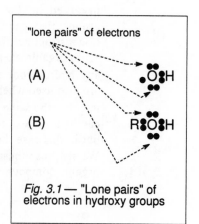

Fig. 3.1 — "Lone pairs" of electrons in hydroxy groups

tional group, and B, a hydroxy- group bonded to a hydrocarbon radical. The latter formula can be simplified by using bonding lines:

R-O-H or R-OH

In these two formulae, the 'lone pairs' of electrons on the oxygen atom, which are not, here, involved in bonding, are understood to be present.

It is useful to regard a hydroxy-compound, such as R-OH, as a molecule in which a hydrogen atom of the hydrocarbon of which R is a radical has been replaced by hydroxy. For example, the alcohol of formula CH_3-CH_2-CH_2-CH_2-CH_2-OH is a derivative of the hydrocarbon CH_3-CH_2-CH_2-CH_2-CH_3 in which a hydrogen atom bonded to a carbon atom at one end of the chain (a terminal carbon atom) has been replaced by a hydroxy- group. We can now see a limitation to the use of R, in that it does not indicate at which carbon atom along the pentane chain the substitution has taken place; i.e, we do not know where, in the molecule, the hydroxy group is placed. But, of course, R is used purely as a generalization, and has meaning provided its limitation is borne in mind.

Because all atoms of oxygen, and of hydrogen, are respectively chemically identical, the use of R-OH to stand for any hydrocarbon radical bonded to a hydroxy- group could be taken to imply that all compounds of which the molecules contain this as the only functional group should behave, chemically, in the same way. A more accurate view, supported by countless experiments, is that this is generally true, but that the nature of R has some effect, and in some cases a profound effect, on just how an organic hydroxy- compound behaves in a given reaction. The functional group -OH very largely determines the 'family likeness' of chemical behaviour; that is, what kind of rearrangements of atoms take place when different reactions occur, while the structure or geometry of the molecule may influence how readily and how fast the reactions take place. In extreme cases, a hydrocarbon radical of a particular kind can determine that certain reactions occur at a functional group which do not occur at all if the molecular geometry is different.

We are now in a position to distinguish between alcohols and phenols.

As indicated in the first two paragraphs of this section, the chemical family of *alcohols* is characterized by molecules in which a hydroxy- functional group is bonded to a hydrocarbon radical *other than phenyl*. This distinction arises from the nature of the 'benzene ring' of six carbon atoms wherein, as we noted in section 2.10, the electrons bonding the carbon atoms together are delocalized. This delocalization affects the chemical behaviour of a hydroxy- group bonded directly to the ring to such an extent that it undergoes certain reactions which do not occur when the group is bonded to a hydrocarbon radical other than phenyl.

Phenols

The chemical family of *phenols* is characterized by molecules in which a hydroxy- functional group is bonded *directly* to a benzene ring.

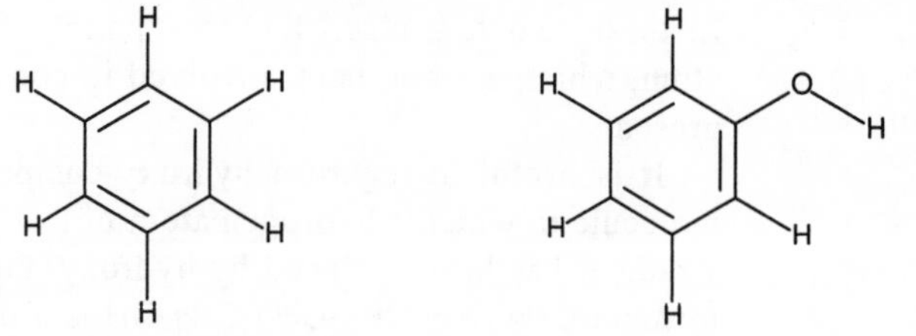

Benzene

Phenol (hydroxybenzene)

Fig. 3.2 — Benzene and Phenol

In the molecule of phenol, the simplest member of the phenol family, one of the hydrogen atoms of benzene is replaced by a hydroxy- group (fig. 3.2).

Phenols which occur in essential oils are *substituted phenols*, in the molecules of which one or more of the remaining five hydrogen atoms of the benzene ring have been replaced by a hydrocarbon radical or functional group of some kind; eugenol, occurring in Clove, Cinnamon Leaf, Pimento and Ylang-Ylang oils, is an example (fig. 3.3).

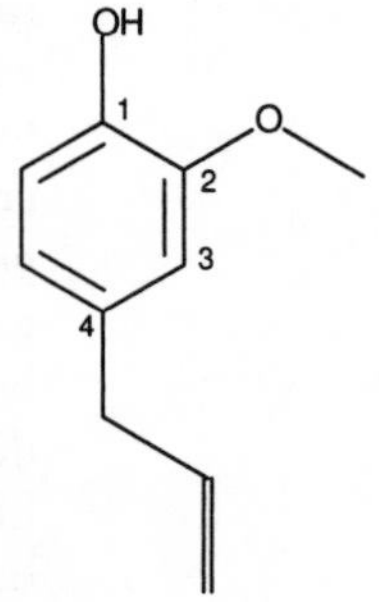

It will be useful, now, for us to illustrate a similarity, and an important difference, between the chemical behaviour of an alcohol and a phenol.

Experiment shows that metallic sodium reacts with water very vigorously, with any alcohol less vigorously and with a phenol very much less vigorously. The reactions are similar in that in all of them a hydrogen atom is replaced by a sodium ion.

Fig. 3.3 — Eugenol 2-methoxy-4-allyl-phenol

Reaction between sodium and water, where HOH = a water molecule:

$$2\,Na_{(s)} \; + \; 2\,HOH_{(l)} \longrightarrow 2\,Na^+\,OH^-{}_{(aq)} \; + \; H_{2(g)}$$

Reaction between sodium and an alcohol:

$$2\,Na_{(s)} \; + \; 2\,ROH_{(l)} \longrightarrow 2\,Na^+\,OR^-{}_{(aq)} \; + \; H_{2(g)}$$

Reaction between sodium and a phenol, where Ph = a phenyl or substituted phenyl radical:

$$2\,Na_{(s)} + 2\,PhOH_{(l)} \longrightarrow 2\,Na^+\,OPh^-_{(aq)} + H_{2(g)}$$

Now to differentiate between an alcohol and a phenol:

Testing for phenols and alcohols

If a few drops of an alcohol of the kind that occurs in essential oils, e.g. citronellol, geraniol or linalöl, are added to a strong, aqueous solution of an alkali, such as potassium hydroxide, and the mixture is stirred, the drops of the alcohol do not dissolve but float on the solution and no reaction occurs.

If a few drops of a phenol that occurs in essential oils are similarly treated, the phenol dissolves, because a reaction takes place with the formation of a water-soluble, organic product:

$$PhOH_{(l)} + K^+\,OH^-_{(aq)} \longrightarrow PhO^-\,K^+_{(aq)} + H_2O_{(l)}$$

Notice that in this reaction the phenol, PhOH, acts as an acid, donating a hydrogen ion to the hydroxide ion of the potassium hydroxide to form a water molecule; the familiar neutralization reaction:

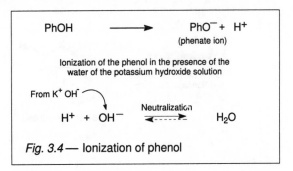

Fig. 3.4— Ionization of phenol

The drops of the phenol dissolve in the alkali solution because the phenate ion, PhO^-, is soluble in water.

A further important difference between an alcohol and a phenol is that a phenol, particularly if liquid (some, such as phenol and thymol, are colourless, crystalline solids) is readily attacked by oxygen in the air, whereas an alcohol resists this form of attack. Phenol itself slowly turns pink if stored in a bottle from which amounts are regularly withdrawn; eugenol, when pure a colourless liquid, turns yellow fairly quickly, then darkens, eventually becoming reddish brown, and the same darkening occurs in essential oils containing eugenol or other phenol. Solutions of phenates suffer atmospheric oxidation much more readily than the parent phenols, with the formation of dark-coloured oxidation products.

A third difference between alcohols and phenols is readily seen in the presence of compounds of iron (specifically iron III ions), to which alcohols are chemically indifferent; phenols react to form intensely reddish coloured, complex compounds. Thus if an essential oil containing a phenol as one of its constituents were to be shipped in a rusty steel drum, the contents would quickly become unusable or would need redistillation before use. A moist, phenol-containing oil shipped in a non-rusty steel drum would suffer the same fate, for reasons we have discussed.

Both alcohols and phenols form *esters* by direct or indirect reaction with organic acids. Esters are discussed in sections 3.6 and 3.7.

Many of the alcohols that occur in essential oils, or that are used in perfumery as aroma chemicals, possess soft, sweet flowery, green, herbaceous or woody odours. The odours of volatile phenols are typically 'medicated' in character, as with thymol and carvacrol (and phenol itself), or pungent and spicy, as with eugenol. The names of both alcohols and phenols carry the suffix '-ol'.

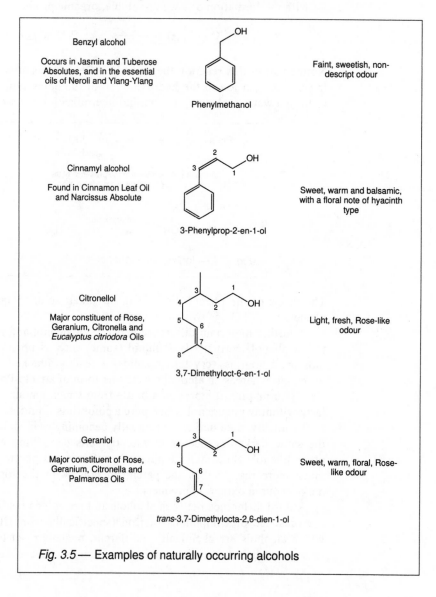

Benzyl alcohol		
Occurs in Jasmin and Tuberose Absolutes, and in the essential oils of Neroli and Ylang-Ylang		Faint, sweetish, non-descript odour
	Phenylmethanol	
Cinnamyl alcohol		
Found in Cinnamon Leaf Oil and Narcissus Absolute		Sweet, warm and balsamic, with a floral note of hyacinth type
	3-Phenylprop-2-en-1-ol	
Citronellol		
Major constituent of Rose, Geranium, Citronella and *Eucalyptus citriodora* Oils		Light, fresh, Rose-like odour
	3,7-Dimethyloct-6-en-1-ol	
Geraniol		
Major constituent of Rose, Geranium, Citronella and Palmarosa Oils		Sweet, warm, floral, Rose-like odour
	trans-3,7-Dimethylocta-2,6-dien-1-ol	

Fig. 3.5 — Examples of naturally occurring alcohols

Linalōl

Major constituent of
Rosewood, Coriander
and Ho Oils

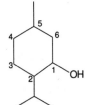

Light, floral, woody and spicy
(in relation to Coriander) odour;
very slightly citrus

3,7-Dimethylocta-1,6-dien-3-ol

Menthol

Major constituent of
Peppermint and *Mentha
arvensis* Oils

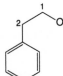

Cool, refreshing odour,
recalling Peppermint

5-Methyl-1,2-iso-propylcyclohexanol

Phenylethyl alcohol

An important constituent
of Rose, Geranium, Neroli
and Ylang-Ylang Oils

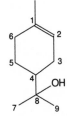

Warm, Rose-like and honey-
like odour

2-Phenylethyl alcohol

alpha-Terpineol

Occurs as a major constituent
of Pine oils and as a minor
constituent of many other
essential oils

When very highly purified
possesses a sweet and delicate,
floral, Lilac-like odour

1-Methyl-4-isopropyl-cyclo-hex-1-en-8-ol

Fig. 3.5 *(contd.)* — Examples of naturally occurring alcohols

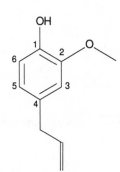

Carvacrol

Occurs widely in essential
oils of plants of Labiatae
family – Thyme and Sage Oils

Phenolic and spicy odour

2-Methyl-5-isopropylphenol

Eugenol

Major constituent of Clove,
Cinnamon Leaf and Pimento
Oils; minor constituent of
Rose and Ylang-Ylang Oils

Pungent, spicy, characteristic
of Clove

4-Allyl-2-methoxyphenol

Thymol

Major constituent of Thyme
and Origanum Oils

Powerful, "medicated" and
herbaceous odour

3-Methyl-6-isopropylphenol

Fig. 3.6 — Examples of naturally occurring phenols

3.3 Aldehydes: Functional Group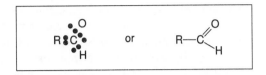

The carbon atom of this functional group is joined to the oxygen atom by a double bond and to the hydrogen atom by a single bond:

A reaction typical of all aldehydes is their ready oxidation to the corresponding organic acids. This can be effected by means of a suitable oxidizing agent, such as alkaline potassium permanganate solution or, in many cases, simply by exposure to air:

Aldehyde   Organic acid

where [O] represents an oxygen atom from an oxidizing agent (such as one of the two oxygen atoms of an oxygen molecule).

Notice that the carbonyl group (>C=O) of the aldehyde is unaffected by this reaction. The organic acid produced is known as a *carboxylic acid*.

The functional group, a carboxyl group (*see right*), is characteristic of all organic acids (but remember that phenols also can act as acids in the presence of an alkali; phenols are not, however, carboxylic acids). The carbonyl group (>C=O) must
be carefully distinguished from the aldehyde group (-CHO) and the carboxyl group (-COOH), of both of which it is a part. As we shall see in section 3.4, the carbonyl group can be a functional group on its own: it then has properties different from those that it shows as part of an aldehyde or carboxyl group.

A range of aldehydes is manufactured synthetically for use in perfumery. These are classified by perfumers into two groups according to odour properties and applications as perfume ingredients:

(a) *fatty aldehydes*, related chemically to natural fats;
(b) *other aldehydes*, having a wide diversity of molecular structure.

The fatty aldehydes are few in number, and are closely related in molecular structure, odour qualities and applications. Their hydrocarbon radicals consist of chains of from 7 to 12 carbon atoms bonded to hydrogen and all of them are readily oxidized by atmospheric oxygen to produce unpleasant-smelling carboxylic acids known as fatty acids. The odours of fatty aldehydes are very powerful, fatty, waxy and generally unpleasant, becoming acceptable, and even pleasant, when the aldehydes are diluted with an odourless solvent to 0·1% or less. Most of these aldehydes occur in nature as minor constituents of citrus and other essential oils, and as major constituents of a few tropical oils, such as Keesom Oil. We shall discuss their interesting applications in perfumery in Chapter 8.

Naturally occurring aldehydes other than the fatty aldehydes include the citrals neral and geranial found in Lemon and Lemongrass Oils, citronellal in Citronella and *Eucalyptus citriodora* Oils and vanillin in Vanilla extracts. The vanillin molecule is polyfunctional, having more than one functional group in its molecule (aldehyde, hydroxy- and ether). The odours of non-fatty aldehydes display a whole spectrum of odour qualities, ranging from powerful, sharp, lemony (citrals) through floral (anisaldehyde, 'Lilial' [Givaudan-Roure], amylcinnamic aldehyde) to intensely green (several hexenals and heptenals).

Fatty aldehydes are commonly named according to the total number of carbon atoms in their molecules, or with a root denoting the parent hydrocarbon, with the suffix '-al' as, for example, 'aldehyde C8', or octanal. Other aldehydes are named with one or more words referring to molecular structure or association with a natural source,

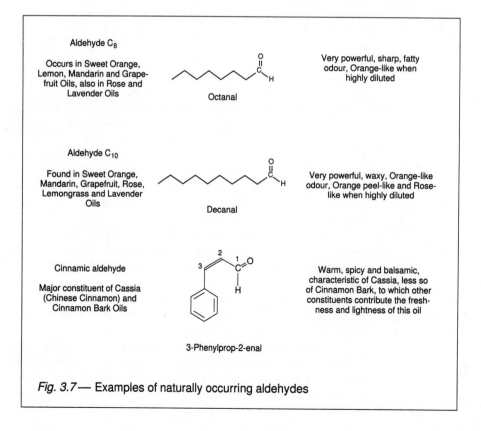

Fig. 3.7— Examples of naturally occurring aldehydes

Citronellal

Major constituent of Citronella, Melissa and *Eucalyptus citriodora* Oils

Strong, citrus and coarsely Rose-like odour, characteristic of Citronella

3,7-Dimethyloct-6-en-1-al

Geranial

This is alpha-citral which, with neral, occurs as a major constituent of Lemongrass and *Litsea cubeba* Oils, also in Lemon, Lime, Melissa and Verbena Oils

Light, sharp, fresh odour, characteristic of Lemon

trans-3,7-Dimethylocta-2,6-dienal

Neral

Neral is beta-citral. It occurs, with geranial, as a major constituent of Lemongrass and *Litsea cubeba* Oils, also in Lemon, Lime, Melissa and Verbena Oils

Light, sharp odour of Lemon, somewhat less fresh than geranial

cis-3,7-Dimethylocta-2,6-dienal

Vanillin

Major constituent of dried and cured Vanilla fruits. Occurs also in Benzoin, Styrax and Balsams of Peru and Tolu

Soft, sweet, powdery, typical of Vanilla, but lacking the richness of odour of natural Vanilla

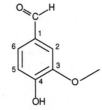

4-Hydroxy-3-methoxybenzaldehyde

Fig. 3.7 (contd.) — Examples of naturally occurring aldehydes

followed by the word 'aldehyde'. Examples, here, are phenylacetaldehyde, anisic aldehyde and cinnamic aldehyde. A few aldehydes, such as vanillin and heliotropine, retain their original, trivial names for everyday use. Chemically, all aldehydes are named according to their hydrocarbon skeleta, followed by '-al', as in octanal,

4-methoxybenzaldehyde (= anisaldehyde) and the citrals (*cis-* and *trans-*3,7-dimethylocta-2,6-dienals). Some examples of naturally occuring aldehydes are shown in figure 3.7.

The 'pseudo-aldehydes'

Certain powerfully odorous and, as it transpired, extremely useful, aroma chemicals were, at the time of their introduction to perfumery many years ago, named by their originators as aldehydes, though in fact they belong to other chemical classes. The reason for concealment of the true identity of these materials was to prevent, at least for some considerable time, their synthesis by competitors, so preserving a commercial advantage for their originators.

Trade names are today applied to new fragrance materials in preference to disclosure of their true nature simply for ease of identification and memorization since, in contrast to the situation in earlier times, the analysis of a volatile product to determine its composition is, if costly, a simple matter, occupying hours rather than weeks.

Three well-known 'pseudo-aldehydes' are shown in table 3.1.

Table 3.1 — 'Pseudo-aldehydes'

Name in common use	Chemical name	Odour character
'Aldehyde C_{14}, Peach, so-called'	gamma-Undecalactone	Powerful, Peach-like
'Aldehyde C_{16}, Strawberry, so-called'	Ethyl methyl phenyl glycidate	Soft, sweet, persistent, Strawberry-like
'Aldehyde C_{18}, Coconut, so-called'	gamma-Nonalactone	Powerful, Coconut-like

A structural formula for 'Coconut lactone', named as nonanolide-1,4, appears on page 71. The 'Peach lactone' has an identical molecular ring structure, but has seven carbon atoms in the side-chain instead of the five present in 'Peach lactone'. The structural formula for 'Strawberry ester' (*see* name suffixes: -yl -yl -yl -ate, indicating a member of the ester family of chemicals) is as follows. Note the small ring of two carbon atoms and one oxygen atom in the glycidate radical (fig. 3.8).

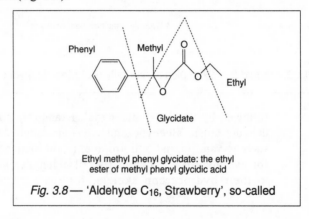

Ethyl methyl phenyl glycidate: the ethyl
ester of methyl phenyl glycidic acid

Fig. 3.8 — 'Aldehyde C_{16}, Strawberry', so-called

3.4 Ketones: Functional Group $-\overset{\overset{\displaystyle O}{\|}}{C}-$

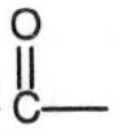

We have already noted the existence of this group of atoms as part of the aldehyde and carboxyl functional groups, wherein its individuality is considerably modified by bonding to a hydrogen atom in aldehydes and to a hydroxy- group in organic acids. In a ketone, the carbonyl group is bonded to two hydrocarbon radicals, and so, unlike the aldehyde or carboxyl groups, cannot be situated at one end of a molecule; that is, it cannot be a terminal functional group. Thus a ketone has the following general formula:

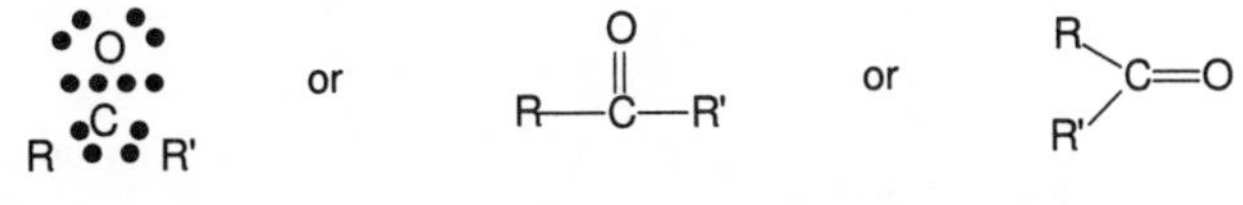

It is a matter of convenience as to which of the last two formulae is used. Note that in neither of these formulae can R or R′ stand for a hydrogen atom, otherwise we would have:

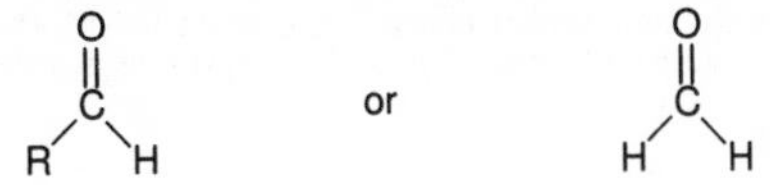

An aldehyde

Formaldehyde or methanal - the simplest aldehyde

The family of ketones exhibits a wide range of different odour types, but relatively few ketones occur as important constituents of essential oils. Examples of those which do are the celery-like *cis*-jasmone, in Jasmin Absolute, the violet-smelling ionones of Boronia Absolute and the alpha-irone present as the main odorous constituents of Orris Oil, also methyl amyl (pentyl) ketone in Clove oils.

Ketones are named either by reference to the hydrocarbon radicals bonded to the carbonyl group as, for example, in figure 3.9, or, in the case of simple ketones only, to the total number of carbon atoms in the chain of which the carbonyl carbon atom is a part (fig. 3.10).

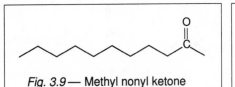

Fig. 3.9 — Methyl nonyl ketone (major constituent of Rue Oil)

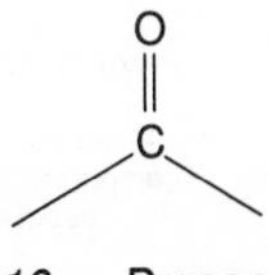

Fig. 3.10 — Propanone: dimethyl ketone or acetone

Some ketones retain their older, trivial names, or are known by abbreviated chemical names, e.g. alpha-ionone (fig. 3.11).

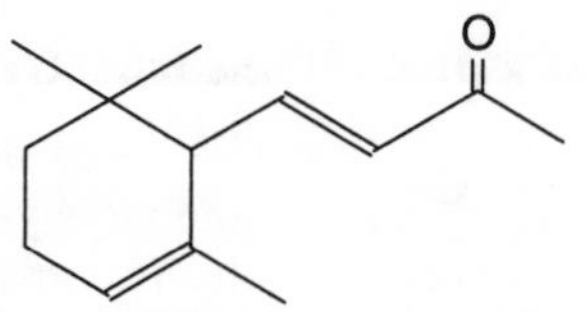

Of ketones manufactured synthetically for use as perfume ingredients, the ionones are the most outstanding; their odours are very highly appreciated and they are of great versatility in the range of their applications. Some examples of other naturally occurring ketones are given in figure 3.12.

Fig. 3.11 — alpha-ionone

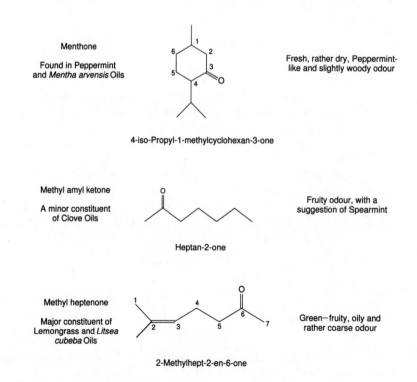

cis-Jasmone

Important constituent of Jasmin Absolute

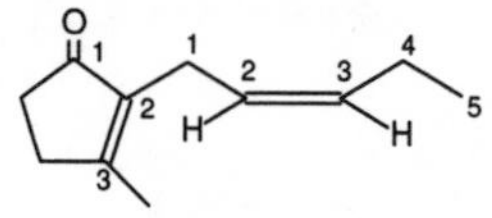

Warm, spicy, celery-like and floral odour

3-Methyl-2-(*cis*-pent-2-en-1-yl)-cyclo-pent-2-en-1-one

This compound is named by first numbering the positions of the substituent groups of the cyclopentene ring, starting with the ketone carbonyl group bonded to C_1. The C_2 of the ring is bonded to a pentene side chain, of which the carbon atoms are numbered separately, as shown. The side chain is regarded as a radical, and is of *cis*- arrangement, hence "-(*cis*-pent-2-en-1-yl)". The position of the methyl group bonded to the ring is given by "3-methyl", and "-2-en-" gives the position of the double bond in the ring.

Menthone

Found in Peppermint and *Mentha arvensis* Oils

Fresh, rather dry, Peppermint-like and slightly woody odour

4-iso-Propyl-1-methylcyclohexan-3-one

Methyl amyl ketone

A minor constituent of Clove Oils

Fruity odour, with a suggestion of Spearmint

Heptan-2-one

Methyl heptenone

Major constituent of Lemongrass and *Litsea cubeba* Oils

Green–fruity, oily and rather coarse odour

2-Methylhept-2-en-6-one

Fig. 3.12 — Further examples of naturally occurring ketones

3.5 Carboxylic Acids: Functional Group —C⟨=O / OH⟩

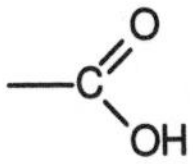

The functional group -COOH, carboxyl, is characteristic of all organic acids known as carboxylic acids. It consists of a hydroxy group and an oxygen atom bonded to the same carbon atom, which is itself bonded to a hydro-carbon radical in molecules of organic acids. A carboxylic acid has the following general formula:

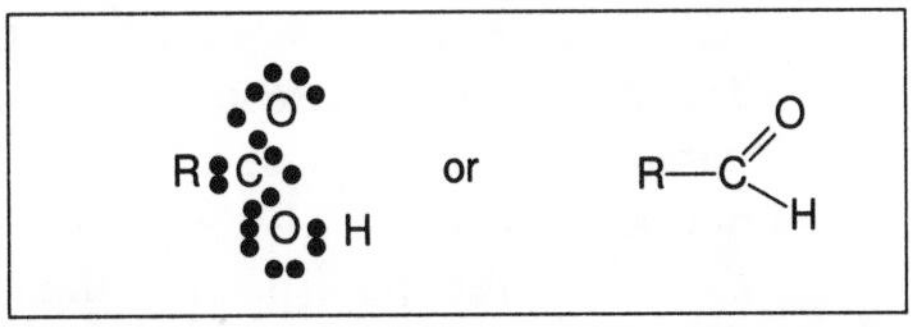

The carbonyl group and the hydroxy- group of a carboxylic acid influence the chemical properties of each other to such an extent that the carboxyl group as a whole possesses its own unique set of properties, of which two are of particular importance:

3.5.1 Ionization in the Presence of Water

Acids such as vinegar and lemon juice are typically sour-tasting, a sensory impression that results from the behaviour of their carboxyl groups in the presence of water. This may be expressed in the form of an equation:[1]

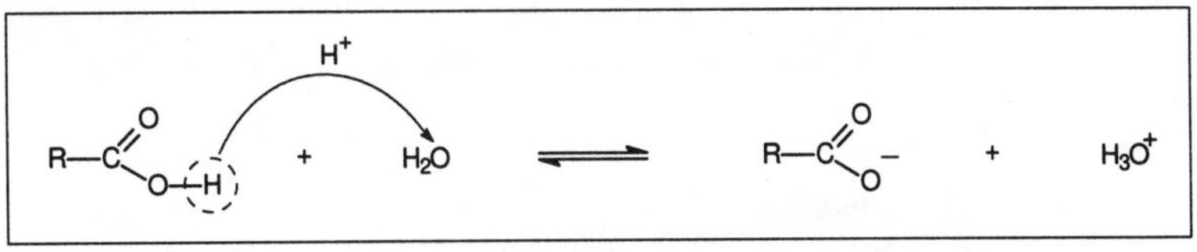

Note that the above reaction is reversible, as indicated by the reverse half-arrows. This means that if an organic acid is mixed with water the forward reaction will take place, but that, as increasing numbers of ions are formed by the forward reaction, these ions increasingly react together to produce the original acid and water. Thus in the solution of the acid a state of balance (or equilibrium) is quickly established in which the speed or rate of the forward reaction is exactly matched by the speed of the reverse reaction. The strength

---

1. In this reaction, the hydrogen atom of the carboxyl group is transferred to the water molecule as a hydrogen ion (a proton) because the negative charges on the lone pairs of electrons on the oxygen atom of the water molecule are strong enough to overcome the attractive force of the pair of electrons bonding that hydrogen atom to oxygen in the carboxyl group. Once released, the hydrogen ion bonds to one of the lone pairs of electrons on the oxygen atom of the water molecule. The bond so formed is an ordinary covalent bond but the water molecule, having gained a proton, becomes a positively charged oxonium ion. It is the oxonium ion that is the causative agent of acidity in aqueous solution.

of the acid solution clearly depends on the concentration of oxonium ions present, which in turn depends on two factors:

a) the extent to which the pure acid will release hydrogen ions to form oxonium ions with water. Weak acids do this only to a small extent; strong acids to a large extent;

b) how much of the acid is dissolved in a given quantity of water. The acid of vinegar, acetic (or ethanoic) acid, and the acid of lemon juice, citric acid, are both weak acids, though strong enough to taste extremely sour if undiluted. Three drops of lemon juice in a glass of water gives a solution of scarcely noticeable acidity, whereas neat lemon juice is just too unbearably sour for most people, though some will suck a lemon with impunity! This goes to show that taste sensations are every bit as subjective as odours, a subject to which we shall return later in this book.

Inorganic acids, that is, those whose molecules are not based on skeletons of carbon atoms, are, in some cases, very strong acids; sulphuric acid and hydrochloric acid are examples. When added to water their molecules ionize completely, producing enormous and highly dangerous concentrations of oxonium ions which can quickly and severely damage living cells.

Most organic acids are weak acids, producing low concentrations of oxonium ions in aqueous solution. Those organic acids that are volatile usually possess unpleasant odours.

3.5.2 Formation of Esters

Organic acids react with alcohols to form esters, the properties of which, including odour, are different from those of the acids and alcohols from which they are derived. This type of reaction, known as *esterification*,[2] may be expressed as follows:

| Organic acid | Alcohol | Ester | Water |

As shown, the esterification reaction is reversible; it is important in the synthesis of esters for use as solvents and as perfume ingredients.

---

2. Note that in the esterification reaction the hydroxy- group of the carboxylic acid forms a molecule of water with the hydroxy hydrogen atom of the alcohol.

The reverse reaction, called *hydrolysis* (*hydro*-:water; *lysis*: a splitting) can occur in an ester-containing essential oil containing a proportion of dissolved water resulting from the process of steam- or water-distillation used for separating it from its natural source. Any significant degree of hydrolysis occurring in an essential oil will inevitably lead to spoilage from the unpleasant odours of the carboxylic acids formed. These acids will ionize to a small extent in the presence of the water dissolved in the oil, producing oxonium ions, which act as a catalyst to the hydrolysis reaction, causing it to proceed faster than it would in their absence. We should remember, also, that organic acids are produced by the oxidation of aldehydes (sect. 3.3); hence the acid content of an aldehyde-containing essential oil can be increased by oxidation, with consequent acceleration of the hydrolysis of any esters present if the oil is moist.

Clearly, since most essential oils have at least some content of both aldehydes and esters, they should be both dry and protected from oxidation by correct storage (sect. 3.13).

Essential oils of good quality frequently contain traces of free organic acids arising, in all probability, from the hydrolysis of esters during distillation, which would be encouraged by the hot conditions involved. These normal traces of acids contribute faint odour nuances which have long been accepted as desirable features of the odour profiles of the oils in which they occur. The acidity, and hence the likelihood of serious deterioration, of an aldehyde-containing and/or moist, essential oil increases with the age of the oil.

3.6 Esters: Functional Group

The ester functional group appears in the general formula for an ester given in section 3.5.1. The molecular structure of an ester in the region of the functional group is as follows:

Typical of the ester group is its reaction with water, when hydrolysis occurs with cleavage of the —C—O— single bond (fig. 3.13). Hydrolysis is, as we have noted, the reverse of esterification.

Members of the chemical family of esters are widely distributed in nature, many occurring as the volatiles of fruits, such as raspberry, strawberry, banana and pineapple. We refer, here, to volatiles rather than essential oils because the volatile flavour principles are present in such minute proportions that it is simply not feasible to isolate them by distillation or otherwise as commercial products; the cost

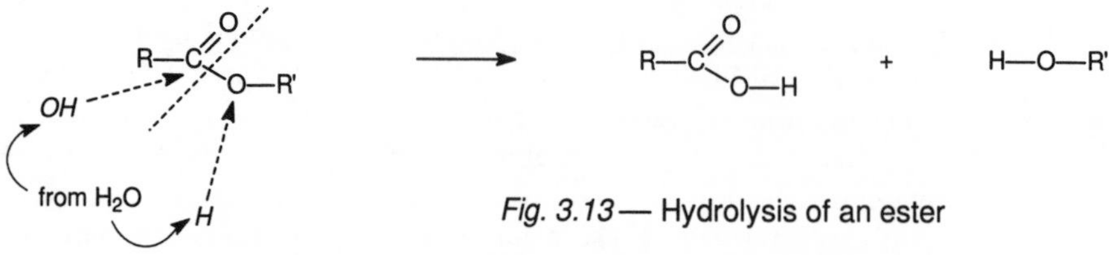

Fig. 3.13 — Hydrolysis of an ester

would be prohibitive. For flavour purposes, the juices of fruits are concentrated under conditions which, as far as possible, preserve their flavour qualities, whereafter unavoidable losses are made up with minute amounts of synthetic materials, all of which are chemically identical to naturally occurring flavour constituents, and which are known as 'nature identical' aroma chemicals.

The odour notes of fruits and fruit juices are important minor contributors to the fragrance profiles of modern perfumes, and are supplied by a range of mostly inexpensive aroma chemicals, some of which have not been reported as occurring in nature.

One of the few essential oils in regular supply having a non-citrus fruity note as a distinctive feature of its odour profile is 'Roman' Chamomile Oil produced in England and elsewhere in Europe by steam distillation of the flowers of *Anthemis nobilis*. The constituents of this oil mainly responsible for its fruitiness are the iso-amyl esters of the unsaturated carboxylic acids angelic acid (found also in the Angelica root) and tiglic acid (derived from the fixed oil of *Croton tiglium* — Croton Oil). These acids are *cis-trans* isomers (*see* fig. 3.14). The structural formulae for the iso-amyl (isopentyl) esters of these acids are as follows:

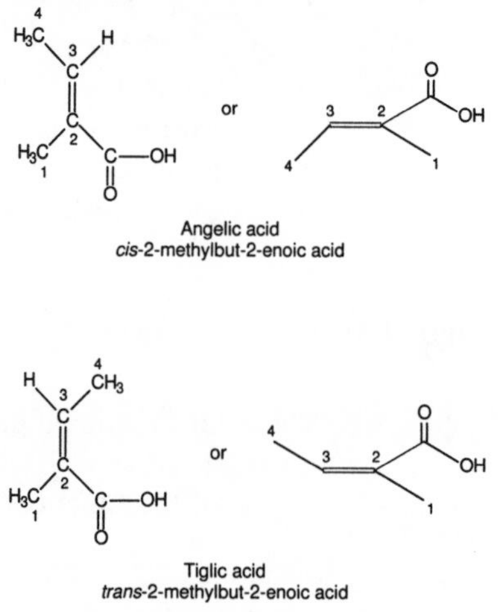

Fig. 3.14 — Angelic and Tiglic Acids

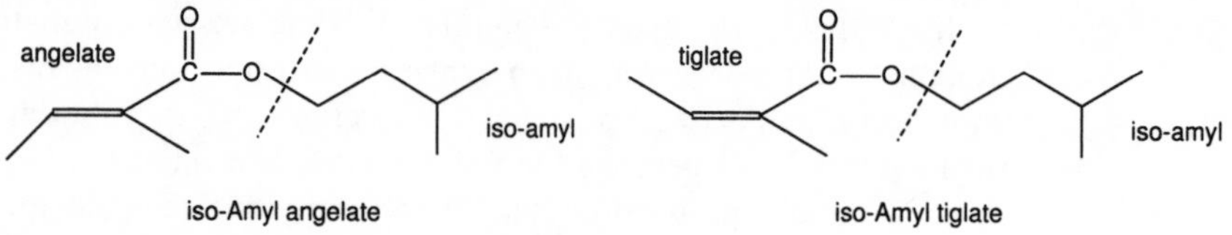

Fig. 3.15 — iso-Amyl Esters of Angelic and Tiglic Acids

Benzyl acetate

Major constituent of Jasmin Absolute. Occurs also in Ylang-Ylang and Neroli Oils

Floral and somewhat fruity odour of Jasmin character

Citronellyl acetate

Found in Citronella and Geranium Oils

Fresh, floral, Rose-like and fruity odour

3,7-Dimethyloct-6-en-1-yl acetate

Citronellyl formate

A constituent of Geranium Oil

Light, floral, Rose-like and fruity odour

3,7-Dimethyloct-6-en-1-yl formate

Geranyl acetate

Occurs as a minor constituent of Geranium, Citronella, Lavender, Petitgrain and many other essential oils

Sweet floral, Rose-like, somewhat fruity and green odour, having a suggestion of Lavender

trans-3,7-Dimethylocta-2,6-dien-1-yl acetate

Linalyl acetate

An important constituent of Bergamot, Lavender, Lavandin, Spike Lavender, Clary Sage, Neroli and Petitgrain Oils

Sweet, herbaceous and somewhat floral and fruity odour, reminiscent of Bergamot and Lavender Oils

3,7-Dimethylocta-1,6-dien-3-yl acetate

Fig. 3.16 — Other examples of naturally occurring esters

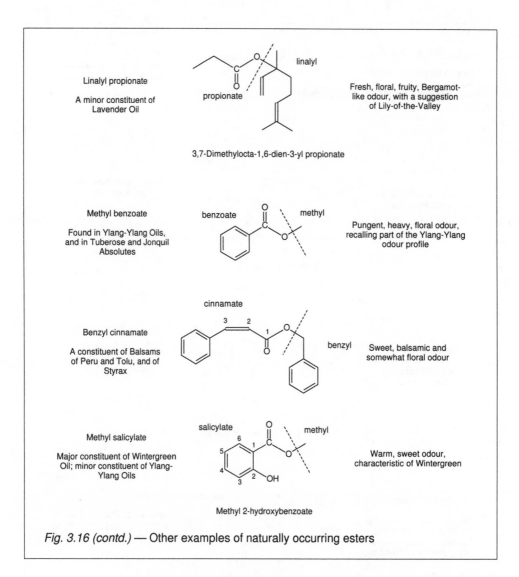

Linalyl propionate

A minor constituent of
Lavender Oil

propionate   linalyl

Fresh, floral, fruity, Bergamot-
like odour, with a suggestion
of Lily-of-the-Valley

3,7-Dimethylocta-1,6-dien-3-yl propionate

Methyl benzoate

Found in Ylang-Ylang Oils,
and in Tuberose and Jonquil
Absolutes

benzoate   methyl

Pungent, heavy, floral odour,
recalling part of the Ylang-Ylang
odour profile

Benzyl cinnamate

A constituent of Balsams
of Peru and Tolu, and of
Styrax

cinnamate   benzyl

Sweet, balsamic and
somewhat floral odour

Methyl salicylate

Major constituent of Wintergreen
Oil; minor constituent of Ylang-
Ylang Oils

salicylate   methyl

Warm, sweet odour,
characteristic of Wintergreen

Methyl 2-hydroxybenzoate

Fig. 3.16 (contd.) — Other examples of naturally occurring esters

The odour of Roman Chamomile Oil may be described as fruity, richly herbaceous and agrestic, an agrestic note being an odour of the countryside — of field, meadow, hayloft and (with certain reservations) farmyard.

The very important consequences of the hydrolysis of esters have been discussed in section 3.5.2.

3.7 Lactones: Functional Group —C(=O)—O— **as Part of a Ring Structure**

A lactone is an ester in which the ester functional group is part of a ring system, the other atoms of the ring being carbon atoms. An example of the formation of a lactone will help to make this clear.

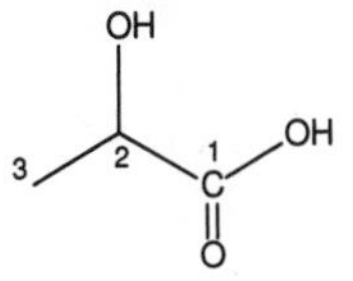

Fig. 3.17— Lactic acid
2-hydroxypropionic acid

Lactic acid, occurring in sour milk, is a hydroxy- acid (fig. 3.17). Hydroxy-acids in which the hydroxy- functional group is neither too near to, nor too far from, the -COOH carboxyl group undergo a chemical change when heated with a dilute acid or alkali in which, as in the formation of chain-type esters from alcohols and carboxylic acids, the product is formed with the elimination of water. In the case of a hydroxy-acid, a lactone is formed by interaction of the hydroxy- group and carboxyl group of the *same molecule*, as with 4-hydroxynonanoic acid lactone, prepared from 4-hydroxynonanoic acid, a derivative of the 9-carbon nonanoic acid (L. *nonus:* ninth), as in figure 3.18.

Many lactones, like many esters, possess fruity odours, and some occur in nature, contributing to the flavours of fruits. Some examples of naturally occurring lactones are given in figure 3.19.

The chemical name of a lactone is derived from the name of the hydroxy-acid from which it is formed, followed by the word 'lactone', or from the number of carbon atoms in a molecule of this acid, followed by the suffix '-olide', together with figures denoting the positions of the carboxyl and hydroxy- groups of the parent acid. Thus 4-hydroxy-nonanoic acid lactone (fig. 3.18) is systematically named nonanolide-1,4.

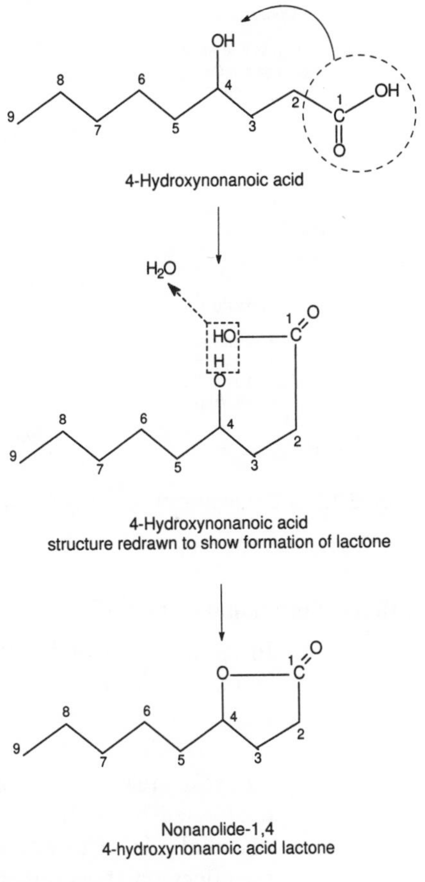

4-Hydroxynonanoic acid

4-Hydroxynonanoic acid
structure redrawn to show formation of lactone

Nonanolide-1,4
4-hydroxynonanoic acid lactone

Fig. 3.18 — Formation of a lactone

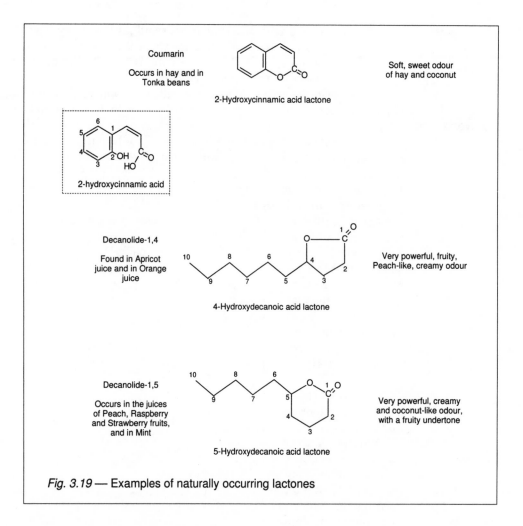

Fig. 3.19 — Examples of naturally occurring lactones

3.8 Ethers: Functional Group —O—

In the molecule of an ether, two hydrocarbon radicals are bonded to an oxygen atom:

R-O-R′

Most ethers are stable, relatively unreactive compounds, being unaffected by boiling water or steam as used in the distillation of essential oils, or by acids or alkalis. Atmospheric oxygen has little or no effect on those ethers which occur as constituents of essential oils, and consequently essential oils rich in ethers, such as Aniseed and Fennel Oils, do not pose storage problems if kept cool and protected from light. As a family, ethers display a variety of odours, from the sweet, characteristically Aniseed note of anethole (4-methoxypropenylbenzene) to the pungent, almost 'medicated' odour of methyl *para*cresol (*para*-cresyl methyl ether, or 4-methoxytoluene).

Anethole

Major constituent of
Aniseed, Star Anise and
Fennel Oils

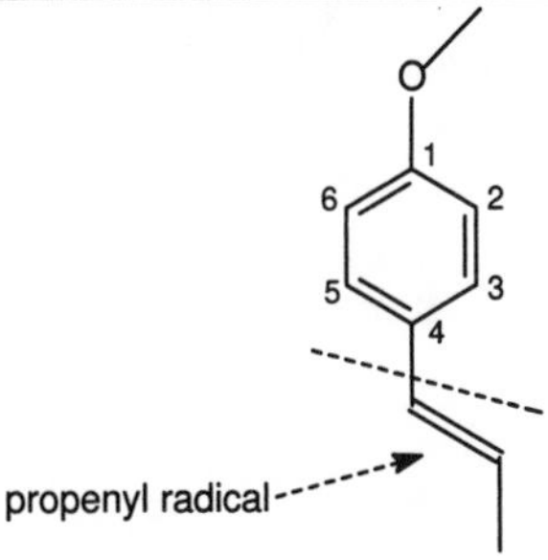

Sweet odour, characteristic
of Aniseed

propenyl radical

4-Propenylphenylmethyl ether

Estragole

Major constituent of Basil
and Estragon (Tarragon)
Oils

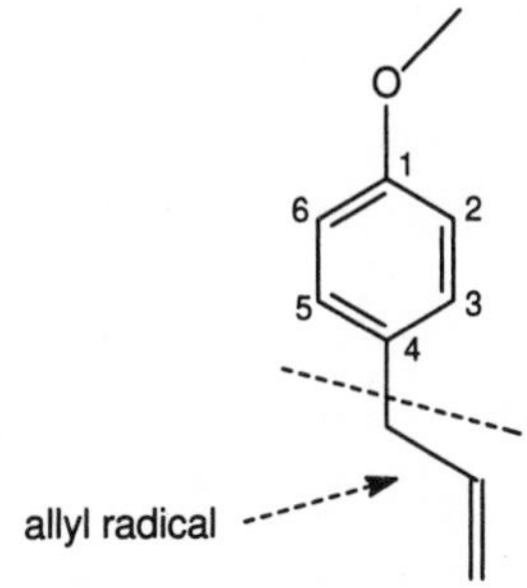

Sweet, anisic, herbaceous
odour

allyl radical

4-Allylphenylmethyl ether

Methyl *para*-cresol

Occurs in Ylang-Ylang Oil

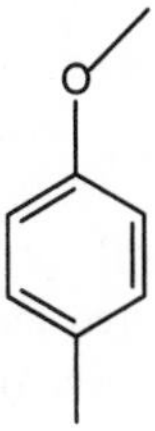

Pungent odour, reminiscent
of Ylang-Ylang Oil

para-Cresyl methyl ether

allyl radical

Safrole

Major constituent of
Sassafras Oil; minor
constituent of Nutmeg
and Camphor Oils

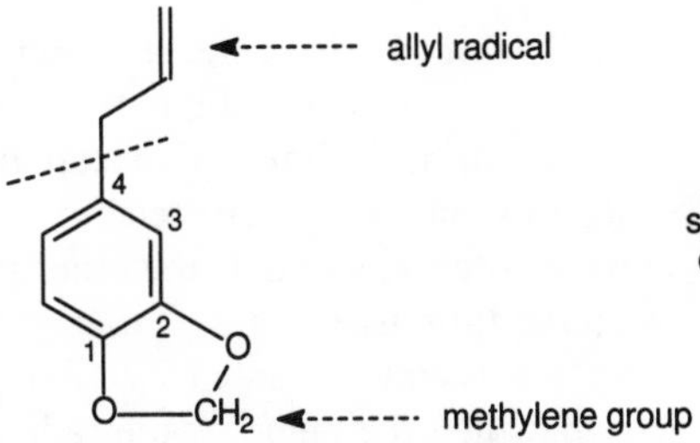

Sweet, warm, woody and
spicy odour with some floral
character. Odour is typical
of Sassafras Oil

methylene group

4-Allyl-1,2-methylenedioxybenzene

Fig. 3.20 — Examples of naturally occurring ethers

The names of simpler ethers specify the hydrocarbon radicals bonded to the oxygen atom, followed by the word 'ether', as in diphenyl ether and *para*-cresyl methyl ether, or make use of the syllable '-oxy-', as in 4-methoxytoluene. Many ethers retain trivial names which are simply easier to use in conversation than their chemical names. Figure 3.20 shows examples of some naturally occurring ethers.

3.9 Acetals: Functional Group

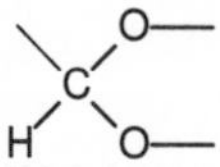

Few acetals occur as constituents of essential oils. We include them in this chapter more in reference to aroma chemicals used in perfumery.

An acetal is produced by a reaction between an aldehyde and an alcohol in the molecular proportions of 1:2, with the elimination of water:

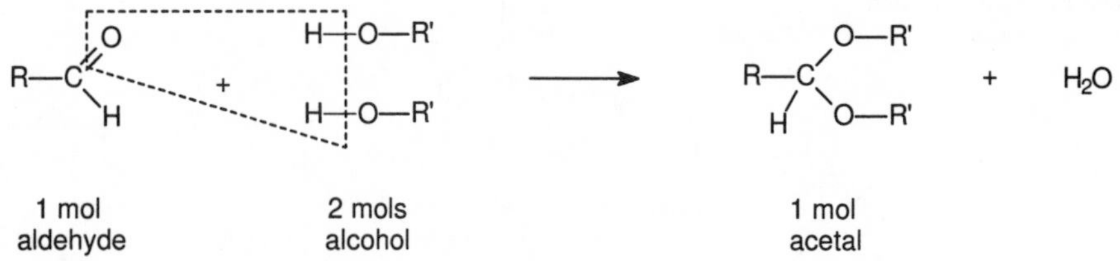

| 1 mol aldehyde | 2 mols alcohol | 1 mol acetal |

Fig. 3.21 — Formation of an acetal (simplified)

A glance at the general formula for an acetal shows that members of this family are branched-chain di-ethers: ethers having two ether functional groups per molecule, and so it is reasonable to suppose that they may be stable compounds, resistant to chemical attack. Acetals are, in fact, stable towards alkalis, but suffer partial decomposition, to the original aldehyde and alcohol, in the presence of acids.

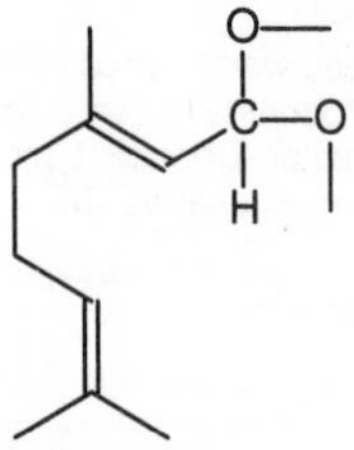

Fig. 3.22 — Citral dimethylacetal

The odour of an acetal is related to the odours of the aldehyde and the alcohol from which it is formed. Thus citral forms a dimethyl acetal having a somewhat oily, lemony odour, closely related to that of the parent aldehyde. Methyl alcohol (the other parent of this acetal) possesses little true odour.

An acetal is named by first naming the parent aldehyde, then the name of the radical bonded to each of the two oxygen atoms, prefixed by 'di-'. It is worth noting that commercial citral dimethyl acetal is a mixture of the dimethyl acetals of the two isomers of citral (sect. 3.3).

3.10 Amines: Functional Group –NH₂ and Imines: Functional Group >NH

A nitrogen atom has three unpaired electrons in its outer electron shell and one lone pair of electrons. In the amino- functional group, -NH₂, two of the unpaired electrons form bonding pairs with the single electrons of the two hydrogen atoms, while the third is available for bonding with an unpaired electron of a carbon atom to form an amine (*see* diagram, right).

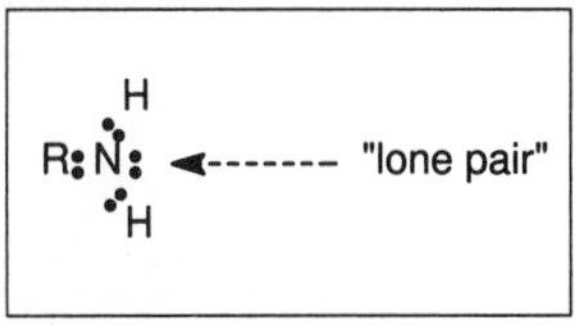

$$R\!:\!\overset{\overset{\textstyle H}{\cdot}}{\underset{\underset{\textstyle H}{\cdot\cdot}}{N}}\!:\quad \longleftarrow\text{------ "lone pair"}$$

Simple amines, where R comprises a small number of carbon atoms, possess fishy or other unpleasant odours, some exceedingly revolting. The only amines of major importance as constituents of essential oils are also esters, and are known as anthranilates; derivatives of anthranilic acid, of which methyl anthranilate is most frequent occurrence (fig. 3.23).

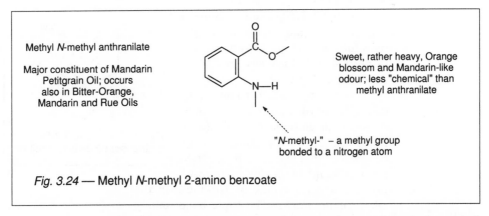

Methyl anthranilate

Found in Sweet Orange, Lemon, Mandarin, Bergamot, Neroli and Ylang-Ylang Oils, and in Jasmin and Tuberose Absolutes

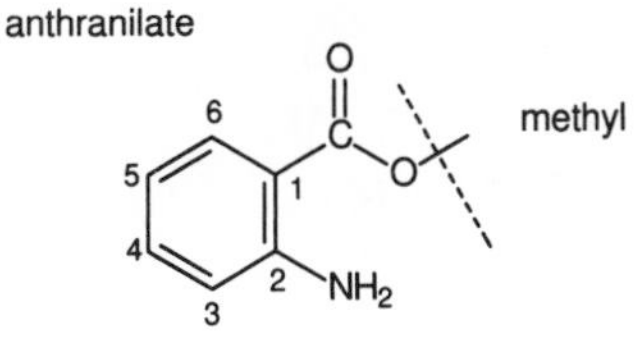

anthranilate

methyl

Rather "chemical" odour of Orange blossom and Neroli

Fig. 3.23 — Methyl 2-aminobenzoate

An interesting derivative of methyl anthranilate has a methyl group substituting for one of the two hydrogen atoms of the amino-group:

Methyl *N*-methyl anthranilate

Major constituent of Mandarin Petitgrain Oil; occurs also in Bitter-Orange, Mandarin and Rue Oils

Sweet, rather heavy, Orange blossom and Mandarin-like odour; less "chemical" than methyl anthranilate

"*N*-methyl-" – a methyl group bonded to a nitrogen atom

Fig. 3.24 — Methyl *N*-methyl 2-amino benzoate

This compound is an example of an imine ester. Both methyl anthranilate and methyl *N*-methyl anthranilate possess Orange Blossom-type odours, though rather coarse and 'chemical' in character; they illustrate the fact that potentially malodorous functional groups can, when associated with other groups in the same molecule, give rise to odours which are at least not unpleasant.

The cyclic imines indole and methyl indole, or skatole, possess odours that are disliked by most people, quite possibly in anticipation of sensory experiences far worse than either of these substances actually produces, for both occur in human faeces. Indole, if pure, smells of naphthalene — old-fashioned moth balls; skatole is less naphthenic and more faecal. Indole occurs, at several per cent, in the absolutes of Jasmin and Orange Flower, lending to these products their heaviness of odour and animalic odour character; skatole is found in the glandular secretion of the civet which, in the fresh condition, possesses an odour which will clear a laboratory of its denizens in seconds. Strangely, both indole and skatole, as aroma chemicals, can, in skilled hands, produce very beautiful fragrance effects in floral perfumes, but only if used with great discretion. They have the following formulae:

Indole   Skatole

Fig. 3.25 — Indole and skatole

3.11 Nitriles: Functional Group   —C≡N

Nitriles do not occur as constituents of essential oils, but are mentioned here for their importance as substitutes for the corresponding aldehydes in perfumery. Aldehydes are alkalisensitive, and so in alkaline products, such as toilet soaps, perfumes containing aldehydes are likely to deteriorate with consequent spoilage of fragrance. Citral, for example, may be replaced in a perfumes by geranonitrile, though with due compensation for a certain lack of freshness in the odour of the nitrile. The triple bond joining the carbon and nitrogen atoms of the nitrile functional group is very strong, being formed from three bonding pairs of electrons:

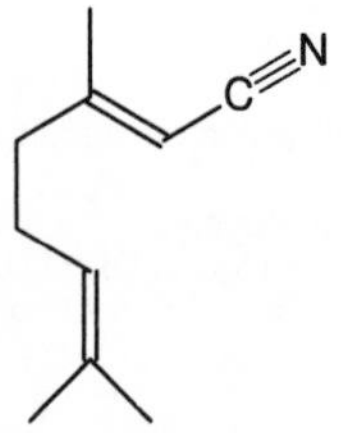

Fig. 3.26 — *trans*-3,7-Dimethyl-octa-2,6-dien-1-nitrile

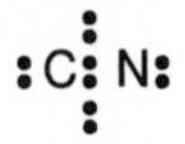

3.12 Sulphur-Containing Constituents

Organic sulphur compounds have an unenviable reputation with regard to odour, some of the simpler examples possessing truly stupefying smells. Various sulphides and disulphides form the chief constituents of the essential oils of Leek, Onion and Shallot, while others are present, in trace amounts, in many essential oils and in the still notes produced during the distillation of essential oils. Their odours are both powerful and diffusive. Some examples are shown in figure 3.27.

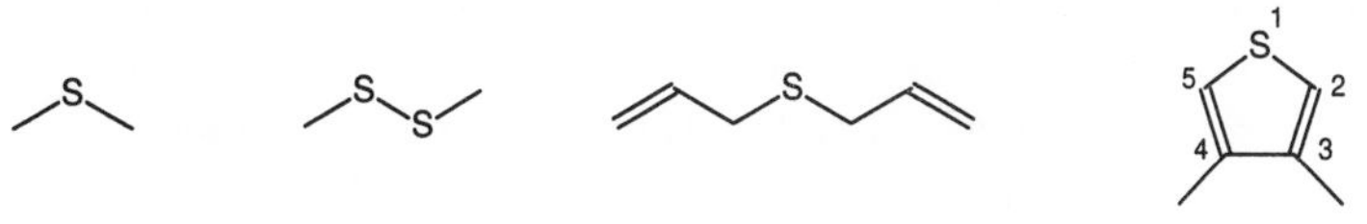

Dimethyl sulphide   Dimethyl disulphide   Diallyl disulphide   3,4-Dimethylthiophene

Fig. 3.27 — Some odorous organic sulphur compounds

3.13 Some Chemical Reactions Relating to the Stability of Essential Oils

All essential oils are prone to deterioration simply by ageing and by exposure to environments which cause chemical changes to their constituents to take place. The same is true of perfumes and perfumed products. If a freshly produced and dried essential oil were to be confined in a container of high-quality glass under a headspace of nitrogen or other inert gas, and protected from light, then the only chemical changes that could occur to the oil would be those caused by reactions between constituents. The lower the storage temperature, the more slowly would these reactions proceed; but proceed they would, over successive years, until eventually no further perceptible change would occur. Among possible reactions would be those between aldehydes and alcohols to form acetals, between traces of organic acids and alcohols and between alcohols and esters (alcoholysis). Because all of these reactions and others likely to occur are reversible, the final molecular state of the oil would be very far from one of complete inactivity, but one of dynamic equilibrium, or balance, in which the rate of each of the forward reactions would be equal to the rate of the reverse reaction. How fascinating it would be to open a sample of an essential oil stored for a hundred years under such conditions, for analysis in comparison with a fresh sample of the same oil produced under the same conditions.

But we do not take such extremes of trouble with the storage of essential oils — there is simply no need under good conditions of stock-keeping, when a supply of any given essential oil will have been used long before it begins to show detectable signs of deterioration. In the practical situation, essential oils are kept under conditions which will preserve their quality for the foreseeable maximum period of their storage, plus a good margin of time to accommodate unforeseeable circumstances of reduction of demand. If stored under poor conditions, then deterioration will be inevitable, and costly.

The following are the main reactions involved in the spoilage of essential oils through poor storage. Some of them are catalysed by traces of metal compounds, for example those of copper; all are hastened by exposure to light and elevated temperatures.

3.13.1 Oxidation
a) Oxidation of terpenes
Terpenes are, in general, readily oxidized by exposure to oxygen of the air, with the formation of oxidation products having odours of quite different character. These give rise to the spoilage of essential oils, not only in respect of odour, but also because certain of them have been found to possess allergenic properties.[3]

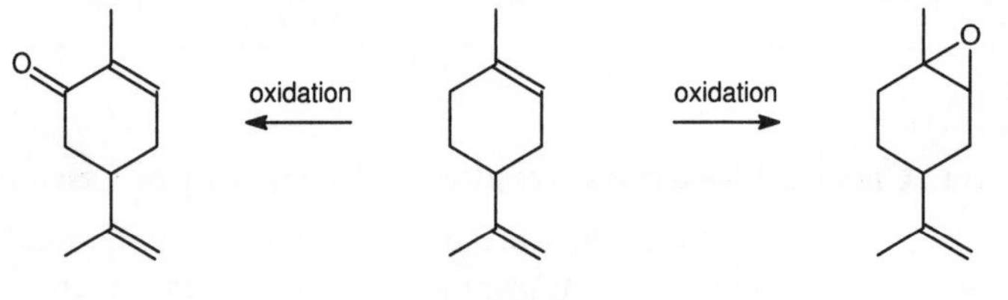

Carvone
(strong odour of caraway)

Limonene
(little characteristic odour)

Limonene oxide
(piney, rather harsh odour)

Fig. 3.28 — Oxidation products of Limonene

b) Oxidation of phenols
Phenol turns pink, and many other phenols darken, with increasing age, especially if their containers are opened from time to time. The same result of oxidation is seen in essential oils containing phenols, such as the Clove oils (bud, stem and leaf), which contain high proportions of eugenol. Phenate ions (PhO⁻; *see* p. 55) are, as we have noted, much more readily oxidized.

c) Oxidation of aldehydes
This subject has been discussed in section 3.3. Sufficient, here, to add that essential oils containing both aldehydes and monoterpenes, such as the citrus oils, are *very* prone to oxidation.

---

3. Ann-Therese Karlberg, Kerstin Magnusson and Ulrika Nilsson, Air oxidation of *d*-limonene (the citrus solvent) creates potent allergens. *Contact Dermatitis,* **26,** No. 5:332-340 (1992).

3.13.2 Hydrolysis of Esters
See section 3.5.2, page 66.

3.13.3 Ionization of Carboxylic Acids
This is discussed in section 3.5, page 65.

3.13.4 Polymerization of Unsaturated Compounds
Old citrus oils, stored under experimentally poor conditions, become thick and smelly. In more scientific terms, their viscosity increases and their odours deteriorate. This form of spoilage is caused largely by the polymerization of terpenes, particularly monoterpenes, such as the pinenes and limonenes. It may be readily demonstrated by pouring a little Sweet Orange Oil into a largish bottle of colourless glass, plugging the neck of the bottle loosely with cotton wool and then leaving the experiment on a sunlit window-sill. The experiment simulates in a week or two what would happen under far less drastic conditions over a much longer period of time — an 'accelerated storage test' based on the same principle as the stability tests used for estimating the 'shelf lives' of perfumes in consumer products.

Polymerization is easier to illustrate than it is to define. If the gas ethene (ethylene) is heated under pressure and in the presence of a suitable catalyst, the unsaturated molecules link together to form long, saturated chains. This may be expressed in the form of an equation, as shown in figure 3.29.

The product of this reaction, the familiar polythene, is one of the most versatile of plastics. The ethene is termed a *monomer*, the polyethylene a *polymer*. The process is known as *addition polymerization* because, effectively, ethene molecules 'add on' to one another to form the product, in which n is a large number.

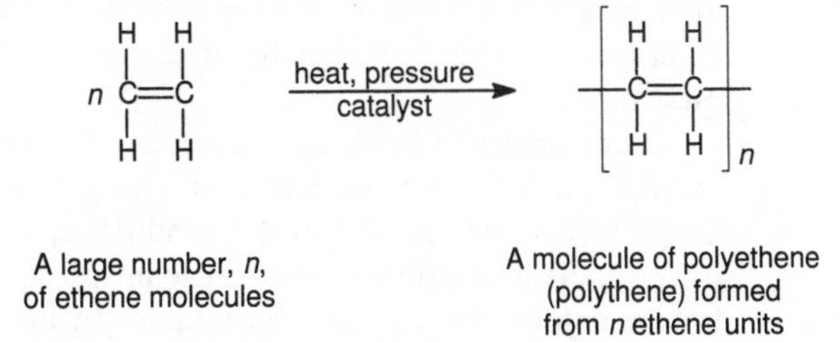

A large number, n, of ethene molecules	A molecule of polyethene (polythene) formed from n ethene units

Fig. 3.29 — Formation of polyethene

The alternative to addition polymerization is *condensation polymerization* in which, in its simplest form, two different kinds of molecules react together with the elimination of water.

An example is provided by the manufacture of a variety of nylon, employing a dicarboxylic acid and a di-amine, each of six carbon atoms (fig. 3.30). The equation of figure 3.30 shows the reaction between just one of each kind of molecule; further reactions occur between the molecule of the condensation product and (a) another molecule of the acid at the amino- group, marked *, and (b) another molecule of the di-amine at the carboxyl group, marked **. Both reactions are repeated many times to form a long, puckered chain. Countless numbers of such chains, when stretched by pulling the softened plastic, form a single 'Nylon 6/6' thread of parallel 'straight' chains. The thread is enormously strong, showing the great strength of the bonds linking the atoms of the chains together.

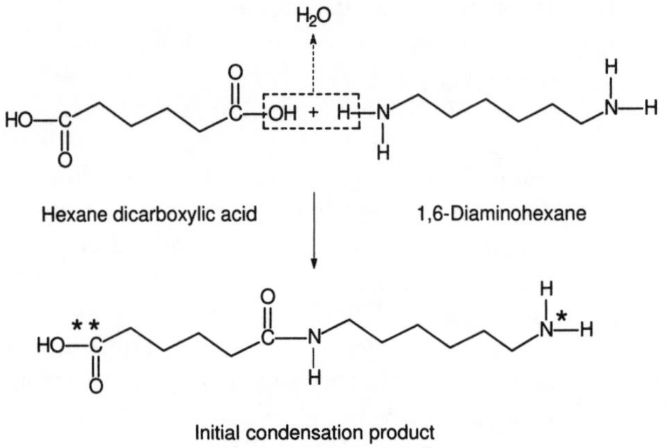

Fig. 3.30 — Initial step in the preparation of nylon

Under oxidizing conditions, such as can exist in a poorly stored essential oil rich in terpenes, resinous polymers form with increasing age of the oil. This is evidenced by the previously mentioned increase of viscosity, and the development of haziness in the oil, long after loss of freshness in the top note has given warning of incipient deterioration; thus it is usually seen only in elderly and useless samples of oil.

Occasionally, surprising instances of deterioration occur as, for example, a fifty-year old bottle of Ylang-Ylang Oil, a product which keeps well under good storage conditions, exhumed from the cellar of an ancient pharmacy; this museum piece was of a deep, golden brown colour and as thick as treacle. In another case, a sample of Patchouli Oil (or so the container was labelled) turned black and solidified within six months of normal storage.

3.14 Storage of Essential Oils

Essential oils should be stored under the following conditions:

a) in a cool place of even temperature. Citrus and other essential oils rich in monoterpenes should be stored in a refrigerator at about 10°C. Sandalwood, Vetivert and Guaiacwood Oils do not need to be refrigerated, but kept in a cool place. Cedar-wood Oils deposit crystals of cedrol, a sequiterpene alcohol, if refrigerated, and these are very difficult to redissolve; Rose Otto behaves similarly, but the crystals can be, and should be, redissolved by the warmth of the hand, or by allowing the oil to stand in a warm place for a short period of time. Neither of the last-mentioned oils need be refrigerated;

b) under a *small* headspace of air, to minimize oxidation;

c) protected from light, particularly sunlight, which accelerates deterioration (photocatalytic effect);

d) in securely closed containers, to prevent loss of top notes by evaporation and the inward diffusion of oxygen to replace that absorbed by the oil as it oxidizes;

e) never in plastic containers, the material of which may leak reactive monomer into the contents, with disastrous results, or may absorb small molecules from the contents, or allow them to pass clean through, with loss of their contributions to the odour of the oil, and whatever aromatherapeutic effect they may have.

Meticulous attention to the handling and storage of essential oils will be repaid in full by preservation of their valuable properties.

3.15 Fire

Essential oils are flammable, and although their vapours will not ignite in air below 40°C, the highest temperature ever likely to be encountered even in a heat wave, they will burn at a wick, meaning that an essential oil-soaked tissue or rag is a dangerous fire hazard. Furthermore, terpene-rich essential oils absorbed onto paper tissue or rag have been known to ignite spontaneously by rapid oxidation occurring over the large surface area presented by the fibres of the material. This can occur under quite cool atmospheric conditions, and its likelihood increases with temperature rise. Oxidation is always accompanied by increase of temperature, which when high enough causes ignition.

Sensible precautions are to store all essential oils that are not kept in a refrigerator, and that are not required for immediate use, in a cool place where no other flammables are kept, and to keep the door to this place locked shut. This will also ensure that children do not have access. Spills of essential oil should be mopped up with tissue or rag, which is then soaked in water containing a little dishwashing detergent; it is then disposed of in an external waste bin. This precaution applies also to smelling strips impregnated with essential oils, unless required to be retained for sensory evaluation.

3.16 Safety in Use

If an essential oil should come into accidental contact with the skin it should be washed away with soap and plenty of warm water. In the unlikely event of an essential oil entering the eye, it should be washed away with large volumes of warm water only, and advice sought from a doctor, pharmacist or optician.

Detailed information on the safety of essential oils is given in the publication *Plant Aromatics: A Data and Reference Manual on Essential Oils and Aromatic Plant Extracts* by Martin Watt, obtainable from the author, at 7 Elm Court Park, Chelmsford Road, Blackmore, Essex CM4 0SE.

Chapter 4

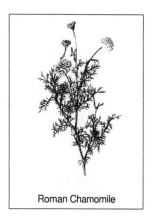

Roman Chamomile

Essential Oils and Carrier Oils

4.1 How to Smell

Careful smelling, followed by written recording of sensory impressions perceived, should become automatic for anyone involved with essential oils or any other aromatic materials of fragranced products, for by disciplined use of the nose much information on their quality may be gained. Although the human nose is always the final court of judgment of odour quality, it has limitations, and in a fragranced product manufacturing situation, sensory evaluation is accompanied by physico-chemical analysis for purposes of quality assessment.

Some information on the top note of an essential oil or perfume may be obtained by smelling directly from the container, but not by spraying a perfume into the air, which does nothing but give a totally false impression of the fragrance. The personal testing of perfumes is discussed in Chapter 10.

For the evaluation of odour quality, one end of a paper smelling strip, labelled with the name or reference mark of the sample to be smelled, is dipped into the liquid to be tested to a depth of about half a centimetre. Solids and very viscous semisolids are dissolved in a solvent, such as pure alcohol, for odour evaluation. Immediately after dipping, the strip is briefly touched against the inner rim of the container to remove excess liquid and is then smelled. It is important always to try to standardize smelling procedure, particularly when checking a sample by comparison with an odour standard representing the odour quality required. The smelling strip should therefore be held horizontally beneath the nose, with a flat side, not an edge, presented to the nostrils. The strip must not be allowed to touch the nose, otherwise traces of odorous liquid will be transferred to the end of the nose, rendering further smelling useless until the nose has been washed free from contamination. Each odour-laden intake of air through the nostrils should occupy no more than a second or two, to avoid olfactory fatigue, and should be followed by a brief resting period before smelling is resumed. When an impregnated smelling strip is to be retained for a time, it should be set aside so that it cannot fall, and with its impregnated end well clear of any surface.

The odour of almost every aromatic material, and certainly every perfume, changes as it evaporates, and so for a complete profile of the odour of a sample a dip will need to be smelled at intervals until no further odour change is observed. The odour properties of essential oils will be discussed in Chapter 5 of this book.

4.2 Carrier Oils

There is one property that all of the materials we call oils have in common, which is that they do not mix with water to form clear solutions unless a third ingredient of the mixture, a solubilizer, is present in sufficient proportion. In scientific terms, the molecules of water and of an oil do not become mutually dispersed in one another to form a mixture which will not separate on standing. Even if a suitable solubilizer is present, the result of shaking a mixture of oil and water is not to form a true solution, but a liquid in which the particles of oil are so small that it is transparent to light — a colloidal solution, or sol, in which the part played by the solubilizer is to prevent the dispersed, colloidal particles from coalescing.

Many oily-looking liquids are not in fact oils, and will form true solutions with water. Glycerine is a viscous liquid of oily appearance, but when it is mixed with Rose Water, a solution of traces of Rose Otto in water, a clear solution is produced which does not separate into its constituents on standing. Glycerine is not, therefore, an oil. Similarly treated, a mixture of any essential oil, vegetable oil, or mineral oil such as liquid paraffin, with water does separate and so, on the basis of their immiscibility with water, these products are classified physically as oils.

All oils from natural sources are mixtures of organic compounds, and the same is true of most synthetic oils, such as isopropyl myristate, an odourless cosmetic oil purified to retain small proportions of other oils of similar composition which enhance, rather than impair, its emollient properties. The importance of synthetic oils is that they are of far less variable quality than natural oils and do not go rancid, and that in certain instances they possess better properties for their purposes than any natural fixed oil. Some synthetic oils are also cheaper than any equivalent natural oil.

One useful classification of oils is by reference to their chemical composition:

1. Essential oils are mixtures of terpenes and oxygenates, together with certain organic compounds of other types.

2. Vegetable oils are, in most cases, mixtures of esters of glycerine (glycerol) and long-chain fatty acids, together with some proportion of free fatty acids.

3. Mineral oils, such as liquid paraffin, are almost entirely mixtures of hydrocarbons of high molecular weight.

Carrier oils are highly purified vegetable oils where purification refers to the removal of all constituents that are unsuitable for their intended purpose, and not to chemical purity, which refers to a substance consisting of atoms or molecules of one kind only. Vegetable oils are, as we have noted, mixtures, and so cannot be chemically pure. A further consideration in relation to the composition of carrier oils is that they are not completely odourless, a result of the presence of very small proportions of volatiles, which are responsible for their usually faint, characteristic odours.

In figure 4.1, a formula for the type of ester typical of the composition of a carrier oil follows formulae for the glycerol and fatty acids from which it is derived.

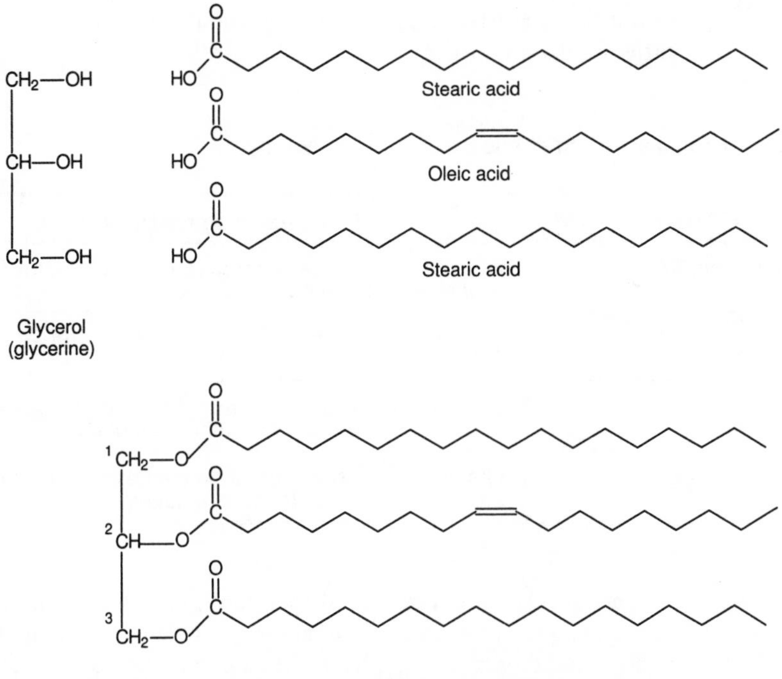

Glycerol
(glycerine)

Example of a triglyceride:
2-oleo-1,3-distearin

The structures of the above molecules are written conventionally; as they exist in nature, each of them is free to take up an almost infinite variety of shapes within the limitations of the bonding and their molecular environment; i.e. any restricting effects of other, nearby molecules

Fig. 4.1 — Structure of a triglyceride

Vegetable oils, mineral oils and synthetic cosmetic oils are known as *fixed oils*, for when absorbed into paper they leave a permanent, oily stain. Fixed oils, unlike essential oils, are nonvolatile, or rather almost nonvolatile, since they are not entirely odourless and so must contain some proportion, however small, of volatile matter, as do all odorous materials. In contrast, an essential oil does not leave a permanent oily stain on paper if it is totally volatile. The presence or absence of nonvolatile matter in an essential oil is easily confirmed by weighing a smelling strip on a sensitive balance, impregnating it with two drops of the essential oil under examination, weighing again, and then leaving the strip for the oil to evaporate until there is no further loss in weight. This experiment may be usefully repeated, using two drops of any carrier oil.

Some essential oils are of such low volatility, however, that one has to live long enough to complete the test. Results of such tests with the citrus oils soon reveal the presence, and proportion, of nonvolatile matter, because these oils evaporate relatively quickly. The balance used must be a sensitive one, preferably weighing to an accuracy of 0·001 g or less. There is a possible flaw in this kind of experiment, which will be left to the reader to consider. [*Hint:* How would the result be affected if the essential oil on the strip were to suffer oxidation during exposure to the air?]

Table 4.1 — Examples of carrier oils used in aromatherapy

Carrier oil	Source and properties
Avocado Pear Oil	Obtained by expression from the dried fruits of *Persea gratissima*. Has emollient properties.
Olive Oil	Expressed from the ripe fruits of *Olea europaea*. Emollient and soothing to the skin.
Sesame Oil	Extracted by expression from the seeds of *Sesamum indicum*. Has properties similar to those of Olive Oil.
Wheat Germ Oil	Obtained by expression or solvent extraction from the embryos of wheat, *Triticum aestivum*.

Carrier oils should be stored in a cool place, where the temperature undergoes only small fluctuations, protected from light and in tightly closed, almost completely filled containers to prevent the onset of rancidity.

There are many carrier oils in use in aromatherapy other than those exemplified, some containing vitamins once thought to be of benefit to the skin by external application. The dermatological literature should be consulted for up-to-date information on the properties of vegetable oils when applied to the skin.

4.3 Natural Sources of Essential Oils

The earth's biosphere comprises all regions of the earth supporting living things; it is richly endowed with odour-producing plants, of form ranging from simple bacteria, yeasts and microscopic fungi, such as those responsible for fermentation, to flowering plants of great complexity, where essential oils are manufactured and stored only in particular locations, or are distributed more generally throughout the aerial parts or root system. The total number of known plants is estimated at about 250,000, of which about one-tenth have been found to be essential oil-bearing. Certain plants, such as *Cistus ladaniferus*, from which the highly aromatic preparations of Cistus and Labdanum of perfumery originate, manufacture and exude sticky, resinous products which coat the surfaces of the leaves and stems. Others, such as the trees of Boswellia and Commiphora species yielding Frankincense (Olibanum) and Myrrh, respectively, do so only slowly, but much faster in response to injury to the cambium, the thin, green region of living, conducting tissues just beneath the inner bark, thereby effectively preventing water loss and invasion by pathogenic micro-organisms.

The natural sources of some examples of essential oils are given in the following table (table 4.2). Not all of the sources listed yield products used in aromatherapy; all of them are, however, in use as perfume and/or flavour ingredients. The following abbreviations appear in the right-hand column, to indicate the processes used to obtain the various types of product available: Exp. = Expression; SD = Steam distillation; WD = Water distillation; Ext. = Extraction with volatile solvents.

Table 4.2 — Sources of essential oils

	Name of Product	*Natural Source*	*Part of Plant Used*	*Process*
1	Ambrette Seed Oil	*Hibiscus abelmoschus*	Seeds	SD
2	Amyris Oil	*Amyris balsamifera*	Comminuted heartwood	SD
3	Aniseed Oil	*Pimpinella anisum*	Dried, crushed fruits	SD
4	Basil Oil	*Ocimum basilicum*	Flowering tops	SD
5	Benzoin, Siam, Resinoid	*Styrax tonkinensis*	Exudate from tree-trunk	Ext.
6	Bergamot Oil	*Citrus bergamia*	Outer rind of fruits	Exp.
7	Caraway Seed Oil	*Carum carvi*	Ripe fruits, dried and crushed	SD
8	Cedarwood Oil, Virginian	*Juniperus virginiana*	Sawdust	SD
9	Chamomile Oil, German	*Matricaria chamomilla*	Flowers	SD
10	Chamomile Oil, Roman	*Anthemis nobilis*	Flowers	SD

Table 4.2 (contd.) — Sources of essential oils

	Name of product	Natural source	Part of plant used	Process
11	Cinnamon Bark Oil	*Cinnamomum zeylanicum*	Dried, inner bark of coppiced trees	SD
12	Cinnamon Leaf Oil	*Cinnamomum zeylanicum*	Partly dried leaves and twigs	SD
13	Cistus Oil	*Cistus ladaniferus*	Aerial parts of plant, covered with exudate	SD
14	Clove Bud Oil	*Cyzygium aromaticum*	Crushed, unopened, dried flower-buds	WD
15	Clove Leaf Oil	*Cyzygium aromaticum*	Dried leaves	WD
16	Clove Stem Oil	*Cyzygium aromaticum*	Sun-dried stems	SD
17	Coriander Oil	*Coriandrum sativum*	Dried and crushed fruits	SD
18	Cypress Oil	*Cupressus sempervirens*	Needles and twigs	SD
19	*Eucalyptus citriodora* Oil	*Eucalyptus citriodora*	Leaves	SD
20	Eucalyptus Oil	*Eucalyptus, globulus et al.**	Leaves	SD
21	Fennel Oil	*Foeniculum vulgare*	Crushed fruits	SD
22	Frankincense Oil	*see* Olibanum Oil		
23	Frankincense Resinoid	*see* Olibanum Resinoid		
24	Galbanum Oil	*Ferula galbaniflua*	Exudate from aerial parts of plant	SD
25	Galbanum Resinoid	*Ferula galbaniflua*	Exudate from aerial parts of plant	Ext.
26	Geranium Oil	*Pelargonium graveolens*	Leaves and green branches	SD
27	Guaiacwood Oil	*Bulnesia sarmienti*	Finely comminuted wood	SD
28	Jasmin Absolute	*Jasminum officinalis*	Freshly picked flowers	Ext.
29	Juniper Berry Oil	*Juniperus communis*	Partly dried and crushed, ripe berries	SD
30	Labdanum Resinoid	*Cistus ladaniferus*	Oleo-resin, obtained by treating leaves and twigs with boiling water	Ext. of crude oleo-resin
31	Lavandin Oil	*Lavandula hybrida*	Flowers and stalks	SD
32	Lavender Absolute	*Lavandula officinalis*	Flowers and stalks	Ext.
33	Lavender Oil	*Lavandula officinalis*	Flowers and stalks	SD
34	Lavender Spike Oil	*Lavandula latifolia*	Flowers and stalks	SD
35	Lemongrass Oil	*Cymbopogon citratus* and *Cymbopogon flexuosus*	Partially dried leaves	SD
36	Lemon Oil	*Citrus limonum*	Outer rind of fruit	Exp.

*Species other than *globulus*, yielding essential oils rich in eucalyptol (cineole), are mostly used.

Table 4.2 (contd.) — Sources of essential oils

	Name of product	Natural source	Part of plant used	Process
37	*Litsea cubeba* Oil	*Litsea cubeba*	Fruits	SD
38	Marjoram Oil	*Origanum marjorana*	Dried leaves and flowering tops	SD
39	*Mentha arvensis* Oil	*Mentha arvensis*	Dried aerial parts	SD
40	Myrrh Oil	*Commiphora spp.*	Exudate from tree trunk	SD
41	Myrrh Resinoid	*Commiphora spp.*	Exudate from tree trunk	Ext.
42	Neroli Oil	*Citrus aurantium* var. *amara*	Freshly gathered flowers from cultivated trees	WD
43	Oakmoss Absolute	*Evernia prunastri*	Entire lichen	Ext.
44	Olibanum Oil	*Boswellia spp.*	Exudate from tree trunk	SD
45	Olibanum Resinoid	*Boswellia spp.*	Exudate from tree trunk	Ext.
46	Orris Oil (known also as Orris 'Concrete')	*Iris pallida*	Dried, finely comminuted rhizome	SD
47	Patchouli Oil	*Pogostemon patchouli*	Dried, lightly fermented leaves	SD
48	Petitgrain Oil, Bigarade	*Citrus aurantium* var. *amara*	Leaves and green twigs	SD
49	Pimento Berry Oil	*Pimenta officinalis*	Dried, crushed fruits	SD
50	Pine Oil, Sylvestris	*Pinus sylvestris*	Needles and twigs	SD
51	Rose Absolute	*Rosa centifolia*	Freshly gathered flowers	Ext.
52	Rose Otto (Rose Oil)	*Rosa damascena*	Freshly gathered flowers	SD with cohobation
53	Rosemary Oil	*Rosmarinus officinalis*	Aerial parts of plant	SD
54	Rosewood Oil	*Aniba rosaeodora*	Chipped wood	SD
55	Sage Oil, Clary	*Salvia sclarea*	Flowering tops and leaves	SD
56	Sage Oil, Dalmatian	*Salvia officinalis*	Dried leaves	SD
57	Sandalwood Oil, East Indian	*Santalum album*	Comminuted heartwood	SD or WD
58	Sandalwood Oil, West Indian	*see* Amyris Oil		
59	Tarragon Oil (Estragon Oil)	*Artemisia dracunculus*	Aerial parts of plant	SD
60	Thyme Oil	*Thymus vulgaris*	Dried herb	SD
61	Ti-Tree Oil	*Melaleuca alternifolia* *Melaleuca linariifolia*	Leaves	SD or WD
62	Tonka Absolute	*Dipteryx odorata*	Seeds ('beans')	Ext.
63	Tuberose Absolute	*Polyanthes tuberosa*	Freshly gathered flower buds, just about to open	Ext.

Table 4.2 (contd.) — Sources of essential oils

	Name of product	Natural source	Part of plant used	Process
64	Vanilla Absolute	*Vanilla planifolia; Vanilla tahitensis*	Cured fruits ('beans')	Ext.
65	Vetivert Oil	*Vetiveria zizanoides*	Chopped rootlets	SD
66	Violet Leaves Absolute	*Viola odorata*	Leaves	Ext.
67	Ylang-Ylang Oils 'Extra' and Nos. 1 to 3	*Cananga odorata*	Freshly gathered flowers	Fractional SD

4.4 Geographical Distribution of Essential Oils

The number of aromatic plants from which essential oils are obtained for use in perfumery and flavouring, which are the main areas of their application, is only a small fraction of those that could be so exploited, at least on an experimental basis. Nature is replete with fragrance, and the ingenuity of the human species is such that, given time and the necessary physical resources, any odorous source can today be made to yield its secrets, with the possibility that its essential oil might become of value as food flavour, perfume ingredient or therapeutic agent. The economics of essential oil production are, however, based on the existence of a firm demand for unfailing supplies of oils of unvarying, acceptable quality — ideals earnestly striven for but, in view of the many variable conditions attending the cultivation, harvesting and processing of crops, never fully attainable. To speculate from current trends and the ever-accelerating progress of scientific research and technological development, the time may not be too far in the future when tightly standardized essential oils are produced under conditions least damaging to their composition from genetically engineered plant material cultivated in ideally controlled environments.

The growth to healthy maturity of a plant demands those conditions of soil composition, texture and moisture, and of environmental suitability in which the innumerable chemical reactions which find expression in the life of the plant can proceed without damaging deviation from the pathways ultimately determined by the genetic code peculiar to that plant. Given favourable soil conditions, the fate of the plant will depend on how close the environmental conditions of temperature, sunlight and humidity, among others, in which it exists match those which promote its optimum growth and development. Plants such as *Ferula galbaniflua*, from which Galbanum Oil is obtained, which are adapted to arid conditions, will not grow well, if they will grow at all, in tropical locations where flourish other plants, such as Ylang-Ylang, which would perish in the desert. Cultivated essential oil-yielding plants need expert husbandry to be grown successfully.

Thus there is, in general, a natural geographical distribution of plants, which reflects the limitations of their ability to grow successfully over a wide range of soil and climatic conditions. A plant species introduced into a new growing area can be expected to thrive only if its individual environmental requirements are met, usually within fairly narrow limitations of variation.

The main areas of geographical distribution of some important essential oil producing plants are shown on the map (fig. 4.2). The areas indicated are not necessarily those where the plants are also processed to obtain their essential oil. Dried plant materials, spices, for example, are commonly shipped from the growing areas to Europe for processing. Most flowers, however, need to be processed as soon as possible after harvesting, otherwise much of their essential oil would be lost by evaporation.

4.5 Processes for Obtaining Essential Oils

The process chosen for obtaining an essential oil from its natural source has to be one which will give a maximum, economic yield of a product of the quality demanded by customers, who are perfume and flavour manufacturers, and by major pharmaceutical companies using essential oils as flavouring and therapeutic agents. Purchasers of essential oils quite naturally aim to pay a minimum price for a product which is fully compliant with the sensory and analytical standards set for it, which will remain constant within predetermined limits of variation from one supply to the next, and which will be available when required for the foreseeable future. The processes used in the essential oils industry are those which, over generations of experience, have been found to be the most reliable for obtaining oils of the required quality.

4.5.1 Expression Processes

Expression processes are applied to citrus fruits, to release the essential oil contained in the oil cells of the outer, coloured rind, and to the production of vegetable oils, certain of which are used as 'carriers' in the formulation of aromatherapeutic preparations (sect. 4.2). The oil glands of citrus fruits may easily be seen with the naked eye when an orange, lemon or grapefruit is cut into halves, and if these glands are large enough, and the rind not too hard, a little of the essential oil may be expressed by pressing the rind with a fingernail, when the true odour of the natural oil may for a moment be smelled.

The production of citrus essential oils involves harvesting the fruit from cultivated trees at the correct stage of maturity, and either scraping the rind (scarification) or applying lateral surface pressure to release the oil. Each oil gland contains a collection of oil-producing cells filled with protoplasm — the proteinaceous living matter within which the chemical processes constituting the life of the cell take place. These reactions are, ultimately, under the control of the

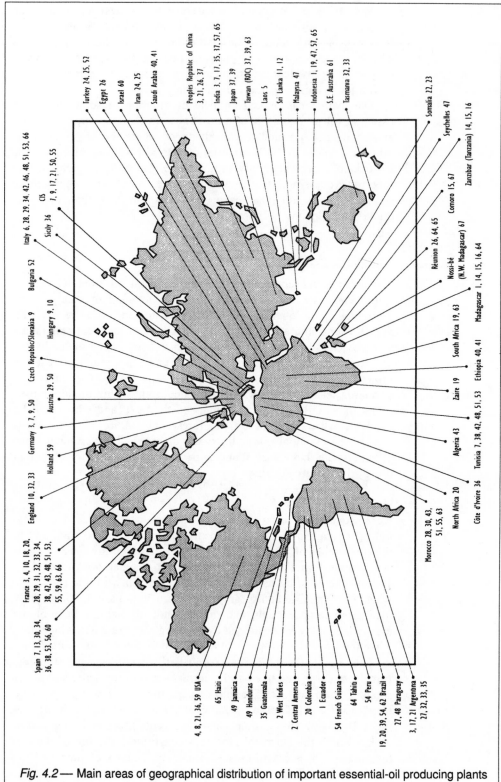

Fig. 4.2 — Main areas of geographical distribution of important essential-oil producing plants

Key to geographical distribution of essential oils as shown on map opposite

	Name of source material	Examples of geographical sources
1	Ambrette seeds	Ecuador, Indonesia, Madagascar
2	Amyris wood	West Indies, Central America
3	Aniseed fruits	France, Germany, Argentina, PRC, India
4	Basil herb	France, USA
5	Benzoin resin	Laos
6	Bergamot fruits	S. Italy
7	Caraway fruits	Germany, Spain, CIS, Tunisia, India
8	Cedar wood, Virginian	USA
9	Chamomile herb, German	Hungary, Germany, CIS, Czech Republic, Slovakia
10	Chamomile herb, Roman	England, France, Hungary
11	Cinnamon Bark	Sri Lanka
12	Cinnamon leaves	Sri Lanka
13	Cistus herb	Spain
14	Clove buds	
15	Clove leaves	}Madagascar, Zanzibar (Tanzania)
16	Clove stems	
17	Coriander fruit	CIS, India, Argentina
18	Cypress needles and twigs	France
19	*Eucalyptus citriodora* leaves	Brazil, Indonesia, South Africa, Zaire
20	*Eucalyptus, globulus et al.* leaves	Brazil, North Africa, France, Colombia
21	Fennel fruits	Argentina, PRC, CIS, USA
22	}Frankincense oleo-gum-resin	Somalia
23		
24	}Galbanum oleo-gum-resin	Asia Minor, Iran
25		
26	Geranium herb	Réunion, Egypt, PRC
27	Guaiac wood	Argentina, Paraguay
28	Jasmin flowers	Italy, Morocco, France
29	Juniper berries	N. Italy, Austria, France
30	Labdanum oleo-resin	Spain, Morocco
31	Lavandin herb	France
32	}Lavender herb	France, England, Tasmania, Argentina
33		
34	Lavender Spike herb	Spain, France, Italy
35	Lemon grass	Guatemala, Cochin (India), Argentina, India
36	Lemon fruits	Sicily, USA, Spain, Côte d'Ivoire
37	*Litsea cubeba* fruits	Côte d'Ivoire, PRC, Taiwan (ROC), Japan
38	Marjoram herb	Spain, Tunisia, France
39	*Mentha arvensis* herb	Brazil, Japan, Taiwan (ROC)
40	}Myrrh oleo-gum-resin	Saudi Arabia, Ethiopa
41		
42	(Neroli) Bitter-Orange flowers	S. France, Tunisia, Italy

Key to distribution of essential oils (contd.)

	Name of source material	Examples of geographical sources
43	Oakmoss lichen	France, Hungary, Morocco, Algeria
44	}Olibanum oleo-gum-resin	*see* Frankincense oleo-gum-resin
45		
46	(Orris) Iris rhizome	Italy
47	Patchouli leaves	Indonesia, Malaysia, Seychelles
48	(Petitgrain) Bitter-Orange leaves and green twigs	S. France, Tunisia, Italy, Paraguay
49	Pimento fruits	Jamaica, Guatemala, Honduras
50	Pine (sylvestris) needles and twigs	Central and Southern Europe, CIS
51	Rose (centifolia) flowers	Morocco, France, Tunisia, Italy
52	Rose (damascena) flowers	Bulgaria, Turkey
53	Rosemary herb	Spain, Tunisia, France, Italy
54	Rosewood	Brazil, Peru, French Guiana
55	Sage, Clary, herb	France, CIS, Morocco
56	Sage, Dalmatian, herb	Spain
57	Sandalwood, East Indian	India, Indonesia
58	Sandalwood, West Indian	*see* Amyris wood
59	Tarragon (Estragon) herb	France, USA, Holland
60	Thyme herb	Spain, Israel
61	Ti-Tree leaves	S.E. Australia
62	Tonka seeds, cured	Brazil
63	Tuberose flowers	S. France, S. Africa, Morocco, Taiwan
64	Vanilla fruits, cured	Madagascar, Réunion, Tahiti
65	Vetivert rootlets	India, Indonesia, Réunion, Haiti
66	Violet leaves	S. France, N. Italy
67	Ylang-Ylang flowers	Comoro Islands, Nossi-Bé (N.W. Madagascar)

nucleus of the cell, and would proceed extremely slowly — far too slowly to maintain the life of the cell — were it not for the presence of enzymes. Enzymes are biochemical catalysts the functions of which are to control the speeds or rates of biochemical reactions, maintaining each one at an optimum level, to coordinate with other reactions in the cell. Greatly simplified, this means that if, in some part of the protoplasm a substance, E, is to be produced from another substance, A, the reaction sequence A→B→C→D→E, known as a reaction pathway, occurs in that order, each individual reaction being controlled by an enzyme specific to that reaction. It is through such pathways that the many different constituents of an essential oil are produced.

Citrus oils are expressed mechanically, by either scarification or compression of the outer rind. Either of these processes releases a mixture of the essential oil and protoplasm from the disrupted oil glands, which is washed away by a stream of water to centrifugal separators for recovery of the oil. Thus, during production, the constituents of an expressed citrus oil inevitably come into contact with water, air containing oxygen and enzymes capable of enormously accelerating oxidative and hydrolytic reactions. This is certain, at least to some small extent, to affect the composition of the oil.

Producers of citrus oils commonly add minute, but effective, proportions of antioxidants to their products immediately following expression, to minimize the onset of oxidation during storage and transport. The identity and content of any antioxidant present are not, however, disclosed and so, as regards storage conditions to be adopted, a user without access to means for detecting the presence of an antioxidant has to assume that none has been added. In addition to volatile constituents, nonvolatiles present in citrus oils include waxy material from the cuticle of the rind, pigments from the outer rind and, in some oils, phototoxic compounds called furanocoumarins which we shall discuss later in this chapter. Natural Bergamot Oil is particularly rich in its content of furanocoumarins (pp. 107–8) which form a white deposit if the oil is chilled in a refrigerator.

Distilled citrus oils, which are useful ingredients for cheap, industrial odour-masking agents and perfumes, are not recommended for use in aromatherapy.

4.5.2 Distillation Processes

Basically, distillation involves heating a liquid or solid material to a temperature sufficiently high to produce a vapour, and then cooling the vapour to cause it to condense to a liquid or solid distillate. Two main types of distillation are applied to the production of essential oils: these are *water distillation* and *steam distillation*.

In *water distillation*, the source material is placed in a glass or metal-walled vessel (copper is traditional, stainless steel is used for the construction of modern distillation plant) resembling a large, cylindrical kettle, but having a vapour pipe fitted at the top in place of a spout at the side. The vapour pipe curves over to lead downward through a tank of circulating cold water, in which region the pipe is usually coiled to allow a long length of it to be cooled with economy of space. The tank of cold water and associated vapour pipe form the condenser; the coiled part of the vapour pipe is called the 'worm'. A vertical extension of the worm continues downward to pass out at the bottom of the condenser, where its open end is suspended over a receiving vessel (the *receiver*) for the products of distillation, known as the *distillate*. The entire set of equipment for distillation is known as a *still*. The lid of the still, clamped tightly to the body of the distillation vessel during the process, together with its attached va-

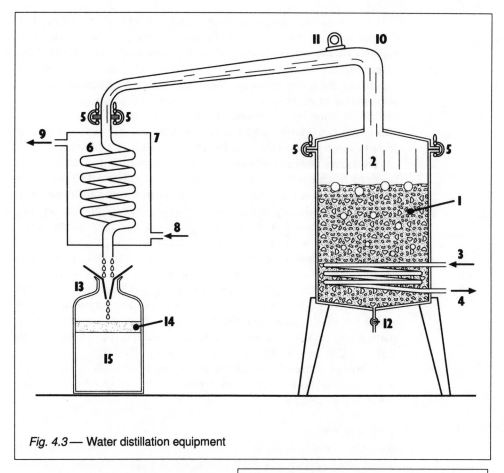

Fig. 4.3 — Water distillation equipment

pour pipe, is called the *still head*, which can be unclamped and lifted clear of the distillation vessel and worm by means of a pulley system (fig. 4.3).

To operate the still, the distillation vessel is charged with the material to be distilled, together with a sufficient quantity of water. The still head is clamped tightly to the distillation vessel and to the worm and the flow of cold water to the condenser turned on. Heat is then applied to the distillation vessel by means of a coiled pipe through

Key to figure 4.3

1. Source material and boiling water
2. Steam and essential oil vapours
3. Steam, at well above 100°C, from boiler to heating coil
4. Steam from heating coil to waste heat boiler
5. Clamps
6. "Worm": coiled part of condenser pipe
7. Water-cooled condenser
8. Cold water to condenser tank
9. Water to waste, carrying heat from "worm"
10. Still head
11. Lug for lifting still head
12. Drainage cock
13. Receiver
14. Essential oil
15. Distillation water

which steam flows under pressure, or by simply lighting a fire beneath the vessel — a traditional means of heating using dried, spent material from a previous distillation as fuel. Eventually, the water in the distillation vessel boils. By the same processes of hydrolysis that causes vegetables to become softened, permitting release of the essential oil contained in the oil glands that it supports. The oil vaporizes, and its vapour is carried over into the condenser in the current of steam produced by continuous boiling of the water in the distillation vessel. In the condenser, both steam and essential oil vapour condense to the respective liquids which are collected in the receiver.

Essential oils less dense than water separate as an upper layer, floating on the distillation water; those few that are denser than water (Clove, for example) form a lower layer. Once the essential oil has separated completely from the water it may, if necessary, be freed from dissolved water by treatment with anhydrous sodium sulphate:

$$Na_2SO_4 \quad + \quad 10\,H_2O \quad \rightleftharpoons \quad Na_2SO_4 . 10H_2O$$

The dried oil is then filtered bright and filled into suitable containers for storage and transport. The sodium sulphate does not in any other way affect the composition of the essential oil.

It should be noted that there is no connection between the vapour pipe of the still and the condenser water: neither can vapours from the still get into the cooling water, nor cooling water pass into the receiver.

Hard fruits, seeds and woods are comminuted, that is, reduced to small pieces or powder, before distillation to render their oil cells accessible to the boiling water, while some other materials, e.g. dried Patchouli leaves, are allowed a brief period for the onset of fermentation to break down cell walls for the same purpose.

In *steam distillation*, steam from a separate boiler is injected into the distillation vessel through jets in a ring-shaped pipe secured beneath a perforated support, upon which rests the charge of material to be distilled.[1]

A modern theory of steam distillation, advanced by E.F.K. Denny, of the Bridestowe Estate, Tasmania, proposes that injected steam condenses around the margins of essential oil droplets which have diffused from oil glands in particles of the charge onto the surface of the particles. In condensing, the steam gives up latent heat, which vaporizes the oil. Presumably the same thing happens in water distillation, by condensation of steam within bubbles onto particles of the charge as the water boils. This theory was put forward to explain why essential oils do, in fact, distil in steam efficiently when their generally low volatility suggests that they should not.

---

1. Note that if, in water distillation, the water in the distillation vessel is heated by a steam coil, there are no jets in this coil to provide steam for the process (fig. 4.4). If steam jets were provided, the process would be one of steam distillation.

Key to figure 4.4

1. Source material and steam
2. Steam and essential oil vapours
3. Steam under pressure to jets in distillation vessel
4. "Live" steam issuing from jets in annular steam pipe
5. Clamps
6. Perforated support for charge
7. Drainage cock

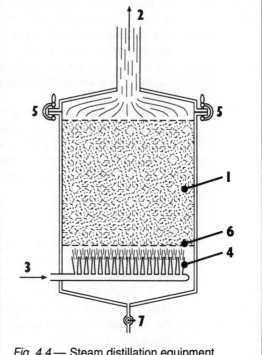

Fig. 4.4 — Steam distillation equipment

The conditions of steam distillation promote a much faster rate of distillation of an essential oil than those pertaining to water distillation, because the flow of steam from the boiler is much faster than that produced by boiling water in the distillation vessel. The advantage is that the essential oil being distilled is exposed to the risk of hydrolysis for only a relatively short period of time. Thus essential oils such as Lavender, which would be seriously damaged by the long contact with hot water and steam necessary for water distillation, survive steam distillation with minimum hydrolysis of those esters which greatly contribute to the quality of the oil.

Latent heat

The fact that, in condensing, steam does give up latent, or 'hidden', heat on condensing the liquid water, is painfully demonstrated if steam from a kettle is accidentally allowed contact with the skin: a nasty scald results. In contrast, the short-lived burn inflicted by touching the side of the kettle for the same period of time is trivial, because the metal wall is simply a hot surface at a temperature of about 100°C and has no latent heat to release. Latent heat is the energy that fast-moving molecules of a vapour must give up in slowing down sufficiently to condense to the liquid state, in which they move about more slowly. A further quantity of latent heat is evolved when a liquid solidifies. The two quantities of heat are known, respectively, as the *latent heat of vaporization* and the *latent heat of fusion*.

Certain essential oils contain constituents that are slightly soluble in water, and which become lost to the distillation water to an appreciable extent when the oils are distilled. This does not matter in the case of very cheap oils, such as Lemongrass, because the financial loss is negligible, and because it would cost more to recover the loss than the recovered oil would be worth. The situation is quite different with costly oils, such as Rose Otto, obtained by water distillation, the phenylethyl alcohol content of which dissolves in the distillation water to a considerable extent (1·5% at 20°C), so depleting the oil of the fragrance effect of this constituent and reducing the yield of the oil. In such instances the distillation waters collected in the receivers are continuously returned to the distillation vessel, so retaining water-soluble constituents within the system. This process is called cohobation. Alternatively, the waters are extracted by thorough admixture with a pure, water-immiscible, volatile solvent, such as hexane. Being more soluble in the organic solvent than in water, constituents of the essential oil dissolved in the water tend to pass through the water/solvent interfaces of the countless hordes of small solvent globules produced by the churning action of the extractor, with only a small tendency to return to the water. In this way, the solvent captures dissolved oil, though never completely, a proportion of the oil always remaining dissolved in the water. Several extractions or, alternatively, the use of a continuous extraction process, may therefore be necessary for effective and economic recovery of the oil. The passing of a dissolved substance from one to another of two immiscible solvents is known as *partition*.

The large, yellowish white and highly fragrant flowers of the tree *Cananga odorata* are water-distilled to produce the Ylang-Ylang oils of commerce. Distillation is stopped and restarted three times, and the receiver changed on each occasion, to yield four fractions of the complete oil. The first fraction, Ylang-Ylang Oil 'Extra', contains the most volatile constituents of the oil (i.e., almost all of the top notes) together with smaller proportions of constituents of lower volatility. The second and third fractions, constituting Ylang-Ylang Oils Nos. 1 and 2, contain larger proportions of less volatile constituents, while the final fraction, Ylang-Ylang Oil No. 3, is composed of the least volatile constituents of the oil, together with small proportions of those of higher volatility. This process of fractional steam distillation does not, as we have indicated, by any means effect any complete separation of constituents, but yields Ylang-Ylang oils of different grades for different purposes in the composition of perfumes.

In some of the most recently developed steam distillation equipment, herbaceous material is crushed within a novel type of still and is transported through wide, horizontal pipes by Archimedean screw action. Steam under regulated pressure flows within the pipes in the opposite direction, yielding essential oils reputed to be of high quality.

It is important to remember that an essential oil produced by water or steam distillation must, for reasons we have discussed, suffer at least some alteration to its composition during the process, and this notion is completely supported by the results of analysis. If half of a quantity of a source material is steam distilled, and the other half extracted with a pure, volatile solvent, which is subsequently recovered, marked differences in the composition of the two products, one an essential oil and the other an extract, are observed on subsequent analysis. These differences are caused, in the first process but not the second, not only by the hydrolysis of volatile esters, but also by hydrolysis of nonvolatile constituents of the protoplasm known as *glycosides*. A glycoside, on being hydrolysed, undergoes partial decomposition to form a sugar, such as glucose, which is nonvolatile, and another compound called an *aglycone*. The aglycones of certain glycosides present in essential oil-yielding plant matter are volatile, and so enter into the composition of distilled essential oils. Examples of such 'bound' volatiles, released during distillation, are proportions of the 'Rose alcohols' geraniol and citronellol, also linalöl and the two citrals neral and geranial. It is therefore inaccurate to refer to distilled essential oils as natural products, but more correct to describe them as products prepared from their natural sources by distillation — an academic point, really, but one worth bearing in mind (fig. 4.5).

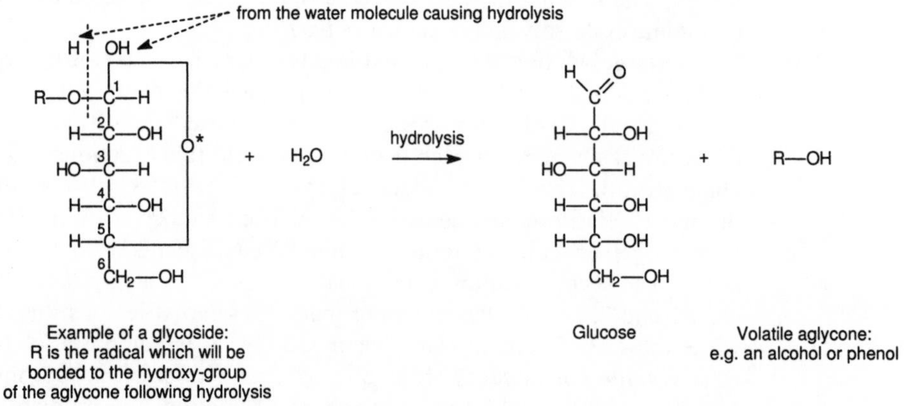

Example of a glycoside:
R is the radical which will be
bonded to the hydroxy-group
of the aglycone following hydrolysis

Glucose

Volatile aglycone:
e.g. an alcohol or phenol

Notice that the glucose molecule has a skeleton of six carbon atoms; it is a hexose sugar (Greek: *hex*, six; *-ose* = family name-ending of all sugars). Also notice that it is an aldehyde, and a polyhydric alcohol in reference to the several hydroxy- groups in the molecule.

In the glycoside molecule, five of the six carbon atoms form a ring structure of six atoms with the oxygen atom marked *. However, because the glycoside is a sugar derivative, we write the structural formula as shown so that this relationship can be clearly seen.

A further important feature of the formula for the glycoside is that O* is bonded directly to C_1 and C_5; the angled bonds between C_1 and O* and between C_5 and O* do *not* indicate that there are extra carbon atoms interposed between these atoms. An alternative way of showing the bonds between C_1 and O*, and C_5 and O*, would be to used curved lines.

Fig. 4.5— Hydrolysis of a glycoside

A further reaction which takes place during the distillation of essential oil-bearing plant material is the partial hydrolysis of protein forming the living matter of the cells. Weakly bonded fragments of the molecules split off to form highly odorous, sulphur-containing products of hydrolysis of very small molecular size, which distil over with the vapours from the still and dissolve in the condensed essential oil, imparting to it an obnoxious smell, known as a 'still note'. Still notes present in an essential oil can be eliminated by exposure to air for several hours or by blowing air into the oil for a short period of time. This promotes the evaporation of the responsible compounds and possibly also to some extent their oxidation to odourless products.

Certain essential oils, German Chamomile, for example, are blue, due to the presence of chamazulene, a dark-blue, volatile, odourless hydrocarbon of interesting molecular structure (fig. 4.6).

Chamazulene is rather unstable, and so blue chamomile oils slowly lose their blue colour, becoming green and finally yellow with age.

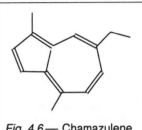

Fig. 4.6 — Chamazulene

4.5.3 *Extraction with Volatile Solvents*

The principle of solvent extraction is illustrated every time a pot of tea is made. The hot water dissolves flavour principles (volatiles and nonvolatiles having flavour properties), pigments and other extractable matter from the tea leaves, forming an extract solution. Following a period of infusion with the pot insulated against heat loss, which is the purpose of the tea cosy, the aqueous solution delivered from the pot is subjected to colation (passed through a strainer) to remove particles of insoluble matter (bits of leaf) and is then consumed. Tea granules are produced by evaporating the water from an extract solution of tea leaves, by a process which retains the flavour principles as well as the pigments.

Solvent extraction is applied to those parts of plants whose essential oils are too far degraded by distillation to be of any use as perfume ingredients, of which Jasmin and Tuberose flowers are examples, or to prepare extracts (absolutes or resinoids) from parts of plants which are, alternatively, distilled (Rose, Ylang-Ylang, Galbanum, etc.) to provide perfumers with products from the same sources having different odours.

Jasmin flowers provide a typical example of a process of solvent extraction. The flowers, freshly hand-picked in the early morning, are as soon as possible washed in a closed vessel with a purified, volatile hydrocarbon solvent, such as hexane. As it flows over the flowers, the solvent dissolves essential oil from the oil glands, together with natural petal wax and small amounts of pigment from the calices which support the corollas of the flowers. The extract solution so produced is filtered, and the filtrate subjected to low-pressure distillation to recover the solvent for further use. The residue, containing about 55% of essential oil, takes the form of a brownish, waxy mass and is known as *Jasmin Concrete* (fig. 4.7).

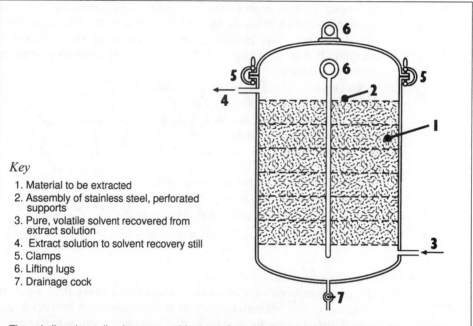

Key

1. Material to be extracted
2. Assembly of stainless steel, perforated supports
3. Pure, volatile solvent recovered from extract solution
4. Extract solution to solvent recovery still
5. Clamps
6. Lifting lugs
7. Drainage cock

The volatile solvent dissolves extractable matter from the charge as it slowly passes upward in the extraction vessel, which may be heated or operated cold, according to the requirements of each material treated.

The solvent is recovered from the extract solution by distillation and is recycled to the extraction vessel. Thus the extracted matter is not distilled but remains as the final product in the distillation vessel of the solvent recovery still.

Once extraction has been completed, any remaining solvent is steamed out of the charge. The extraction vessel is opened, and the assembly of perforated supports, together with the exhausted charge, lifted out for removal of the charge and cleaning ready for the next extraction process.

Fig. 4.7 — Solvent extraction equipment

For most present-day purposes the waxes present in concretes are unwanted, serving merely to dilute the essential oil the product contains; they are also poorly soluble in other aromatic materials and in ethanol, a disadvantage difficult to overcome. The waxes do, however, help to preserve the essential oil contained in a concrete. Concretes are for this reason often stored and transported as such. To remove the waxes from Jasmin Concrete the product is warmed and vigorously stirred with pure alcohol (ethanol) at a temperature of from 45 to 60°C, whereupon the concrete melts and the liquid mass is broken up into minute globules, the combined surface area of which is vastly greater than the surface area of the original mass.

Taking place over this enormous area, the partition of essential oil from the wax into the alcohol, in which it is more soluble, is efficient. Several similar extractions of the same quantity of concrete are required for economic transfer of the essential oil into the alcohol. In practice, to avoid having to use very large quantities of alcohol for the extraction of a concrete, a system is employed in which weaker alcoholic extract solutions from the final stages of the extraction of one batch of concrete are used in the early stages of the extraction of the next batch.

The wax of the concrete is not totally insoluble in ethanol, and so some dissolves. To remove most of it finally, the bulked alcoholic extract solutions are chilled to −12°C, with stirring, and these conditions are maintained for several hours. During this time much of the wax is precipitated. Final cold filtration gives a dewaxed extract solution from which the alcohol is recovered for further use by gentle distillation under reduced pressure. The distillation temperature is therefore lower than it would be at normal atmospheric pressure, protecting delicate constituents of the dissolved essential oil from thermal decomposition, and ensuring that the more volatile constituents of the essential oil do not distil over with the alcohol.

Several stages of alcohol recovery are necessary to concentrate finally the extract solution ready for vacuum stripping of the last traces of alcohol. The residual extract is *Jasmin Absolute*, a somewhat viscous, brownish liquid possessing a fragrance closely recalling natural Jasmin, yet rendered less than natural by reason of its enormous concentration relative to the greatly diluted condition of the fragrance as smelled from the living flower. Jasmin Absolute, like other absolutes, contains some proportions of residual flower wax, also traces of pigments not removed by treatment of the concrete with alcohol, in which they are soluble.

Certain absolutes, especially those from chlorophyll-rich plant matter, such as hay, are too highly coloured for use as ingredients of perfumes for white products, which they would visibly tint at the concentrations used. These absolutes may be decolorized by treatment with activated charcoal, which selectively adsorbs the most intensely coloured pigments, leaving more weakly coloured ones, such as tannins, in the product at acceptable levels of intensity.

The resinous exudates of certain plants as, for example, Myrrh, Frankincense, Benzoin and Labdanum, contain essential oil, resins and, in some cases, gums. As exuded, they also contain fragments of tree bark, bits of leaf, earth and the corpses of unfortunate insects, and so need to be purified. They are treated by solvent extraction and subsequent filtration of the extract solution to remove insoluble matter, usually employing purified, volatile hydrocarbon solvents, with final recovery of the solvent by vacuum distillation. The products of the process are the resinoids of perfumery. Alternatively, the crude material is steam-distilled to produce an essential oil, the nonvolatile and odourless resins and gums remaining in the distillation vessel.

Benzoin is exceptional in yielding no essential oil to distillation, because its aromatic constituents are insufficiently volatile. Benzoin Oil does not, therefore, exist.

4.5.4 Short-path, or Molecular, Distillation

This is a process for preparing completely volatile products from delicate materials containing some proportion of nonvolatile matter, such as the absolutes of perfumery. The basic principle involved is gentle evaporation of a thin film of the material to be treated from a surface over which the film is continuously replenished, under almost total vacuum conditions. Molecules of evaporating volatiles have only a short distance to travel before encountering a cooled surface on which to condense, and can freely pass to this surface under the vacuum conditions used (no molecules of air gases to impede their progress). Only very gentle heating is employed to cause efficient evaporation of the volatiles, molecules of which therefore remain intact during the process. Molecular distillates of costly absolutes are even more expensive than the products from which they are prepared, and so are necessarily reserved for use in the fine fragrance sector of perfumery. The extraction of aromatic plant matter with hot fat, and the absorption of flower fragrances by *enfleurage*, are both obsolete processes of historical interest.

4.6 Applications of Essential Oils

Until the entry into perfumery, in the later years of the nineteenth century, of synthetic chemicals having useful odours, essential oils and extracts of aromatic source materials were the only ingredients available to the perfumer for the composition of perfumes. They numbered about 400 different items, and with this palette, severely limited, as it transpired, in comparison with the 'perfumery organ' of no more than twenty years later, the artist in fragrance composed his symphonies, in almost total darkness as to the chemical composition of the materials he handled, unsuspecting of the transformation the coming century would visit upon his gentle craft and oblivious of the fact that the best-loved of his creations were forerunners of perfumes to be hailed as masterpieces of fragrance creation, and accorded status in perfumery of no lesser degree than that achieved by the greatest works of the visual arts, music and mathematics.

The exquisite, classic perfumes of the late nineteenth and early twentieth centuries were created with the aid of materials new to perfumery: freshly discovered, synthetic chemicals possessing novel odours, which the more daring and adventurous of perfumers saw as representing creative opportunity rather than intrusion into a time-honoured preserve where only natural materials were believed capable of giving expression to creative inspiration. The twentieth century has witnessed a revolution in perfumery, in which aroma chemicals have become of ever-increasing importance as ingredients of perfumes for thousands of personal-care and household products, inspiration for the creation of many of which having 'trickled down' from original ideas embodied in fine personal fragrances.

Today, the demand for perfume exceeds by far the total available supply of all essential oils added together, yet the demand for essential oils does not diminish, the supply being limited mainly by the cost and availability of land for the growing of crops of aromatic plants. We shall discuss examples of the applications of essential oils in perfumery in Chapter 6.

The flavour industry is a very large user of essential oils, those in greatest demand being the citrus, spice and mint oils. Most of these oils are, in fact, more important as flavour ingredients than they are in perfumery. The culinary spices are also extracted with volatile solvents to produce the extracts known as oleo-resins. These products constitute the total, concentrated flavours of the various source materials, such as Ginger, Nutmeg and Pepper, rather than only the odour part of flavour given by the respective essential oils, because most of the sweet, bitter acidic, salty and pungent principles are nonvolatile, and so do not distil over with the volatiles of the essential oils. The volatiles of Vanilla are insufficiently volatile for the production of an essential oil, and so this natural source of fragrance and flavour is available only as the cured fruits (Vanilla 'beans') or as an absolute or oleo-resin. Oleo-resins are suitable for use only as flavour ingredients.

By the 1930s, every pharmacy held stocks of some twenty or thirty essential oils; these were used mainly for medicinal purposes or flavouring. Some pharmacists of this era made their own perfumes, for which they kept a much wider selection of oils and a range of aroma chemicals, as well as materials for the manufacture of cosmetics. When wartime conditions caused depletion of supplies of well-known personal-care products, these worthies were in an excellent position to make up the deficiencies with preparations formulated in blacked-out laboratories behind their dispensaries. Some of their concoctions were rather strange, and were rarely the same from one batch to the next. But, being much more concerned with other matters, nobody seemed to mind, and when one ingredient became unobtainable another would be substituted following a little experimentation.

Today, many pharmacies stock small bottles of essential oils or dilutions of essential oils in carrier oils for aromatherapy in the home.

4.7 The Composition of Essential Oils

A genuine distilled essential oil is a mixture of organic chemicals, some of which were present as constituents of the oil before the source plant was subjected to processing, others having been formed during processing by the hydrolysis of glycosides and by unavoidable, partial decomposition of delicate, natural constituents unable to withstand the ravages of hot steam. Such artifacts are accepted as normal constituents of a genuine oil, as they contribute to the properties by which the oil is recognized and identified.

Essential oils delivered to perfume and flavour companies are frequently found to be adulterated with cheaper materials, such as similar oils of lower cost, cheap terpenes and aroma chemicals. The purposes of adulteration are, basically, to render a poor quality oil saleable, to 'stretch', or 'extend', a good quality oil for sale as a 'natural' product and, quite ethically and with the knowledge of customers, to adjust the physico-chemical properties of an essential oil by blending oils of the same kind from different geographical sources, so that the product conforms to customers' specifications. Essential oils of guaranteed, unadulterated quality are available, but they cost more than the corresponding 'regular' oils which are completely acceptable as ingredients of perfumes for personal-care and domestic cleaning aids, in which applications fine quality oils would be wasted, even if they could be afforded.

The constituents of an essential oil are, as we have noted, usefully classed into terpenes or oxygenated constituents and certain compounds which do not fall into either of these categories. Subdivision of the terpenes into monoterpenes and sesquiterpenes, and the 'oxygenates' into chemical families by reference to the functional groups which characterize the chemical behaviour of their molecules, are first steps in the direction of understanding the nature and properties of essential oils.

Analysis shows that a typical essential oil, such as Geranium, is composed of a small number of *major constituents*, present at levels down to 1% of the oil, and a larger number of *minor constituents*, present from 1% down to 0·1%, which together comprise more than 99% of the oil. Since, today, most of these constituents are available as aroma chemicals of high quality, it is possible to 'reconstitute' an oil by mixing together synthetic representatives of its natural composition in the proportions prescribed by the results of analysis of the genuine oil. If this is done, however, the result is invariably disappointing as regards the odour quality of the resulting mixture, for the reason that the experiment will have taken no account of the *trace constituents* of the essential oil, present at levels below 0·1% down to a few parts per trillion, i.e. per million million, certain of which can and do, even at this infinitesimal dilution, contribute noticeably to the quality of the oil. An example, here, is the trace constituent of Grapefruit Oil, thioterpineol (alpha-terpineol with a sulphur atom replacing the oxygen atom in its molecule), which currently is the record-holder among odorous chemicals in being the most intensely powerful known to science. This glowing testimonial some time ago inspired one devotee of smells to calculate that if 10 grams of the vapour of the stuff could be evenly distributed in the Earth's atmosphere everyone inhabiting the planet would smell it: a worthy candidate for inclusion in a modern perfume, one might think; but too late! The perfumers have been using a derivative of the synthetic version as a perfume ingredient for some years!

The citrus peel oils, the only essential oils produced by expression, contain small proportions of dissolved, nonvolatile matter, consisting of waxes and colouring matter from the rind and, much more importantly, certain derivatives of coumarin which are phototoxic. Lime Oil, exceptionally, is mostly steam-distilled and used mainly as a flavour ingredient. The subject of the composition of essential oils is further discussed in Chapter 6, section 4 *et seq.*

4.8 Phototoxicity of Citrus Oils

The term *phototoxicity* refers to damage to tissues, specifically those of human skin, resulting from contact with certain substances, called *photosensitisers*, in the presence of ultraviolet light. One form of this condition, known as *berloque dermatitis,* is caused by a coumarin derivative, bergaptene, occurring at about 0·3% in Bergamot Oil and at lower levels in Orange, Mandarin and Lemon Oils.

The proportion of crystalline derivatives of coumarin found dissolved in Bergamot Oil amounts to about 2%, but of these only bergaptene is phototoxic. It is a member of the chemical family of furanocoumarins, or psoralens, derived from coumarin as shown in the following structural formulae (fig. 4.8).

Note the presence of a methoxy- (methyl ether) group at C_5 in the highly phototoxic bergaptene, and the absence of this group in the nonphototoxic furanocoumarins bergaptal and bergamottin.

Bergamot Oil is an important ingredient of fine Eaux de Cologne and of the top notes of countless other toilet waters and extrait perfumes. To reduce the proportion of bergaptene to a safe level in these and other fragranced products, the International Fragrance Association (IFRA: *see* Chap. 7) recommends a maximum limit of this phototoxic agent in products for application to skin exposed to sunshine. To obviate completely the possibility of exposing users to the risk of photoxicity, natural Bergamot Oil in a formula may be replaced by furanocoumarin-free Bergamot Oil or, if fragrance considerations permit, by an equivalent proportion of the terpeneless oil — a product concentrated with respect to oxygenates by removal of most of the terpenes.

Regarding the use of Bergamot Oil in aromatherapy, consideration should be given to the calculation shown below.

The maximum safe level of bergaptene, as recommended by IFRA is 0·0015%;
i.e: 100 g product must not contain more than 0·0015 g bergaptene   (i)
If Bergamot Oil contains 0·3% of bergaptene
then 0·3 g bergaptene is present in 100 g of Bergamot Oil
∴ 0·0015 g bergaptene is present in $\dfrac{100 \times 0.0015}{0.3}$ = 0·5 g of the oil
From (i) 100 g product must not contain more than 0·5 g of Bergamot Oil.

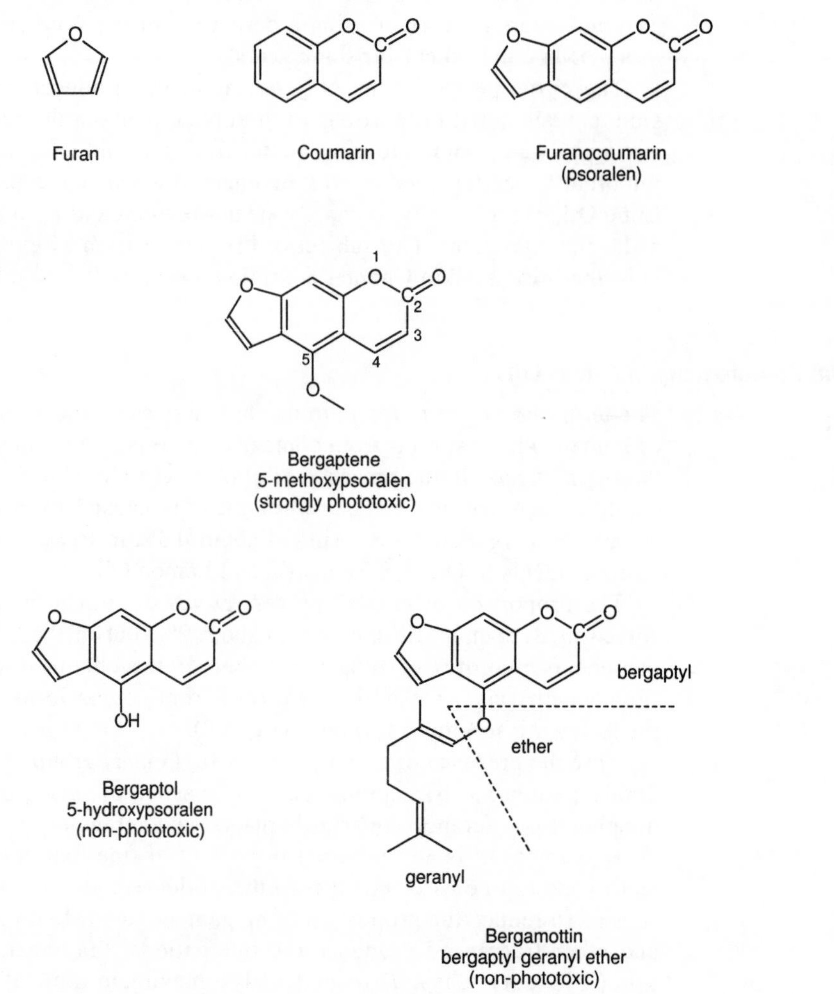

Fig. 4.8 — The family of furanocoumarins (psoralens)

On the basis of the above calculation, the maximum safe strength of a solution of Bergamot Oil in a carrier oil for use in aromatherapy is 0·5%, or 1 g Bergamot Oil in 200 g of final solution.

In the case of a blended oil for use in aromatherapy, i.e. a preparation containing more than one essential oil dissolved in a carrier oil, account must be taken of the additive phototoxic effect of combined phototoxic agents. Hence if Bergamot is combined with another phototoxic essential oil, the maximum safe proportion of Bergamot Oil in the preparation will be less than 0·5%. There would seem to be no good reason why natural Bergamot Oil should not be totally replaced by the furanocoumarin-free oil for all purposes.

Chapter 5

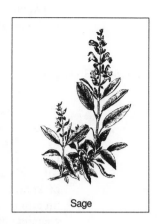

Sage

Odour Properties of Essential Oils

5.1 The Evocative Property of Odours

An exceptionally sensitive nose is an effective aid to the survival of many animals, and has undoubtedly saved many relatively defence-less species from extinction long ago. In comparison with the nose of the domestic cat or dog, the human appendage is a poor affair indeed, permitting perception of a far narrower range of odours, and then only at levels of concentration much higher than is necessary for their detection by most other mammals.

We humans take little notice of smells, excepting those which arouse our curiosity, pleasure or disgust, or which evoke sudden, and perhaps temporarily overwhelming, yet always fleeting, recall of feelings and situations of marked pleasure or pain, long consciously forgotten, on encountering the same smell, or a very similar one many years later. It is a thought-provoking possibility that a complete record of all personal experience lies buried in the mind, awaiting just the right trigger for recall. The present writer, no doubt in common with many other people, finds it possible, on smelling a certain odour source, to recapture what seems to be the totality of his experience when using the same material many years ago in a learning situation of intense interest and pleasure. The instantly evocative smell on entering a school can induce a unique kind of pleasure and mental refreshment. The odour-evoked experience is usually but a flash of memory which cannot be held in the mind for contemplation, but which can be so real as to be much more than a momentary return to the past. Perhaps the infinitesimal duration of the experience concentrates its effect to the brink of reality.

The evocative property of odours may be involved, in a more general way, in the application of aromachology, the sensory aspect of aromatherapy, to the inducement of mood benefits.

At the conscious level, an odour has certain properties which we shall now discuss.

5.2 Odour Strength

Until the recent introduction of instrumental means for the objective measurement of odours, the odour strength of a chemical, which would, of necessity, have to be highly purified, could be found only by the use of trained observers using rigorously standardized procedures of sensory estimation. Basically, these techniques involve dissolving a subject material in an odourless solvent to form a solution of known strength. This solution is then further diluted with measured quantities of the same solvent until any greater dilution of the chemical cannot be smelled at all. For a given person used as a tester, the highest dilution of the chemical which he or she can just smell is recorded as a personal 'odour threshold' for that material. From the results obtained by as large a number of other testers as reasonably possible, a figure representing an average 'minimum perceptible' concentration of the material is calculated. To obtain valid results, statistical methods have to be used to eliminate errors resulting from the subjectivity which plagues all attempts at accuracy in work of this kind.

Here are some examples of minimum perceptible values from tests using aqueous solutions of the test chemicals.

Table 5.1 — Minimum perceptible values for some materials

Test material	Odour threshold: number of grams substance dissolved in 10^{12} grams (1000 000 000 000 = 1 trillion grams) water at 20°C*
Ethyl alcohol (ethanol)	10^8 = 100 000 000
Butyric acid (found in rancid butter)	240 000
Amyl acetate (odour of 'pear drops')	5000
Methyl mercaptan (CH_3SH; odour of rotting cabbage)	20
beta-Ionone (floral odour of violets)	7
2-Methoxy-3-isobutylpyrazine (intense, earthy-green odour)	2

*One gram amounts of any of the chemicals named in the above table are equivalent to approximately one fifth of a teaspoonful. One trillion grams of water occupy, approximately, 200 million gallons — the volume of a New York skyscraper. It is not, of course, necessary to use a tank of this size for the experiments. A 'strong' solution of, say, 0·1 g of the test substance, accurately weighed, is prepared in pure water sufficient to make 1000 g of solution using, if necessary, an odourless co-solvent for a substance poorly soluble in water, and known dilutions of this solution are made under standardized conditions. Eventually, a dilution is reached beyond which a tester is unable to perceive any odour sensation. The tester's personal odour threshold is that previous dilution which can be just be smelled.

The odour threshold of an essential oil would depend on the odour strengths of its constituents, and the proportions in which they are present in the oil, but since these are both variable among different samples of the same oil, the property of odour threshold also is variable. Weakly odorous major constituents of essential oils, limonene in Lemon Oil, for example, are of odour weakening effect, whereas strongly odorous minor constituents as, for example, citral in Lemon Oil, together with intensely odorous trace constituents such as fatty aldehydes, contribute largely to the odour strength of the oil.

Human sensitivity to odours is weakened under cold conditions, or if the air is very dry, and so odour evaluations should be made in warm, sufficiently humid surroundings.

5.3 Odour Character

Until very recently, the measurement of odour character without recourse to the human nose was no more than a dream of the future for researchers working in the field of sensory perception. Today, that dream has been brought closer to realization by the invention of detectors capable of distinguishing between certain odorous substances. These instruments do not, however, 'smell' the air dilutions of vapours presented to them, but measure the energy changes produced when the molecules of odorous vapours stick, temporarily, to specially prepared surfaces which are selective as to which molecules they will adsorb and which they will not. *Ad*sorption differs from *ab*sorption in that it is a 'sticking to' rather than a 'soaking up' process. It is seen on clothing when household detergents fail to remove ink stains, which only certain specially formulated stain removers will dispel, by *de*sorption or chemical action. The minute energy changes which occur during the adsorption of odorous molecules by an 'artificial nose' are transformed into electrical energy signals, which are amplified and fed into a computer programmed to interpret them in terms of an odour profile — in this case a graphical report on the different notes present and their relative intensities and not an evaporation profile of the kind we have discussed with reference to an essential oil.[1]

The advantage of a sufficiently sensitive and discriminating odour detector of this kind would be to eliminate the subjectivity inherent in odour evaluation by use of the nose. To equal the sensitivity of the nose it would, however, have to be able to detect the almost vanishingly small concentrations of intensely odorous constituents which noticeably contribute to the odour profiles of many essential oils and

---

1. Further measurements can, of course, be made during the evaporation of a sample of any mixture of volatiles, to obtain a complete odour profile from an "artificial nose".

perfumes, and the delicate, and sometimes extremely complex, nuances that comprise the indefinable elements of 'quality' associated with fine fragrances for personal use.

At the present time, odour character is mostly described in terms expressive of the distinctive odour impressions, known as odour notes, that are perceived by human observers. Just as a trained musician can name the notes of any musical chord, name the instrument sounding a note of a particular quality and even the instruments playing the different parts of an orchestral score, so a trained and experienced perfumer can name the odour notes present in a fragrance *accord* — the odour equivalent of a musical chord — also those of an essential oil, other raw material or finished perfume absorbed onto a smelling strip and the fragrance elements present in a finished perfume.

To describe, communicate and record information on odours some kind of code is necessary, the most obvious and commonly used being the spoken and written word. Perfumery is about feelings and emotions as much as it is about satisfying consumer needs, and for this purpose anything of a coldly scientific nature is about as useful as an electronic calculator for composing poetry. However, there is a difficulty: where odours are concerned, the English language fails us in its complete lack of a vocabulary of odour-descriptive terms. There are, of course, words such as perfume, scent, aroma, fragrant, putrid, stink and stench, but these are colourless terms, expressive only of like or dislike.

For want of a true odour language, the odour vocabulary used in the perfume industry is made up of words referring to families of related odours, such as floral, woody, fruity and herbaceous, terms naming specific sources of odour, such as jasmin, pineapple, lavender, sandalwood and earthy, together with auxiliary expressions — sweet, dry, fresh, sharp, etc. — which have been adopted from common usage in other contexts for use in reference to odours.

When smelling an essential oil or other aromatic material or perfume for the first time, it is best initially to note the relative strength of the odour perceived, then to try to identify the family of odours to which the odour of the product belongs; then, if possible, the specific odour source to which it relates. The description may then be refined by the use of auxiliary odour terms and finally presented to communicate as simple, yet complete, a description of the odour as words will permit. A touch of restraint, here, may be necessary to eliminate flatulent over-enthusiasm and promote accuracy. Like any other artistic exercise, facility in odour description improves with practice, especially if approached systematically, as it does under the imposed discipline of a training situation. For guidance, section 5.8 includes brief odour descriptions of the examples of essential oils given in Chapter 4.

5.4 Odour Persistence or Lasting Power

As we noted in section 4.1, the odour character of almost every essential oil changes as it evaporates from a smelling strip into the air, for the reasons that its constituents have odours that are different from one another, and because they evaporate at different speeds. This may be illustrated by means of a simple experiment in which a mixture of two aroma chemicals of different volatility and odour character, representing constituents of an essential oil, is allowed to evaporate.

In one demonstration of this kind, using smelling strips, a mixture of equal weights of benzyl acetate and eugenol was dipped to a depth of 1 cm and allowed to evaporate. For comparison, separate ½ cm dips of each of the components of the mixture were set aside to evaporate at the same time under the same conditions. The strips were then smelled at frequent intervals until either no further odour change was observed or the odour had faded to vanishing point. The results were as in table 5.2.

Table 5.2 — Odour persistence

Material	Odour	Time to disappearance of odour of:	
		benzyl acetate (hours)	eugenol (hours)
Mixture	floral, spicy	7	more than 24
Benzyl acetate	floral (jasmin-like)	3	—
Eugenol	spicy (clove-like)	—	more than 24

The above results show that eugenol slows down the speed at which benzyl acetate evaporates. This can be explained, in part, by analogy to the relative freedom of a small crowd of people to disperse from a large, open area, contrasted with the difficulty the same people would find in attempting to disperse from the same area if the individuals were scattered among roughly the same number of other people in a crowd of twice the size. There is, however, evidence that molecules of certain chemical classes attract one another more than can be accounted for by the forces of attraction which cause molecules of all liquids to cohere to form droplets or quantities which do not break up into smaller amounts until disturbed. This is caused mainly by a type of bonding which occurs between molecules of certain chemical families: hydrogen bonding.

5.5 Hydrogen Bonding and its Effects

The molecular weight of water, H_2O, is $(2 \times 1) + 16 = 18$; that of carbon dioxide, CO_2, is $12 + (2 \times 16) = 44$; yet carbon dioxide, with a molecule nearly two-and-a-half times heavier than a water molecule, is a gas at 20°C, and normal atmospheric pressure, while water is a liquid under these conditions. Why?

The anomalous condition of water is explained by the existence of an extra force of attraction between water molecules which is present to only a very much lesser extent between the molecules of carbon dioxide, and which is totally insufficient to maintain the coherence of carbon dioxide in the liquid state at 20°C, except under very high pressure. This attractive force is known as *hydrogen bonding*.

In a water molecule, there is a large difference between the electrical charge on the nucleus of the oxygen atom (eight protons give a charge of 8+) and that on the hydrogen nucleus (one proton; charge = 1+). The effect of this disparity is to displace the mean position of the pairs of electrons bonding oxygen to hydrogen in the molecule away from the hydrogen atoms and towards the oxygen atoms, electrons being negatively charged; that is, their orbitals are distorted towards the oxygen atom. Thus the oxygen end of the molecule gains a little extra negative charge, while the hydrogen ends lose a little of the negative charges neutralizing the positive charges on the hydrogen nuclei. This polarizes the water molecule, a condition we can express by means of the following formula for water (fig. 5.1):

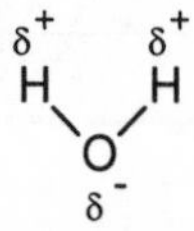

$$
\begin{array}{ccc}
\delta^+ & & \delta^+ \\
H & & H \\
& \searrow O \swarrow & \\
& \delta^- &
\end{array}
$$

where δ^+ means a small increase in positive charge
and δ^- means a small increase in negative charge

Fig. 5.1 — Polarization of the water molecule

The polar water molecules attract one another, forming temporary clumps which, it is deduced, continuously break up and reassemble in liquid water, effectively increasing the molecular weight of water and greatly reducing its volatility.

A hydrogen bond is about 23 times weaker than the chemical bonds joining the oxygen atom to the two hydrogens in a water molecule, but it is about 15 times stronger than the normal forces of cohesion acting between the molecules of a liquid. This explains why water puddles evaporate without decomposition of the water.

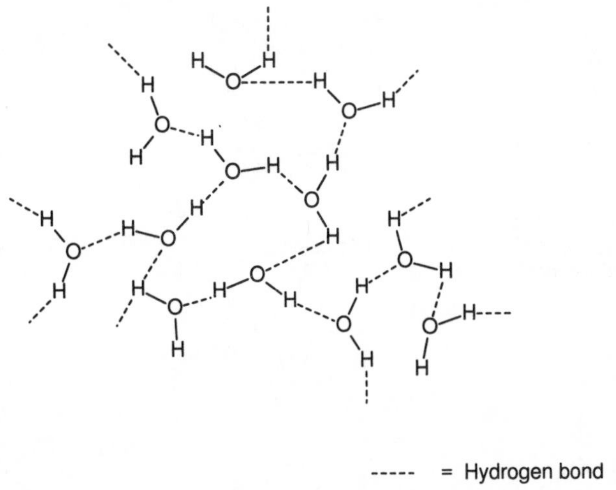

----- = Hydrogen bond

Fig. 5.2 — Hydrogen bonding among water molecules

Without hydrogen bonding, water would be a gas as permanent as neon, and life as we know it here on earth could not exist.

Just as energy is required to break up a mechanical structure, such as a building, so energy is required at the molecular level to decompose a chemical compound. If ordinary sugar is heated it eventually melts, the molten sugar turns yellow, brown and finally black, boiling away and giving off dense, choking fumes. Ultimately, nothing remains but a black cinder of carbon and a strong, caramellic (caramel-like) kind of smell. The sugar has decomposed into one of its elements, carbon, and many odorous volatile products, and this has involved the breaking of bonds. The breaking of chemical bonds requires an energy input. Conversely, when chemical bonds are formed, energy is given out, usually in the form of heat.

Evidence for the formation of hydrogen bonds between molecules of water and alcohol, and between alcohol and glycerol molecules, comes from experiments in which an increase of temperature and a decrease in volume are observed on mixing the liquids. A formula for glycerol appears on page 85 (fig. 4.1).

Table 5.3 — Examples of changes of volume and temperature on mixing certain liquids

Composition of the mixture	Temp. of each liquid before mixing, °C	Temp. after mixing, °C	Temp. change, °C	Final volume at 22°C (cm³)
50 cm³ ethanol + 50 cm³ water	22	29	+7	93·5
50 cm³ ethanol + 50 cm³ glycerol	22	25	+3	96·0

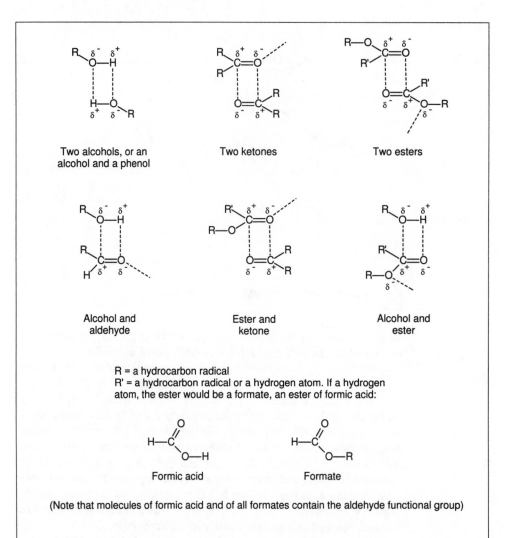

R = a hydrocarbon radical
R' = a hydrocarbon radical or a hydrogen atom. If a hydrogen
atom, the ester would be a formate, an ester of formic acid:

Formic acid   Formate

(Note that molecules of formic acid and of all formates contain the aldehyde functional group)

Fig. 5.3 — Some possibilities for hydrogen bonding among molecules of oxygenates

An oxygen atom bonded to a carbon atom in a molecule is known to have a withdrawing effect on the electrons of the carbon atom, but one very much weaker than that which occurs in a water molecule (an oxygen atom has 8 protons in its nucleus; a carbon atom has 6). Aldehydes, ketones and esters in the liquid state are therefore affected by hydrogen bonding between their molecules, as shown in figure 5.3, even though hydrogen atoms are not involved.

The effect of hydrogen bonding among polar constituents of a liquid essential oil (i.e. the oxygenated constituents) is a tendency for smaller, faster moving molecules of relatively low molecular weight to be held back within the body of the liquid by larger, heavier molecules. We may also speculate that lighter polar molecules moving towards the surface of the liquid exert some pulling effect on heavier, polar molecules, tending to assist their movement towards the surface and so promoting their evaporation.

Hydrogen bonding undoubtedly accounts, at least in part, for the wonderfully coherent odours of flower absolutes, which are much richer in oxygenates than the corresponding distilled essential oils, if the latter exist. Lavender is a good example, here.

On carefully smelling Jasmin Absolute, occasionally, over a period of time, as it evaporates from a smelling strip, its odour is found to change, though almost imperceptibly. This absolute contains no less than 30 to 35% of benzyl acetate, an ester of relatively high volatility, yet at no time during the evaporation of Jasmin Absolute is it possible to identify clearly the floral-fruity and rather coarse odour of benzyl acetate in isolation from the combined effects of the other constituents: a naturally produced blending effect for which hydrogen bonding is doubtless at least partially responsible.

The fixative effect of certain perfume ingredients in prolonging the duration of the fragrance of a perfume can, in part, be attributed to hydrogen bonding, although the presence of larger molecules in a liquid mixture of volatiles must certainly impede the evaporation of smaller ones, so exerting a purely mechanical fixative effect. We shall discuss fixation in perfumes further in Chapter 9.

5.6 Getting to Know Your Essential Oils

The range of essential oils detailed in authoritative works on aromatherapy amounts to almost a hundred different products — about one quarter of the total generally available including aromatic extracts. In the average salon perhaps no more than half this number will be in regular use, yet even a collection of forty to fifty mysterious liquids obscured behind amber glass or completely invisible within aluminium containers can present a daunting challenge to the newcomer faced with the problem of familiarization.

Despite the ever-widening use of the computer for the storage and retrieval of information, the simple card index still has its place if systematically compiled, and can become a personal treasure to the owner, to be updated and used over and over again for many years. Such a system lends itself readily to the making of notes on essential oils, and to adaptation in database form for those who prefer to work with computers.

If adopting a card index system, each card in use should be headed with the name of one of the essential oils in use, with the botanical and geographical sources and main aromatherapeutic uses recorded beneath. Following a brief, physical description of the oil, a note of its chief constituents should be entered, and this should be followed by an odour profile, a most important item of information which we shall consider in section 5.7. Beneath the odour profile, a note of the conditions under which the oil should be stored will afford a constant reminder of the delicate nature of essential oils. The

---

BERGAMOT OIL, FURANOCOUMARIN-FREE

Citrus bergamia, expressed in S. Italy from outer rind of fruits. Processed to remove phototoxic bergaptene.

Sedative, antidepressant   Green to olive green, mobile liquid

Oxygenates	**Terpenes**
Linalöl	Pinenes
Linalyl acetate	Limonene
Aldehyde C_{10}	gamma-Terpinene
Neral	
Geranial	
Citronellal	
Geranyl acetate	
Terpinen-4-ol	

Top notes: Sharp, fresh, citrus (Lemon)
Body notes: Citrus-herbaceous (lavender-like), spicy (peppery)
Dryout: Little characteristic

Fig. 5.4 — Example of index card

---

reverse side of the index card may be used for other data, together with personal notes on results obtained by use of the product in aromatherapy or aromachology. Figure 5.4 shows an example of the most important items of information to record.

Most important among these entries are the odour data which, if accurate, facilitate the recognition and identification of the essential oil, and the storage directions which, if followed, ensure preservation of the properties of the oil for a considerable period of time, the length of which depends very much on the proportion of monoterpenes and aldehydes present.

It is a wise precaution to store all essential oils in a refrigerator, other than those which keep perfectly well if simply stored in a cool place and those producing crystals difficult to redissolve if refrigerated. There is no need to worry about the essential oils of Sandalwood, Cedarwood, Patchouli or Vetivert, which if of good quality to start with will not deteriorate for many years if stored in tightly sealed containers, protected from light and stored in a cool place. Rose Otto will apparently solidify if stored in a refrigerator because it contains odourless, hydrocarbon waxes which are not too soluble in the odorous constituents of the oil and which come out of solution on cooling as a crystalline deposit, called the *stearoptene*, dispersed in the liquid part of the oil, the *olæoptene*. Rose Otto contains about 20% of stearoptene. No harm will come to Rose Otto if stored in a refrigerator, but on removal from storage for use, the crystals must be allowed to redissolve at room temperature or by the warmth of the hand; no other heat source must be used. Citrus oils, with their high content of monoterpenes, chiefly limonene, are particularly vulnerable to attack by oxygen, and suffer immediately and drastically in sunlight and if exposed to elevated temperatures.

Although with good storage conditions in use, the first signs of irreversible deterioration of an essential oil should never be observed, it is useful to know what these are: loss of freshness in the top note, followed by the onset of a general dullness and flatness over the entire odour profile. The odour profile of a high quality sample of each essential oil in use should be memorized, by practice in smelling, by all persons handling or using essential oils.

5.7 Odour Profiling

There are very few essential oils possessing odours which do not change during the period of their evaporation from smelling strips. Exceptions to this general rule include Bitter Almond Oil, consisting almost entirely of benzaldehyde (which, it must be admitted, undergoes oxidation on the strip, but with little odour change, to final dryout) and Wintergreen Oil, composed mainly of methyl salicylate.

Benzaldehyde

Methyl salicylate
(methyl 2-hydroxybenzoate)

Fig. 5.5 — Benzaldehyde and methyl salicylate

It is interesting that both of these constituents occur in the living plants as odourless glycosides, which are accompanied by, though separated from, the enzymes necessary for their hydrolysis. The enzymes are released by exposure of crushed bitter almond (or peach, plum, apricot or cherry) kernels, or the leaves of *Gaultheria procumbens*, respectively, to warm water, which is the treatment to which both are subjected for some time prior to distillation. The benzaldehyde released is accompanied by hydrogen cyanide, a deadly poisonous gas having an almond-like odour, most of which dissolves in the benzaldehyde. It is removed by chemical treatment of the oil before Bitter Almond Oil is offered for sale, making odour evaluation of the product less inconvenient.

All other essential oils display at least some change of odour when evaporating from a smelling strip caused, as we have explained, by the different rates of evaporation and different proportions of their constituents, these changes being 'smoothed out' by the effects of intermolecular forces of attraction.

In general, with exceptions, the order of decreasing volatility of the main chemical families of constituents of an essential oil is as follows:

Table 5.4 — Order of decreasing volatility of an essential oil's main constituents

	Volatility	Molecular weight	Polarity	Odour
Monoterpenes	relatively high	136	low	mostly weak and non-characteristic
Oxygenates	moderate	most in the range 120-220	high	mostly strong and characteristic
Sesquiterpenes	low	204	low	many have characteristic odours of moderate strength

In the perfume and flavour industries it is common usage to refer to derivatives of terpenes, known chemically as terpenoids, as terpenes. In the above table the words monoterpenes and sesquiterpenes refer only to the hydrocarbons, as the figures for molecular weights indicate.

Let us look at some examples of exceptions to the data given in table 5.4.

Oxygenates of low molecular weight include ethanol (mol wt 46) found in Rose Otto, and methyl amyl (pentyl) ketone (mol wt 58) in Clove oils.

The isomeric alcohols alpha- and beta-santalol, important odorous constituents of East Indian Sandalwood Oil, both have a molecular weight of 220; guaiol, the main constituent of the semisolid, semicrystalline Guaicwood Oil of slightly smoky, rose-like odour, has mol wt = 222 (fig. 5.6).

The ketones alpha- and beta-vetivone (fig. 5.7) make important contributions to the odour of Vetivert Oil. They have mol wt = 218.

The macrocylic, musky-smelling lactone ambrettolide, responsible for much of the odour character of Ambrette Seed (Hibiscus Seed) Oil, has mol wt = 252.

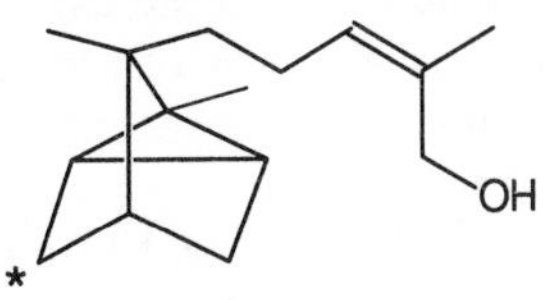

alpha-Santalol

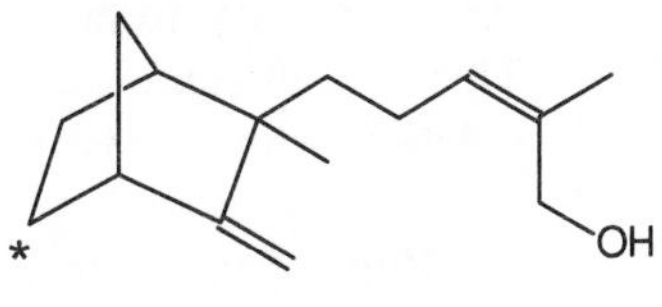

beta-Santalol

In the above diagrams the six-membered ring (indicated by *) is drawn in perspective to make the structures clear

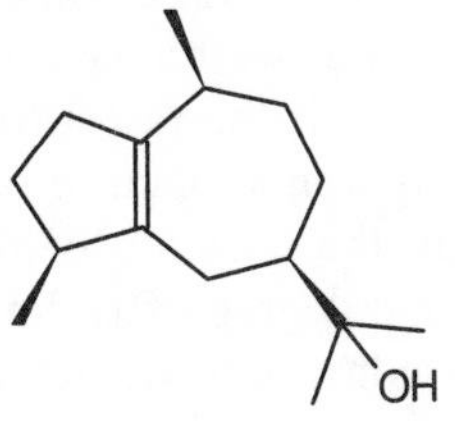

Guaiol

It is worth noting the structural relationship between guaiol (colourless) and chamazulene (blue) [fig. 4.6, p. 101]. Three of the bonds are shown as "wedges", indicating that the carbon atoms at the wider ends are not in the plane of the ring system but above it. See also fig. 2.6 (p. 33).

Fig. 5.6 — alpha- and beta-Santalol and Guaiol

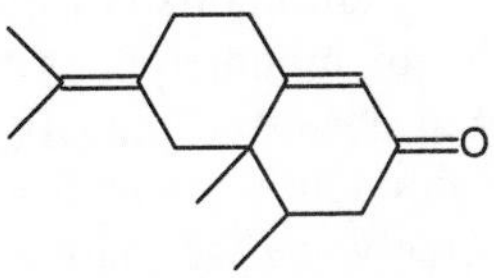

alpha-Vetivone

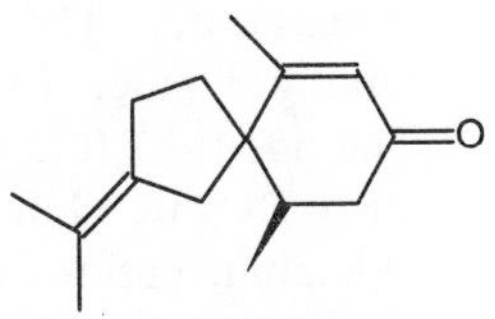

beta-Vetivone

Fig. 5.7 — Vetivones

Fig. 5.8 — Ambrettolide

(Formal structure; the actual molecules can adopt any shape, within the limits of their existence)

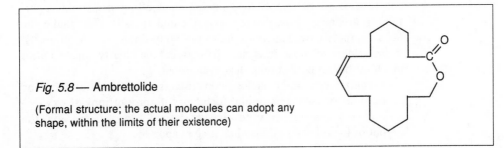

The above structural formulae illustrate something of the molecular complexity found among the constituents of some essential oils. This has, in some instances, resulted in difficulties of structural elucidation which have been overcome only in very recent years with the availability of improved analytical techniques.

With reference to the above table (table 5.4), and to our discussion in section 5.5 of the effects of molecular polarity, we can offer some further explanation of the phenomenon of odour change observed during the evaporation of an essential oil. If the oil is totally volatile, then all of the constituents will begin to evaporate when a sample on a smelling strip is exposed to the air, but they will evaporate at different speeds. Neglecting exceptions, constituents of low polarity, low molecular weight and low odour value, that is, monoterpenes, will evaporate at the fastest rates. Molecules of most oxygenates will tend to hydrogen bond to one another, to a greater or lesser extent, prolonging the duration of the odour notes characteristic of the oil, and to some degree extending the 'life' of less volatile, oxygenated top-note constituents, such as benzyl acetate and linalöl, if present.

Oxygenates of molecular weight around 150 to 200 evaporate quite slowly. The odour of a citrus oil, such as Lemon Oil, will therefore *intensify* on a smelling strip as the monoterpenes evaporate, because they are much more volatile and possess very weak odours in comparison with the very strong odours of the citral, fatty aldehydes, etc., comprising the oxygenates of these oils. This effect may easily be observed by taking a fresh dip of the oil after a first dip has been evaporating for about 15 minutes and comparing the odour intensities of the two samples. Oxygenates of low molecular weight, in addition to monoterpenes, are largely responsible for the top notes of essential oils. The exception among citrus oils is Bergamot Oil, containing a much lower proportion of monoterpenes than the others. The odour of this oil changes, but does not intensify, on a smelling strip. Despite their generally weak odours, monoterpenes make valuable contributions to what we perceive as the 'naturalness and freshness' of the odour of an essential oil.

Oxygenates of high molecular weight evaporate only very slowly, some taking weeks, months or even years to disappear completely. Examples are guaiol, the santalols, ambrettolide, and the vetivones represented in figures 5.6 to 5.8. The essential oils containing these constituents are extremely long-lasting on smelling strips and as perfume ingredients. Oxygenates, as indicated in table 5.4, make the most characteristic contributions to the body notes of essential oils; in the odours of most essential oils they can be clearly smelled after much of the top note content has evaporated.

Sesquiterpenes are tenacious constituents of an essential oil, some proportions of them remaining, together with proportions of oxygenates of very low volatility, to give, as a final odour impression, the dryout of the oil after all else has long evaporated.

It will be useful, here, to summarize some important facts concerning the evaporation of an essential oil.

On first smelling a fresh dip of an essential oil, the top note, consisting of the combined odours of the most volatile constituents of the oil, is perceived. This impression is accompanied by the odours of other constituents, mainly the more volatile components of the body note complex, together with some contributions from less volatile constituents, depending on the intensities of their odours and their proportions in the oil. On smelling the same dip after an interval of time, the body notes may be observed, though always in association with lingering traces of the top note complex. With practice, these latter notes can be ignored. After a further and longer time interval the body notes will have evaporated, leaving a residual odour known as the *dryout*, *dry-down* or *end odour* of the oil. Two question arise:

> *(i) How long does it take for a) top notes and b) body notes to evaporate?*
>
> *(ii) What are the effects of powerful trace constituents on top notes and body notes?*

(i) These periods of time have to be estimated by smelling a genuine sample of each oil. One possible approach would be to evaluate two essential oils of different character (each providing relief from smelling the other) over 14 hours, during the course of a day when interruptions are unlikely and circumstances peaceful.

Take a dip of the essential oil and evaluate the top note complex. Allow this dip to evaporate and re-evaluate briefly every 15 minutes until definite fading of the top note is observed. Allow evaporation to continue for a further 30 minutes, then compare the odour of the dip with that of a fresh dip of the same oil. By comparison, *smelling the original dip first* on each occasion, carefully re-evaluate the top note. Finally, evaluate the body note complex. If possible, allow evaporation to continue until the body notes have completely disappeared, then evaluate the dryout (table 5.5).

Table 5.5 — Evaluation of top and body notes and dryout

Time		Evaluation
hr	*min*	
	0	Take 1 cm dip of essential oil; label strip with name of oil, 'Dip 1' and time of dipping; smell for general impression of top note.
	15	Smell Dip 1 for general impression of any odour changes.
	30	Take second dip of the same oil; label strip with name of oil, 'Dip 2' and time of dipping. Compare odours of Dip 1 and Dip 2, *smelling Dip 1 first*; now top note can be described. Carefully smell Dip 1 for provisional assessment of body notes.
1	00	Smell Dip 1 for final evaluation of body notes. Compare with Dip 2 for any odour differences.
1	30	Smell Dip 1, also thereafter every 30 minutes to final dryout. Evaluate dryout notes.

All of the above evaluations should be recorded in a notebook reserved for this purpose. The body notes of some essential oils, for example, Sandalwood, Vetivert and Patchouli, remain perceptible for days, or even weeks. If the body notes of an essential oil remain strong after 4 hours, evaluate thereafter every hour to a total of 8 hours after dipping, then every 2 hours to 14 hours after dipping. If body notes can then still be clearly smelled, it would be worth taking a fresh dip of the oil, labelled 'Dip 3', and comparing the odours of Dips 2 and 3 after a further 12 hours. A final dryout, different in character from the body notes, may require patience and, as we have noted, a modicum of longevity, to reach. If the body notes simply fade, with no observable odour change, the conclusion must be that the oil exhibits no characteristic dryout notes. If a definite dryout is perceived, but is found impossible to describe, the term 'nondescript' can come to the rescue. A few essential oils, of which Sandalwood is a good example, possess no distinctive top notes.

(ii) The effects of powerful trace constituents depend on the character and intensities of their odours and on their volatilities. The escape of their molecules through the surface of the oil exposed to the air will be impeded by the 'crowding' effect of the much more numerous molecules of other constituents of the evaporating oil, so that whatever their polarity their effects will, to some extent, tend to persist. Trace constituents of relatively high polarity will be subject to hydrogen bonding, with the result that the notes of some of them may persist to the final dryout of the oil. With the aromatic extracts, the absolutes and resinoids of perfumery, the persistence of body notes is extended by the presence of nonvolatile, waxy or resinous constituents. This may be caused by physical entrapment of their molecules or by hydrogen bonding, or both.

5.8 Examples of Terms Used in Odour Description

The descriptive terms in the following list (table 5.6) are those in most frequent general use for describing the odours of essential oils, aroma chemicals and perfumes. A note of the meaning of each term is followed by one or more examples of essential oils to which the term applies.

5.9 Odour Profiles of Essential Oils

The examples of odour profiles of essential oils completing this chapter are given for guidance and to illustrate further the use of odour-descriptive terms. The preparation of an odour profile is, of course, a subjective exercise, the outcome of which depends very much on the personal odour experience, extent of personal odour vocab-

Table 5.6 — Some important terms used in odour description

Term	Explanation	Examples
Animalic	Odours associated with animals	Underlying heavy notes in Jasmin and Orange Flower Absolutes
Balsamic	Sweet and vanilla-like	Benzoin Resinoid
Camphoraceous	Like camphor	Spike Lavender Oil
Citrus	Odours of citrus fruits	Lemon and Orange Oils
Coniferous	Fresh, green and resinous notes of cut, green pine cones	Rosemary Oil, Pine and Fir Oils
Earthy	The smell of rain-moistened earth	Patchouli Oil
Floral	Odours of fragrant flowers	1% Rose Otto or 1% Jasmin Absolute in a carrier oil
Fruity	Odours of edible fruits	Any of the citrus oils; 'Roman' Chamomile Oil
Green	Odours of crushed, green leaves	No common example; Violet Leaf Absolute is typical
Herbaceous, or herbal	Odours of culinary herbs	Thyme and Sage Oils
Medicated	Odours suggesting medication	Wintergreen and Ylang-Ylang Oils
Minty	Notes given by spearmint or peppermint leaves, when stroked	Spearmint and Peppermint Oils
Resinous	Odours of fragrant resins	Myrrh and Frankincense Oils
Spicy	Odours of culinary spices	Clove, Cinnamon and Coriander Oils
Woody	Odours of exotic woods	Sandalwood and Cedarwood Oils

ulary and ability to select from it appropriate descriptive terms, of the evaluator. The given profiles are therefore brief and include terms referring to only the main features of the odours of the essential oils included in the following table (table 5.7). They should be studied critically and compared with personal notes on the odours of the corresponding oils.

The exchange of ideas when working with odours is most profitable for, as in the present writer's experience when working with groups of students, someone very frequently suggests a feature of an odour or odour profile which he has never before considered or realized was present in a sample under evaluation. Whilst it is probably best, in the interest of concentrating contemplative thought, to work alone when first profiling an essential oil, opportunities should be sought thereafter for comparison of notes and re-examining features of profiles with colleagues. This will greatly improve your memory for odours and systematically aid familiarization with all of the essential oils you handle or use.

Table 5.7 — Essential oil odour profiles

	Name of product	Top notes	Body notes	Dryout
1	Ambrette Seed Oil	Fatty, floral	Musky	Rich, sweet, floral, musky, vinous
2	Amyris Oil	Faint	Spicy	Mild, woody, pine-like, balsamic
3	Aniseed Oil	Little distinctive	Sweet, warm, anisic, (characteristic of aniseed)	Warm, not distinctive
4	Basil Oil	Fresh, herbaceous, aniseed-like	Sweet, herbaceous, aniseed-like	Warm, not distinctive
5	Benzoin, Siam, Resinoid	Slightly floral, vanilla-like	Sweet, warm, vanilla-like	Balsamic-powdery
6	Bergamot Oil	Fresh, sharp, lemon-orangey	Herbaceous, orangey, peppery, slightly floral	Warm, like orange pith
7	Caraway Seed Oil	Somewhat 'weedy', typical of caraway	Characteristic of crushed caraway 'seed'	Spicy
8	Cedarwood Oil, Virginian	Woody	Woody, somewhat oily, characteristic of cedarwood	Woody-balsamic
9	Chamomile Oil, German	Sweet, warm, herbaceous, fruity	Sweet, herbaceous, hay-like	Warm, tobacco-like
10	Chamomile Oil, Roman	Sweet, fruity, herbaceous	Warm, herbaceous, somewhat fruity	Warm, herbaceous, tea-like
11	Cinnamon Bark Oil	Sweet, spicy, fruity, floral	Sweet, warm, spicy, fruity	Sweet, 'powdery'
12	Cinnamon Leaf Oil	Warm, spicy, somewhat harsh	Warm, spicy, clove-like	Warm, spicy
13	Cistus Oil	Powerful, warm, ambra-like*	Rich, warm, ambra, balsamic	Dry, balsamic
14	Clove Bud Oil	Fresh, spicy, warm, fruity	Warm, spicy, somewhat woody	Warm, spicy, woody
15	Clove Leaf Oil	Spicy, woody	Dry, woody, spicy	Clove-like
16	Clove Stem Oil	Spicy, of clove	Dry, woody, spicy	Clove-like
17	Coriander Oil	Light, peppery, woody, slightly floral	Woody, spicy, slightly floral	Warm, spicy, rather balsamic
18	Cypress Oil	Fresh, coniferous, camphoraceous	Coniferous, balsamic	Sweet, balsamic
19	*Eucalyptus citriodora* Oil	Fresh, rose-like, lemony	Rose-like, lemony	Nondescript
20	*Eucalyptus globulus* Oil	Powerful, camphoraceous	Warm, camphoraceous	Nondescript
21	Fennel Oil	Sweet, anisic, spicy	Anisic, somewhat spicy	Warm, aniseed-like
22	Frankincense Oil	*see* Olibanum Oil		
23	Frankincense Resinoid	*see* Olibanum Resinoid		
24	Galbanum Oil	Powerful, fresh, sharp, green, earthy, conifer	Green, conifer, balsamic, agrestic	Dry, earthy, spicy

Table 5.7 (contd.) — Essential oil odour profiles

	Name of product	Top notes	Body notes	Dryout
25	Galbanum Resinoid	Green-earthy, somewhat sharp	Green, conifer, balsamic	Aldehydic, agrestic,† floral
26	Geranium Oil	Vegetable, rosey, minty	Rose-like, minty, green	Rich, rose-like
27	Guaiacwood Oil	Soft, sweet, rose-like	Sweet, rose-like, woody, slightly smoky	Nondescript
28	Jasmin Absolute	Floral, fruity, green	Heavy floral, fruity, herbaceous, animalic	Floral, fatty, heavy, animalic
29	Juniper Berry Oil	Fresh, coniferous	Coniferous, woody	Sweet, warm, balsamic
30	Labdanum Resinoid	Little characteristic	Sweet, balsamic, herbaceous, ambra	Dry, woody, ambra
31	Lavandin Oil	Fresh, camphoraceous, herbaceous	Herbaceous, woody, lavender-like	Nondescript, warm
32	Lavender Absolute	Floral, typically lavender-like	Warm, herbaceous, lavender- and hay-like	Woody-spicy, somewhat pungent
33	Lavender Oil	Fresh, floral, slightly fruity	Herbaceous, floral, slightly woody	Nondescript
34	Lavender Spike Oil	Fresh, strongly camphoraceous	Camphoraceous, herbal, lavender-like, woody	Nondescript
35	Lemongrass Oil	Fresh, citrus, slightly oily	Strong, lemony, herbal, green, tea-like	Herbaceous, somewhat oily
36	Lemon Oil	Fresh, light, sharp, citrus	Sweet, fresh, citrus	Warm, nondescript
37	*Litsea cubeba* Oil	Fresh, lemon-like	Sweet, fresh, lemon-like	Lemony, sharp
38	Marjoram Oil	Fresh, camphoraceous, spicy	Warm, spicy, camphoraceous, woody	Warm, spicy, woody
39	*Mentha arvensis* Oil	Fresh, minty	Rather harsh, somewhat minty, woody	Dry, herbaceous
40	Myrrh Oil	Spicy, 'medicated'	Warm, spicy, balsamic	Nondescript
41	Myrrh Resinoid	Light, fresh, spicy	Warm, spicy, balsamic	Warm, spicy, balsamic
42	Neroli Oil	Light, fresh, floral	Light, floral, herbaceous, somewhat citrus	None
43	Oakmoss Absolute	Dry, somewhat 'seashore-like'	Mossy, woody, green, earthy, 'marine'	Warm, woody, balsamic
44	Olibanum Oil	Fresh, lemony, resinous	Resinous, spicy, woody	Balsamic, resinous
45	Olibanum Resinoid	Fresh, lemony, green, resinous	Resinous, balsamic	Little characteristic
46	Orris Oil	Floral, violet-like	Violet-like, woody, fatty	Nondescript
47	Patchouli Oil	Sweet, rich, herbaceous, balsamic	Sweet, earthy, slightly camphoraceous, spicy, woody, balsamic	Dry, woody, balsamic, spicy
48	Petitgrain Oil, Bigarade	Fresh, floral, similar to Neroli	Dry-floral, herbaceous, woody	Dry-herbaceous
49	Pimento Berry Oil	Fresh, sweet, warm, spicy	Sweet, spicy, balsamic, tea-like	Fresh, sweet, spicy

Table 5.7 (contd.) — Essential oil odour profiles

	Name of product	Top notes	Body notes	Dryout
50	Pine Oil, *sylvestris*	Fresh, sweet, coniferous	Coniferous, balsamic	Nondescript
51	Rose Absolute	Sweet, floral, with a beeswax note	Rich, sweet, spicy, waxy, floral	Warm, floral, honey-like
52	Rose Otto (Rose Oil)	Powerful, beeswax-like	Rich, waxy, floral, spicy (clove-like)	Warm, floral, spicy
53	Rosemary Oil	Fresh, strong, camphoraceous, resinous	Resinous, woody, herbaceous, balsamic	Dry, herbaceous
54	Rosewood Oil	Spicy, camphoraceous	Sweet, woody, floral-spicy	Woody-floral
55	Sage Oil, Clary	Sweet, light, herbaceous	Delicate, herbaceous, tobacco-like	Warm, balsamic
56	Sage Oil, Dalmatian	Sweet, fresh, herbal, camphoraceous	Fresh, strong, warm, camphoraceous, herbal	Little characteristic
57	Sandalwood Oil, East Indian	Little distinctive	Soft, sweet, woody, balsamic, fatty-floral	None distinctive
58	Sandalwood Oil, West Indian	*see* Amyris Oil		
59	Tarragon Oil (Estragon Oil)	Sweet, anisic, green	Sweet, aniseed-like, spicy	None distinctive
60	Thyme Oil	Sweet, warm, 'medicated', herbal	'Medicated', herbaceous, spicy, woody	Warm, herbaceous, spicy
61	Ti-Tree Oil	Strong, camphoraceous	Warm, camphoraceous, spicy	Little characteristic
62	Tonka Absolute	Rich, sweet, warm, herbaceous	Warm, sweet, hay-like	Hay-like, coconut-like
63	Tuberose Absolute	Sweet, heavy, floral	Sweet, heavy, floral, with a caramel note	Floral, balsamic
64	Vanilla Absolute	None distinctive	Rich, sweet, balsamic	None distinctive
65	Vetivert Oil	Sweet, earthy, woody	Rich, heavy, woody, earthy, balsamic	Woody, earthy
66	Violet Leaves Absolute	Green, diffusive	Green, floral, violet leaves	Woody, earthy, powdery
67	Ylang-Ylang Oil, 'Extra'	Strong, sweet, 'medicated', floral	'Medicated', floral, fruity, spicy (Clove)	Sweet, balsamic, floral, 'medicated'

* Resembling the odour of ambergris: musty with a note of the sea.

† An odour of the countryside.

Chapter 6

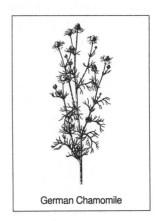

German Chamomile

Quality Control of Essential Oils

6.1 What is Quality Control?

Traditionally, the purpose of quality control has always been to make sure that substandard products do not reach the customer. While the perfection of products offered for sale remains today the ultimate goal of every quality control system, the means whereby this may be achieved, indeed the whole philosophy of quality control, has quite recently been revised, and a new concept, that of total quality management (TQM), introduced.

Before the introduction of TQM, a product, such as a hair shampoo for mass distribution, was designed, developed to satisfactory standards of performance, advertised, manufactured in bulk, filled, capped, labelled, packed and launched into the market. The operations involved were performed by automatic, semi-automatic or hand-operated machines, which were set to carry out their appointed tasks correctly by qualified and experienced persons while others, equally well qualified and experienced in their field of expertise, were concerned with inspection and testing, rejecting substandard units at various stages of manufacture. Whilst this universally-adopted type of system worked well enough, the only *control* of quality resided in the ability of the machine setters to set the machines correctly, in the care with which operatives performed their tasks and in the vigilance of the product inspectors. The machine operators would operate the machines until they were discovered to be producing too many rejects, where upon the machines would be re-set, the rejects consigned to oblivion and production resumed until the number of rejects again became unacceptable.

From time to time a product would reach the customer in a condition unfit for use as, for example, a pressurized shaving foam with a faulty valve. The intending user would then either find it impossible to get the product out or, alternatively, to close the valve once it opened, with results hardly conducive to repeat purchases.

The introduction of computerized control systems for production-line machinery considerably reduced the rate of product rejection, yet never brought the control of quality to the level of perfection achieved by manufacturers of hand-finished products, such as fine fragrances, where the financial return from sales was sufficient to support personal attention to every detail of manufacture. Here, in fact, we have the underlying principle of TQM; that every single individual within a company, no matter what his or her occupation might be, no longer simply carries out the appointed task, but completes it to agreed standards of quality. Thus everyone takes on responsibility for quality control. The system pays for itself from the increased return resulting from improved efficiency, and everyone takes enhanced pride in a job well done and known to have been well done.

In industry, the application of TQM to working and professional inter-relationships is rated as being of equal importance to production tasks and is obviously capable of being extended to services provided for clients or customers.

6.2 Quality Assurance

TQM represents a great advance in the direction of guaranteed product perfection, whether the product is a physical one or a service of some kind. This objective, however, like the absolute zero of temperature, can be approached but never quite reached. That this is so is evidenced by the continuing, though very much reduced, occurrence of faulty products and failures, even where TQM is most willingly and conscientiously practised. Imperfection is a characteristic of human affairs: we can strive only to reduce it to a minimum.

With TQM in force, the exercise of quality *control* at various strategic points in a sequence of manufacturing operations remains an essential safeguard against occasional, inevitable failure of some kind. The aim of TQM and quality control together is quality assurance — the assurance to customers or clients that everything has been done to maximize the compliance of a product or service with the standards of quality expected by the recipient.

Summarizing, quality control is embodied in the practice of total quality management, which comprises:

a) *critical vigilance by every person involved in the manufacture and distribution of a product or provision of a service, to eliminate error and substandard quality;*

b) *the application of physicochemical and sensory tests to evaluate the compliance of products with prescribed quality specifications.*

Thus, regarding products, b) acts as a check on the success of a) for purposes of quality assurance.

The results of quality control tests may be used as feedback to improve the performance of manufacturing processes, so reducing even further the probability of noncompliance of products with their specifications.

6.3 Nonanalytical Physical Tests

Nonanalytical physical tests give information on certain properties of essential oils, though not on their composition.

6.3.1 Appearance

The appearance of an essential oil is no criterion of good quality, but may forewarn of poor quality; it is best judged by observation of a sample in a small test-tube or bottle of colourless glass, in comparison with a standard sample of the same product. Colour, brilliance or transparency, and apparent viscosity are all important aspects of the appearance of an essential oil which should be noted and recorded.

Expressed citrus oils are always coloured, and show natural variations of colour originating from differences in the pigmentation of the outer rind of the fruit. A citrus oil which has been rendered bergaptene-free (or furanocoumarin-free) by vacuum distillation is, or should be, colourless.

Most distilled essential oils of high quality are transparent or only very slightly hazy; a definitely hazy, or cloudy, essential oil is always of questionable quality. Absolutes frequently present a hazy, translucent or even opaque appearance, which is usually caused by particles of poorly soluble, natural wax. Some very darkly coloured, solid absolutes, Hay Absolute, for example, appear to be opaque but may be transparent in very thin layers.

The term *viscosity* is used to refer to the 'thickness' of a liquid or, more scientifically, to its resistance to flow; it is commonly seen in such high viscosity liquids as glycerine and treacle. Water, conversely, is a mobile liquid; one of low viscosity. All expressed and most distilled essential oils used in aromatherapy are mobile liquids; only a few, such as Sandalwood, Vetivert and Amyris, being viscous. Guaiacwood Oil appears as a mass of soft crystals suspended in a brownish, oily liquid; the crystals are of guaiol, a major constituent of this oil. A few essential oils, Orris Oil, for example, are solid at ordinary room temperature. An indication of the viscosity of an essential oil may be obtained by simply moving the oil about in its container, if transparent. If a test sample of an essential oil appears more viscous than a standard sample of the same oil at the same temperature, the test sample is of questionable quality on grounds of the possible polymerization of its terpene content, which can occur under oxidizing conditions (e.g. exposure to the air).

Once a good, critical look has been taken at a sample of an essential oil, the next obvious test is to smell it. We have already discussed in some detail the importance of odour quality in relation to essential oils. Sensory evaluation of purchased essential oils is the only form of quality assessment normally available in the salon, and so it should, for the protection of clients and of the reputations of practitioners, be adopted as a matter of routine.[1]

6.3.2 Specific Gravity (s.g.)

The specific gravity[2] of a solid or liquid is a measure of how much heavier or lighter a given volume of the substance is than the same volume of pure water, measured at a standard temperature. Traditionally, the weighings are made on an analytical balance of high accuracy using, for liquids, a small glass bottle, which is weighed empty before a determination is made. The weight of the bottle is then subtracted from the weight of the bottle plus liquid and from the weight of the bottle plus water. If the liquid is an essential oil, then:

$$s.g. = \frac{\text{weight of a certain volume of essential oil}}{\text{weight of the same volume of water at the same temperature}}$$

Measurements of specific gravity are usually made at 20°C. Most essential oils are 'lighter' (less dense) than water, and have values for specific gravity of less than 1, but a few, for example, Clove oils, are 'heavier' and collect beneath the distillation water during preparation. Here are some examples:

Bergamot Oil	0·882 to 0·886
Clove Bud Oil	1·047 to 1·060
Lavender Oil	0·883 to 0·895
Lemongrass Oil	0·895 to 0·908
Rosemary Oil	0·900 to 0·919
Sandalwood Oil, East Indian	0·973 to 0·985

The specific gravity of an essential oil is, as the examples show, specified as lying within quite a narrow range, lower or higher than the limits of which a figure for specific gravity gives cause for concern and further investigation.

Specific gravity is today usually measured by means of an electronic specific gravity meter which gives the result and the temperature of the sample on a small, liquid crystal display screen. This saves much time and trouble.

---

1. Details of a suggested system of quality assessment for salon use appear in the booklet entitled *Lecture Notes on Essential Oils* (ISBN: 0 9514968 0 8) by the present author, and published in 1989 by Eve Taylor Ltd., 9 Papyrus Road, Werrington Business Park, Werrington, Peterborough PE4 5BH.

2. More correctly called *relative density* but the older term is still in common use.

6.3.3 Refractive Index (R.I.)

On lowering a knitting needle into a bowl of water (fig. 6.1) at an angle of about 60° to the horizontal, the needle appears to bend toward the surface as it enters the water and to unbend as it is withdrawn. This optical effect is called *refraction*, and is caused by a reduction of the speed of light when passing from a less dense medium (in this case air) into a denser medium (water). The refraction of a ray of light passing from air into a transparent liquid or solid medium is expressed numerically as the refractive index of the denser medium with respect to air as, for example, an essential oil:

$$\text{R.I.} = \frac{\text{Sine of the angle of incidence}}{\text{Sine of the angle of refraction}}$$

at a given temperature, both angles being measured at the point of incidence (fig. 6.2).

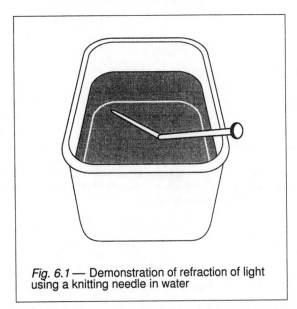

Fig. 6.1 — Demonstration of refraction of light using a knitting needle in water

As in the instance of specific gravity, a specification of refractive index is expressed as upper and lower limits between which, at the given temperature, the refractive index of the test sample should lie.

The property of the refraction of light by a substance can be very responsive to small changes of composition, and so in respect of an essential oil a value for refractive index which is greater or less than the limits of the specified range is regarded as an early warning of the possibility of poor quality, to the extent of adulteration.

Refractive index is measured by means of a refractometer, using a thin film of test sample mounted on a temperature-controlled stage similar to the stage of a microscope. A standard light source gives a visual field, viewed through one of two eyepieces, consisting of adjacent semicircles of coloured light. The field is adjusted by the opera-

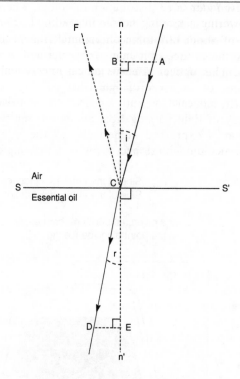

AC is a ray of light incident at *C* at the surface, *SS'*, of a sample of an essential oil, while *nn'* is a normal to the surface (a straight line at right angles to *SS'*). At the point of incidence, *C*, the incident ray, *AC*, is bent towards the normal. *CD* is the refracted ray. Because a liquid is always denser than the air above it, the angle of refraction, *r*, is always less than the angle of incidence, *i*. (*CF* is a weak, reflected ray.)

$$\text{R.I. of the essential oil} = \frac{\text{sine } i}{\text{sine } r} \; *$$

$$\text{sine } i = \frac{AB}{AC} \qquad \text{sine } r = \frac{DE}{DC}$$

$$\text{Hence R.I.} = \frac{AB/AC}{DE/DC} = \frac{AB}{AC} \times \frac{DC}{DE}$$

$$AB = 9 \text{ mm}, \; AC = 35 \text{ mm}, \; DE = 7 \text{ mm}, \; DC = 38 \text{ mm}$$

$$\text{R.I.} = \frac{9/35}{7/38} = \frac{9}{35} \times \frac{38}{7} \qquad = \underline{1.396 \text{ at } t°C}$$

where *t* = temperature of the determination

Fig. 6.2 — Principle of refractive index

---

*This is an expression of a relationship discovered by the Dutch physicist Willebrord Snell (1591-1626), and known as Snell's law:

For a given pair of media at constant temperature, the ratio of the sine of the angle of incidence to the sine of the angle of refraction is constant.

Thus if the angle of incidence is altered, the angle of refraction changes, keeping $\frac{\text{sine } i}{\text{sine } r}$ *constant.*

tor to show an even distribution of colour, whereupon the refractive index of the sample is obtained by reading a scale visible through the other eyepiece. Electronic refractometers give direct readings of refractive index, free from human observational error.

Examples of the refractive indices of essential oils are as follows:

Bergamot Oil	1·464 to 1·467
Clove Bud Oil	1·528 to 1·537
Lavender Oil	1·459 to 1·464
Lemongrass Oil	1·483 to 1·489
Rosemary Oil	1·464 to 1·476
Sandalwood Oil, East Indian	1·500 to 1·510

6.3.4 Optical Rotation

Light waves are analogous to the waves produced in a long length of rope, secured at one end, when the opposite end is moved energetically up and down; they are transverse waves, propagated in a plane perpendicular to the surface to which the rope is secured.

Ordinary white light is composed of transverse waves of different wavelengths, corresponding to the colours of a rainbow, together with invisible rays of shorter and longer wavelength: ultraviolet and infrared rays, respectively. The waves comprising rays of ordinary light move in all planes transverse to the direction of their propagation.

The yellow street lamps seen everywhere today give light which is produced by passing a current of electricity through the vapour of the metal sodium. Under the conditions used, certain electrons of the sodium atoms absorb enough energy to jump from their orbitals into outer orbitals one step further from the nucleus. There they remain for exceedingly brief intervals of time before falling back into their former orbitals, whereupon they each give out a pulse of light energy precisely equal to the quantity they absorbed, and to the difference between the electron energy levels involved. The combined effect of identical energy pulses produced by vast numbers of electrons in the same way is to produce the familiar, yellow 'sodium light', of wavelength 589 nm, which is the same as that given by a positive flame test for the presence of sodium in a substance under analysis. Light of this wavelength may also be produced by filtration from white light, using a yellow optical filter of the correct shade.

A filter of a different kind is that given by a Polaroid™ lens of the kind used for the manufacture of sunglasses of the same trade name. This material absorbs all rays of light passing through it excepting those travelling in one particular plane, called the plane of polarization. Rays emerging from such a filter are plane polarized, meaning that all of them travel in parallel planes. Plane-polarized light of the sodium wavelength is used to measure the optical rotation of essential oils.

To measure optical rotation, a horizontal glass tube, usually 10 cm in length, fitted with plane glass ends, is filled with the liquid under examination. The temperature of the tube and contents is adjusted to a level between 15 and 20°C and the tube is then placed horizontally in a polariscope, which is the instrument used for measuring optical rotation. A beam of plane-polarized light of sodium wavelength is passed through the liquid in the polariscope tube and is viewed at the opposite end through an eyepiece fitted with a second polarizing lens secured to a circular scale marked in angular degrees. The scale is rotated until the two halves of an illuminated field, as viewed through the eyepiece, are equally illuminated, whereupon a reading is taken from the scale.

If the liquid in the polariscope tube is, like water, optically inactive, the scale reading will be zero, and the zero reading of the instrument is, in fact, checked in this way and, if necessary, zeroed before a measurement is made. If the liquid is optically active, its effect on the plane-polarized light waves emerging from the first polarizing lens, the polarizer, is to twist them clockwise or anti-clockwise as they pass through it. Hence to obtain a uniformly illuminated viewing field, the second polarizing lens, the analyser, will have to be rotated by moving the circular scale to which it is attached. The angle of optical rotation is then obtained from the scale reading. The effect of optical activity on a beam of polarized light is shown in figure 6.3.

Liquids which rotate the plane of polarized to the right, i.e. clockwise, are said to be *dextrorotatory*, and the names of organic compounds of this nature are prefixed *d-* as, for example, *d*-limonene. Liquids which rotate the plane of polarized light to the left, i.e.anticlockwise, are *laevorotatory*; the names of laevorotatory compounds are prefixed *l-*, as in *l*-limonene. The explanation of optical activity throws light, so to speak, on the composition of essential oils.

Optical activity is usually caused by a particular feature of molecular structure in which an atom — commonly, though not exclusively, a carbon atom — is bonded to four different atoms or groups of atoms. In such a case there are two, and only two, possible arrangements of these atoms or groups. This is very easily illustrated by means of a model, in which a black sphere, representing a carbon atom, is bonded to spheres of four different colours (fig. 6.4). The carbon sphere then represents an *asymmetric carbon atom*, which is the centre of optical activity of any molecule in which it occurs. A second, similar model is now made, identical with the first. Note that these models have identical arrangements of atoms; they are superimposable. The positions of two of the coloured spheres in one of the models are now reversed, when it is found impossible to superimpose the two models. If one of the models is held in front of a mirror, its reflection is found to correspond with the other model. One of the two models is the mirror image of the other, which explains why they are nonsuperimposable, in the same way as right and left hands are, though similar to one another, nonsuperimposable.

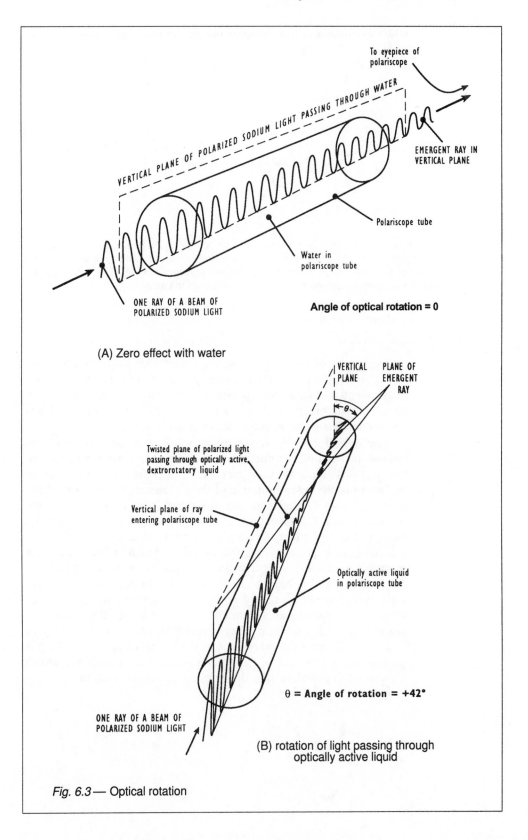

Fig. 6.3 — Optical rotation

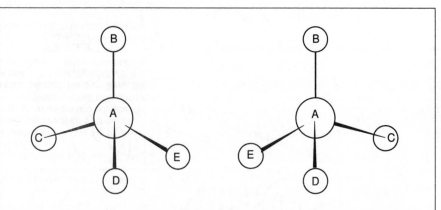

This diagram shows optical isomerism illustrated by means of a molecular model. A is a black plastic sphere representing an asymmetric carbon atom, to which are bonded four spheres of different colours representing different atoms or radicals. These molecules cannot be superimposed, one being the mirror image of the other.

Fig. 6.4 — Optically active molecules

Such pairs of molecules, and the compounds they comprise, are optical isomers or *stereoisomers*; they exhibit stereoisomerism, otherwise known as enantiomorphism (Greek: *enantio* — opposite; *morphos* — shape or form). Some examples of stereoisomers which occur as constituents of essential oils are shown in figure 6.5.

The optical rotation of an essential oil is a summation of the optical rotations of its constituents in relation to their proportions in the oil. Variations of these proportions therefore can give rise to variations of the optical rotation of the oil, bearing in mind the likelihood of 'cancelling' effects due, for example, to an increase in the proportion of a dextrorotatory constituent being balanced, optically, by an increase of a laevorotatory constituent. Measurement of optical rotation is an important aid to the detection of adulteration where, for example, a deficiency of a major, optically active constituent has been 'corrected' by the addition of the corresponding, non-stereospecific synthetic chemical. As normally synthesized in bulk, aroma chemicals containing an asymmetric carbon atom in their molecules are obtained as a mixture of stereoisomers, the optical activity of which is different from that of one of the isomers alone, and which is present in an essential oil. Adulteration of the oil with the aroma chemical will therefore alter the value of its optical rotation.

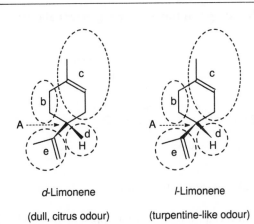

Stereoisomerism in a cyclic mono-terpene, limonene

A is the asymmetric carbon atom in this molecule, while *b, c* and *e* are three different radicals, and *d* a hydrogen atom, bonded to the asymmetric carbon atom, *A*. The molecule *d*-limonene is the mirror image of the *l*-limonene molecule.

Carefully note the difference in the orientation of the radicals *d* and *e* in relation to the plane of the ring.

d-Limonene

(dull, citrus odour)

l-Limonene

(turpentine-like odour)

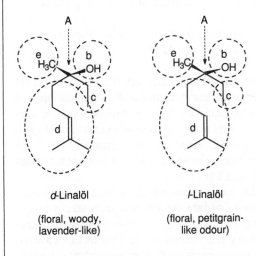

Stereoisomerism in an acyclic mono-terpenoid alcohol, linalöl

A is the asymmetric carbon atom giving rise to optical activity in linalöl, while *b, c, d* and *e* are four different radicals bonded to this atom. The molecule of *d*-linalöl is the mirror image of the *l*-linalöl molecule.

Carefully note the difference in the orientation of the radicals *b* and *e* in relation to *c* and *d*.

d-Linalöl

(floral, woody, lavender-like)

l-Linalöl

(floral, petitgrain-like odour)

Note that the conditions for optical activity in limonene are met, even though the two different radicals, *b* and *c*, are each bonded to the rest of the molecule at two points and not one.

Accompanying the difference of odour character between pairs of certain odorous stereoisomers are differences of odour strength, which in some instances extend to the limit of one of a pair being odorous while the other is odourless.

Study of the literature on stereoisomerism among *pure*, odorous organic compounds reveals in some instances wide differences of opinion on the odour character and strength of the same enantiomer, reminding us of the subjectivity inherent in odour evaluation and description.

The investigation of the odour properties of stereoisomers among constituents of essential oils throws much light on relationships between the odour profiles of the oils and their composition, and between the odours and molecular structures of individual constituents.

Fig. 6.5 — Examples of stereoisomeric constituents of essential oils

Here are some examples of optical rotation among essential oils:

Bergamot Oil	+12° to +24°
Clove Bud Oil	−0° 20′ to −2° 30′
Lavender Oil	−3° to −10°
Lemongrass Oil	−1° to +4°
Rosemary Oil	−5° to +10°
Sandalwood Oil, East Indian	−15° to −20°

6.4 Analytical Chemical Tests

Analytical tests are, basically, of two different kinds:

a) *qualitative*, giving information on *what* is present in a substance;
b) *quantitative*, giving information on *how much* of a constituent
   of a mixture, or element present in a compound, is present.

From the results of qualitative tests on an essential oil, the identity of
one or more of its different constituents may be ascertained after
separation from the oil.

Quantitative information on an essential oil with respect to its
content of single constituents is usually obtained by the technique of
gas–liquid chromatography, to which reference will be made in section 6.5. However, chemical tests also are used to evaluate quality in
respect of all constituents of a particular chemical class present in an
oil as, for example, the total percentage of esters, calculated as linalyl acetate, present in Lavender Oil.

For purposes of research into the composition of individual constituents of essential oils, those of interest are first separated by chromatography, then individually subjected to analysis by mass spectrometry, which also we shall discuss in the next section of this chapter.
From the results of mass spectrometry and other procedures the molecular structure of a constituent may be deduced. The constituent
may then be synthesized for investigation of its properties.

Analytical chemical tests are tests which involve chemical reactions for obtaining the required results; they were, not so long ago,
the only tests available for investigating the composition of essential
oils, either directly or following the separation of constituents by
vacuum fractionation. Analytical physical tests, to be discussed in
section 6.5, are tests in which chemical reactions are not involved for
the purposes of analysis. While not superseding chemical tests, they
have in recent years blossomed in terms of sensitivity and resolving
power to yield a bountiful harvest of analytical information of such
quantity, quality and detail as to be overwhelming were it not for the
data storage capacity of the modern computer. The problem for scientists working in the field of essential oil research is, as it is in medicine and other areas of applied science, how to make effective use of
the mass of continuously updated information which is now avail-

able, even in the more highly specialized regions of human endeavour.

Many analytical chemical tests were developed, along with the simple, physical tests we have outlined, in the nineteenth century. Although now largely automated and computerized for purposes of control and data storage, they remain today the same in principle and in the basic modes of their operation as they have done since they were first applied to industrial quality control many years ago. We can illustrate the kind of procedure involved in a quantitative chemical test by reference to the determination of how much free acid is present in an essential oil, and to the determination of the percentage of esters in an essential oil where these constituents are present in major and quality determining proportions.

6.4.1 Acid Value

With advancing age, the content of free acid in many essential oils tends to increase. This increase results mainly from the oxidation of aldehydes and hydrolysis of esters to form equivalent quantities of organic acids, the stronger of which can, as we have noted previously, catalyse the further hydrolysis of esters. Measurement of the acid content of an essential oil, expressed as its *acid value*, and comparison of the result with the acid value quoted as the maximum acceptable in the specification for the oil, gives an indication of the condition and age of the product and, by inference, its likely rate of deterioration — a guide to whether or not the oil is usable and, if usable, to approximately how long it can be stored under the correct conditions before use as a perfume or flavour ingredient of acceptable quality. In the absence of deterioration, the proportion of free acid to be found in most essential oils is very small. It is measured as the number of milligrams (thousandths of a gram) of an alkali, potassium hydroxide, required to neutralize the free acid in 1 gram of the oil.

To make the determination, 10 g (a quantity more conducive to an accurate result than 1 g) of the essential oil is dissolved in 50 ml of neutral alcohol (ethanol). 1 ml of a standard solution of phenolphthalein indicator is then added. Phenolphthalein is colourless in acid solutions, faintly pink in neutral solutions and bright pink in alkaline solutions, and hence can indicate whether a solution is acidic, neutral or alkaline in reaction. Indicators like phenolphthalein work only in aqueous solution; essential oils, however, are for most practical purposes insoluble in water — hence the use of alcohol, which is miscible with water, to dissolve the 10 g of essential oil. The presence of alcohol keeps the oil in solution when the standard solution to be used for the estimation, which is an aqueous solution, is added. With the alcoholic solution of the essential oil and indicator in a small flask, a solution of potassium hydroxide of known strength is carefully and very gradually added from a burette until the contents of the flask turn, and remain, faintly pink. This method of finding the strength of a solution is known as *titration*, and the point at which an indicator changes colour as the *end-point*.

The alkaline solution has now neutralized the free acid in the essential oil, and since the strength of this solution is known, the acid value of the oil may be easily calculated.

Strength of the potassium hydroxide solution[3] = 0·1 molar = 5·61 g/l
Suppose v ml of 0·1 molar KOH is required to neutralize the free acid in 10 g of essential oil:
1000 ml 0·1 molar potassium hydroxide solution contains 5·61 g KOH
∴ 1 ml of 0·1 molar potassium hydroxide solution contains 0·00561 g KOH = 5·61 mg KOH
∴ v ml of 0·1 molar potassium hydroxide solution contains (5·61 x v) mg KOH
10 g essential oil requires 5·61v mg KOH for neutralization of free acid
∴ 1 g essential oil requires 0·561v mg KOH for neutralization of free acid.

Hence the acid value of any essential oil is given as 0·561 × the volume of 0·1 molar KOH solution required to neutralize the free acid in 1 g.

6.4.2 Determination of Esters

Some essential oils, Lavender Oil, for example, are valued for their content of natural esters (linalyl acetate and other esters in the case of Lavender); an ester value lower than that prescribed in the specification is a certain indication of poor quality.

There are, unfortunately, no chemicals which will react completely and quickly with esters, as potassium hydroxide reacts with acids, and so to estimate the percentage of ester in an essential oil advantage is taken of the facts that a) water will hydrolyse esters to produce *equivalent* amounts of the free acids they yield to hydrolysis, and b) alkalies, such as potassium hydroxide, catalyse hydrolysis and immediately neutralize the resulting free acids.

For a determination, approximately 2 g of the essential oil is accurately weighed, and the free acid it contains is neutralized using the method for the determination of acid value, but without the need for a calculation at this stage. This procedure is necessary so that an error is not introduced by including any free acid already present with the acid produced by hydrolysis of the esters, which would give a high value for ester content and a false impression of the quality of the oil.

The neutralized essential oil is then boiled with 40 ml of 0·5 molar potassium hydroxide solution in a flask fitted with a vertical, water-cooled condenser, the purpose of which is to ensure that none of the essential oil is lost by evaporation during the process. Water

3. The chemical formula for potassium hydroxide is KOH. A molar solution contains 1 mole of a substance dissolved in sufficient solvent (e.g. water) to make 1 litre. A practical definition of 1 mole is a weight of a substance, expressed in grams, equal to its formula weight. Hence mol wt KOH = 39·1 + 16 + 1 = 56·1. A molar solution of potassium hydroxide therefore contains 56·1 g/l KOH, and a 0·1 molar solution 5·61 g/l KOH.

and essential oil vapour rise up the condenser tube, but condense to the respective liquids which run back into the flask beneath: a process called *reflux distillation*. Boiling of the pink liquid is continued for exactly one hour, during which the amount of potassium hydroxide present is proportionately reduced as the acids formed by the hydrolysis are neutralized by the alkali as fast as they are formed. The liquid in the flask is then rapidly cooled, and the residual alkali titrated with 0·5 molar sulphuric acid solution until the bright pink liquid turns pale pink at the end-point. From the volume of 0·5 molar sulphuric acid required to neutralize the excess potassium hydroxide remaining after hydrolysis of the esters, the percentage of esters in the essential oil is calculated. Notice that the 40 ml of potassium hydroxide solution used is very much in excess of the equivalent amounts of the acids that it will be required to neutralize.

This method for the determination of esters cannot distinguish between individual esters, and so the result is expressed with reference to the most important ester present in the oil. This does, of course, introduce errors into the results, but they are errors that are understood by purchasers, who in any case do not rely on analytical figures as the only criteria for the judgement of quality.

Methods that are similar in principle to those used to determine esters are employed for estimation of the percentages of alcohols, aldehydes and ketones in those essential oils containing constituents of these chemical families as important, quality-determining features of their composition, using appropriate reagents.

6.5 Analytical Physical Tests

Tests of this kind are designed to yield information on the nature and proportions of constituents of essential oils. They serve two alternative purposes, the second of which is made possible by the first:

a) separation of the constituents of essential oils, with an absolute minimum of alteration of the composition or molecular structure of individual constituents. In this category we include *gas–liquid chromatography* and other forms of chromatography used in the perfume and flavour industries;

b) elucidation of the molecular structure of individual, separated constituents of essential oils. Important techniques of this kind include *mass spectrometry* and *infrared spectrophotometry*.

6.5.1 Gas–Liquid Chromatography (GLC)

The term 'chromatography' is derived from the Greek words *khroma*, meaning colour, and *graphien*, to write, and referred originally to a technique invented by the Polish botanist, Tswett, in 1927, for separating the coloured constituents of plant pigments, such as chlorophyll.

As originally devised, the apparatus for chromatography was very simple, consisting of a vertical glass tube, plugged at the bottom with glass wool and packed with fine granules of aluminium oxide (called the *stationary phase*) moistened with a solvent, such as alcohol. This arrangement formed the chromatography column. A solution in alcohol (called the *moving phase*) of the pigment to be separated was poured onto the column, in which it slowly descended under gravitation, whereupon the pigments present separated as coloured bands down the column. Sufficient of the solvent was then carefully poured onto the column to transport the coloured bands in different positions down the column, and ultimately out of it at the bottom, a process known as elution. The emerging coloured solutions were collected in different receivers for further investigation.

This kind of procedure, known as *column chromatography*, depends on the property of aluminium oxide to attract molecules of plant pigments and retain them for periods of time which differ according to the composition and structure of their molecules; it involves adsorption ('sticking to') and desorption ('releasing from') of the molecules by the stationary phase. Chlorophyll, as obtained by extraction from grass or other leaves, is a mixture of three pigments: alpha- and beta- chlorophylls (both of similar molecular structure related to the haemoglobin of blood, but each containing a magnesium atom in place of iron) and carotene (related in molecular structure to beta-ionone). The two chlorophylls separate on the column as green bands, while the carotene forms a yellow band.

In GLC, mixtures of gases or vapours[4] are separated into their constituents by an ingenious development of Tswett's process invented in 1942 by Martin and Synge. In 1954 the latter inventors were jointly awarded a Nobel Prize for the invention and development of GLC, in recognition of their major contribution to the advancement of knowledge in the field of physical analysis.

The principle on which GLC depends is different from that of column chromatography using alumina (the old but still retained name for aluminium oxide), being one of partition rather than adsorption of the molecules to be separated. A description, with reference to figure 6.6, will make this clear.

In capillary GLC, which is the form of the technique now mainly used in the perfume industry for its sensitivity, separating power and reproducibility of results, the 'column' takes the form of a narrow silica tube of less than 1 mm. internal diameter and from 30 to 100 m in length. The column is wound into a coil on a former, and is coated on the inside with a very thin film of a nonvolatile substance, as the

---

4. The term *vapour* is normally used to refer to a substance in the gaseous state which exists under ordinary conditions as a liquid or solid. Menthol, for example, normally handled as a colourless, crystalline solid, exists in the dissolved condition in Peppermint Oil. When the oil evaporates, the vapour of menthol passes into the air along with the vapours of other constituents of the oil.

stationary phase, such as a specially prepared silicone polymer. To make an analysis, the column is secured within a temperature-regulated, thermostatically controlled oven, the temperature of which can be computer-programmed to increase, over a period of about 30 minutes, from room temperature to about 300°C. This is important in order to ensure that *all* constituents, from the most to the least volatile, will be vaporized, but not too quickly. A fan ensures an even distribution of heat within the oven, and hence over the entire length of the column, to make sure that once a sample of essential oil has been vaporized all of its constituents *remain* in the vapour state throughout the analysis.

One end of the column is attached to a metal block, the injection block, in which a fine hole leads from the exterior of the block to the beginning of the column. It is through this hole that one minute drop of an essential oil or other volatile material is injected for analysis. The purpose of the injection block is also to cause total evaporation of the sample as soon as it is injected. The block is therefore electrically heated beforehand to a temperature sufficiently high for this to occur, but without causing decomposition of any of its constituents. At the point of evaporation of the sample there is a connection to a cylinder of a gas, usually nitrogen, which is completely chemically inert towards the constituents of any mixture likely to be injected onto the column. This gas is known as the *carrier gas*; its purpose is to carry the vapour of the sample through the column. The carrier gas is the moving phase in GLC analysis.

At the opposite end of the column is a device, called the *detector*, which responds quantitatively to the presence of the truly minute amounts of the vapours of constituents separated by the column. One form of detector is constructed to cause the molecules of the minute amounts of separated constituent vapours flowing through it to decompose by passage through a small flame of burning hydrogen, forming ions. The hydrogen burns at a small metal jet, which is one of a pair of electrodes, the other taking the form of a small metal cylinder surrounding the flame. While no vapour is passing through the detector, the two electrodes are maintained at a high and constant potential difference. The ions formed in the flame, being electrically conducting, cause a small current to flow between the electrodes, which varies between one constituent vapour and another, according to the concentration of ions in the flame on each occasion. The variations in this current, once amplified, are converted into exactly proportional movements of a pen recorder, the pen of which is arranged to draw a line on a sheet of paper moving slowly, at constant speed, in a direction at right angles to its movement across the paper. Hence, as the vapour of each component passes through the detector, the pen draws a peak on the paper as a permanent record of its presence and proportion in the sample.

The electrical signals (changes of current) produced by the detector are fed also into a dedicated computer known as an *integrator*,

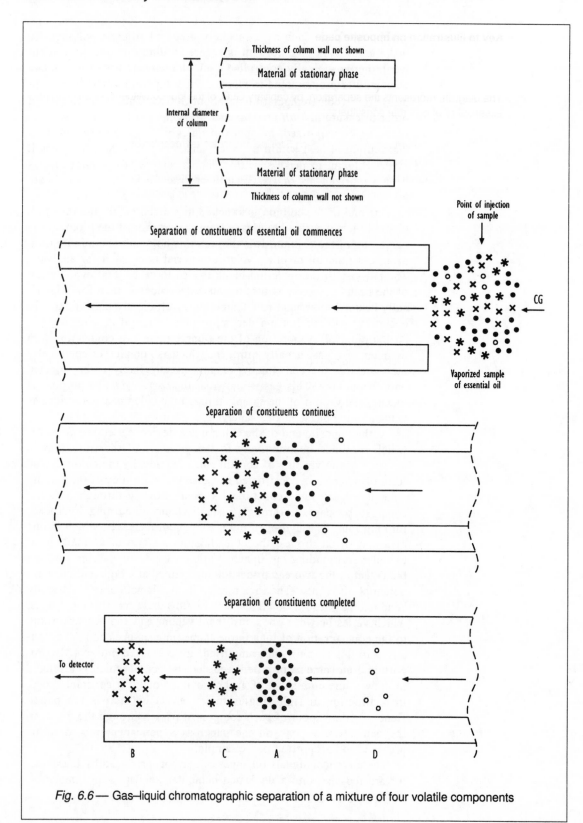

Fig. 6.6 — Gas–liquid chromatographic separation of a mixture of four volatile components

Key to illustration on opposite page

The diagram represents the separation, by capillary GLC, of the four constituents of an imaginary essential oil of only four constituents:

Constituent A:	each 5 trillion molecules represented by ×
Constituent B	each 5 trillion molecules represented by *
Constituent C:	each 5 trillion molecules represented by •
Constituent D:	each 5 trillion molecules represented by °
CG	= carrier gas (nitrogen)

Typical conditions

column length	50 m
column internal diameter	0·5 mm
stationary phase	silicone polymer (type specified)
stationary phase thickness	0·4 micrometre
injection block temperature	105°C
carrier gas	nitrogen
carrier gas rate of flow	0·6 ml/min
oven temp. programming	150° to 210°C at 5°C/min; 210° to 290°C at 3°/min; thereafter held at 290°C to complete elution.
detector	flame ionization (FID)

Readers may be interested in the calculation of the approximate number of molecules per microlitre of essential oil in the sample for GLC.

Assuming s.g. of essential oil	= 0·9
Weight of 0·1 microlitre of essential oil	= 0·1 × 0·9 = 0·09 microgram
	= 0·09 ÷ 1,000,000,000
	= 9×10^{-8} g

Let average molecular weight of constituents = 180

Then by Avogadro's law:

180 g essential oil contains 6×10^{23} molecules, approx.

∴ 1 g essential oil contains $6 \times \dfrac{10^{23}}{180}$ molecules, approx.

∴ 9×10^{-8} g essential oil contains $\dfrac{6 \times 10^{23} \times 9 \times 10^{-8}}{180}$

$$= \frac{54 \times 10^{15}}{180} = 0.3 \times 10^{15} = 3 \times 10^{14}$$

$$= 300,000,000,000,000$$

$$= 300 \text{ trillion, approx.}$$

which on completion of an analysis prints out sets of figures from which constituents of the sample may be identified and their true proportions calculated. For the results of different GLC analyses to be comparable, the column parameters (length, diameter, composition and thickness of the stationary phase, etc.) and conditions of temperature, temperature programming, nature and rate of flow of carrier gas, all have to be standardized and kept the same from one analysis to the next. In practice, the same column is used for very many, successive analyses and, since it is usual to keep a chromatograph working continuously, day and night, for as long as possible, fluctuations in its operating conditions must not be allowed to occur.

A GLC analysis begins with the automatic or manual injection of one accurately measured drop of less than 1 microlitre (one millionth of a litre) through a septum into the injection block of the chromatograph by means of a micro-syringe. The drop is immediately vaporized and the little puff of vapour moved into the column by the carrier gas. What then happens depends on the solubility of each of the constituents of the sample in the material of the stationary phase. The picture we should try to imagine is one in which countless hordes of molecules of the vaporized sample are ceaselessly diving into and shooting out of the stationary phase as they move along the column; smaller, lighter molecules at relatively higher speed and larger, heavier ones more sluggishly. As the sample is propelled along the column, molecules of high solubility in the stationary phase spend much of their time in this phase, and so tend to be left behind, while those of lesser solubility career onward in the carrier gas, remaining in the stationary phase for only short periods of time.

The end result of all this molecular activity is separation of the constituents of the sample in the order of the time that their molecules are resident in the stationary phase, those spending least time in that phase reaching the detector first. The degree of separation achieved during a GLC analysis depends on differences in solubility among the constituents of a mixture separated; differences which are in some cases very small indeed or even zero. The separation of constituents is, however, dependent also on their volatilities, and so two constituents of equal solubility in the stationary phase may, in fact, be separated on the column.

To summarize, the first, almost infinitesimally small, amounts of vapour to reach the detector are those of the least soluble, most volatile constituents of the sample. They are followed by constituents of increasing solubility and decreasing volatility during the course of the analysis, which takes about half an hour to complete under temperature-programmed conditions. The graph produced by the pen recorder consists of a series of peaks the heights of which are approximately proportional to the amounts of the respective constituents in the sample. This graph is known as a *chromatogram* or *GLC trace*. Examples of chromatograms where constituents corresponding to certain of the peaks have been identified appear in figures 6.7 to 6.16.

The area enclosed by the sides of a peak and an extension of the base line (zero response of the detector) forms, almost exactly under ideal conditions, an isosceles triangle, the area of which is approximately proportional to the amount by weight of that constituent in the mixture analysed; that is:

$$\frac{\text{area under a peak, } a}{\text{total area of all peaks, } A} = \frac{\text{weight of constituent, } w}{\text{total weight of all constituents, } W}$$

$$\therefore \quad w = \frac{Wa}{A}$$

$$\text{and \% of constituent} = \frac{Wa}{A} \times 100$$

This is the calculation completed by the integrator in respect of all constituents recorded at the end of an analysis.

There is, however, a snag, which is that the response of the detector is not uniform among constituents of different chemical constitution: it responds almost ideally to some, less perfectly to others. The percentage of each constituent, as calculated and recorded by the integrator, has therefore to be multiplied by a correction factor, obtained by analysis of mixtures of pure constituents of known composition. Modern instruments can be programmed to perform these calculations automatically.

Poor separation of two or more constituents results in overlapping peaks ('shoulders') or even peaks within peaks. Constituents remaining closely associated during analysis may, if necessary, be separated by repeating the analysis under different conditions.

Neither a chromatograph nor the integrator to which it is connected can identify the constituents revealed on completion of an analysis. For this purpose recourse is made to the measurement of retention times of the constituents, which are the times taken from injection of the sample to maximum response of the detector (from the start of the analysis along the chromatogram base line to the middle of a peak, beneath the apex).

As we have noted, the injection block temperature must be high enough to cause 'flash evaporation' of all constituents of a sample to be analysed. At the temperature required, molecules of one or more of the constituents may be caused to vibrate so violently as to suffer partial breakup of their structures; that is, those constituents will begin to decompose, and furthermore the products of their decomposition will be revealed as peaks on the chromatogram — the peaks of artefacts, having nothing to do with the true composition of the sample. Chromatograms of essential oils and other delicate products, such as perfumes, therefore need skillful and experienced interpretation to be of value in quality control or research of a scientific or perfumistic nature.

For purposes of the routine evaluation of deliveries of essential oils arriving at a perfume or flavour company, chromatograms of representative samples are carefully compared with those of corresponding, standard samples which are of known composition and which conform in each case to the quality required. This is done by aligning the traces, one above the other, on evenly illuminated, translucent screens, making any differences clearly visible. Ideally, no differences should be found; however, due allowance has to be made for natural variations of quality resulting from differences in the growing and processing conditions of the source materials which, as we have noted, give rise to differences of composition of an essential oil. Good correspondence with the standard is shown by identity of peak positions and close approximation of the heights of major and minor constituents, also quality-determining trace constituents. The absence of peaks which should be present, and the presence of peaks which should be absent, are both indicative of doubtful quality. For confirmation of the picture presented by the chromatogram of an essential oil, reference is made to the integrator print-out, on which the peak to which each of the sets of figures corresponds is identified by a serial number and the retention time of the vapour constituent on the column. Some examples of typical chromatograms of essential oils are given on pages 152 to 171.

Table 6.1 — List of chromatograms (pages 152–171)

Chromatogram number	Page number	Figure	Chromatogram title
1	152–3	6.7	Bergamot Oil
2	154–5	6.8	Clove Bud Oil
3	156–7	6.9	Geranium Oil, Chinese
4	158–9	6.10	Lavender Oil
5	160–1	6.11	Lemon Oil
6	162–3	6.12	Lemon Oil, oxidized
7	164–5	6.13	Lemongrass Oil
8	166–7	6.14	Rosemary Oil
9	168–9	6.15	Ti-Tree Oil
10	170–1	6.16	Ylang-Ylang Oil, Extra

Chromatograms of Essential Oils

1. On the following chromatograms of essential oils the units of the vertical scale are millivolts (mV), thousandths of a volt, measuring the nett electrical potential difference (p.d.) resulting from the passage of the vapours of individual constituents through the detector. These p.d.'s, after amplification, cause the pen of the pen recorder to move across the paper (itself moving slowly at right angles to the movements of the pen), in proportion to the responses of the detector.

2. The full heights of the largest peaks cannot be shown because they rise further than the width of the paper. These peaks are therefore cut off by the integrator (*see* paragraph 4) at a maximum convenient height. The integrator, however, records their true areas.

3. The units of the horizontal scale are minutes from the start of the analysis, and looking along this scale it is immediately seen that the procedure is very time-consuming, which is its main disadvantage. For this reason the modern chromatograph is fully automated, to run 24 hours a day for as long as reproducible results are obtained. The column then has to be changed for a fresh one and the instrument reset to run under the required standardized conditions. It is then tested for accuracy and reliability using a mixture of pure volatiles of known composition before returning to service. The time at which the middle of a peak appears on a chromatogram is the *retention time* of the corresponding constituent.

4. The figures associated with individual peaks are the areas of the peaks as percentages of the total area of all of them, including peaks of less than 0·01 per cent, the areas of which have not been recorded by the instrument. These figures are calculated by a special computor known as an *integrator*, which works in conjunction with the detector and the pen recorder. If necessary, the sensitivity of the chromatograph can be increased to register accurately and record peaks of the trace constituents of the sample which, as we have noted, can be of great importance in the assessment of the quality of an essential oil.

5. The relative areas of the peaks are not precisely proportional to the percentages of the corresponding constituents in the sample of essential oil, because the detector does not respond uniformly to constituents of different chemical composition and molecular structure. To find the actual percentage of a given constituent, the figure for 'area per cent' has to be multiplied by the *response factor* for that substance. Response factors are obtained from tables prepared from the results of GLC analysis of samples of known constitution under standardized conditions, or the necessary corrections are applied automatically, by a specially programmed computer.

6. Capillary GLC gives very good separation of the peaks corresponding to individual constituents of a sample, but it is not perfect in this respect. Careful examination of one ot the charts of the following series will reveal 'shoulders' on some of the peaks, which result from only partial separation of adjacent peaks. This indicates only partial separation of the corresponding constituents under the particular conditions of the analysis; this may or may not be a disadvantage. Also, if two or more constituents pass through the detector at the same time, they will be recorded as a single peak. If necessary, problems of separation can be solved by replacing the column by one containing a stationary phase of different composition.

7. Peaks identified by name are those of examples of some of the most important constituents, brief comments on which appear in the associated notes.

8. In general, but with exceptions, the order of the peaks from left to right corresponds to decreasing volatility of the corresponding constituents. Thus we find monoterpenes and oxygenates of higher volatility to the left, sesquiterpenes and oxygenates of intermediate volatility in the middle of the chromatogram and all constituents of lower and very low volatility to the right.

9. For clear presentation, each of the chromatograms has been divided to appear on two successive pages, where the point of division is shown by the symbol ↓.

10. Each chromatogram carries a label or 'patch' which contains a sample of the corresponding essential oil, in microencapsulated form. To smell the oil, simply scratch the patch lightly and take a gentle sniff.

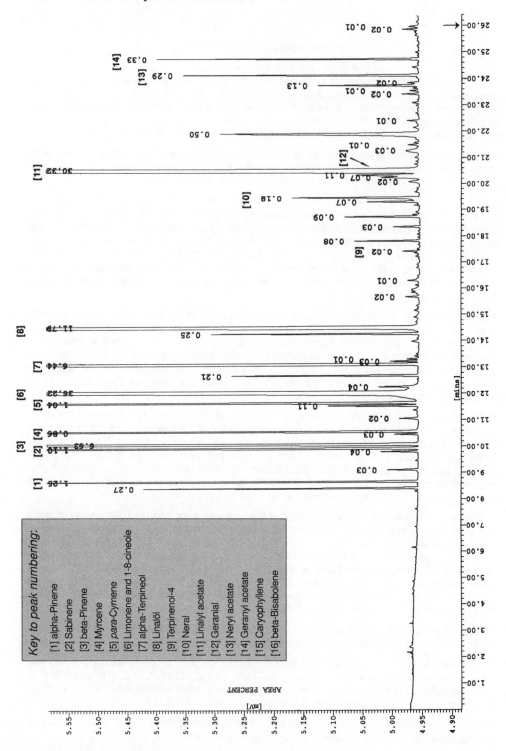

Key to peak numbering:

[1] alpha-Pinene
[2] Sabinene
[3] beta-Pinene
[4] Myrcene
[5] para-Cymene
[6] Limonene and 1-8-cineole
[7] alpha-Terpineol
[8] Linalöl
[9] Terpinenol-4
[10] Neral
[11] Linalyl acetate
[12] Geranial
[13] Neryl acetate
[14] Geranyl acetate
[15] Caryophyllene
[16] beta-Bisabolene

Fig. 6.7 — Chromatogram 1: **Bergamot Oil**

Fig. 6.7 (contd.) — Chromatogram 1: **Bergamot Oil**

Bergamot Oil, like the other citrus oils, is very prone to oxidation. On exposure to air the oil absorbs oxygen by combination with some of the terpenes it contains, the most important of which in this respect are the alpha- and beta-pinenes, sabinene, myrcene and *d*-limonene. Limonene, for example, is oxidized to several limonene oxirides, this chemical reaction, together with others, being the main cause of deterioration of the oil. *d*-Limonene and its oxidation products are indicated on the chromatograms of Lemon Oil (p. 160-1) and oxidized Lemon Oil (p. 162-3). Notice that peaks representing the same constituents appear in the same positions on both chromatograms; this results from both charts having been prepared by analysis of the oils under identical conditions. Notice also the 'shoulders' at the base of the limonene peak on the chromatogram of Bergamot Oil, showing poor separation of some minor and trace constituents having similar retention times under the conditions of analysis. This is a feature of all chromatograms of essential oils, no matter what may be the conditions of analysis.

Regarding other identified constituents, *para*-cymene is not a terpene, but a benzenoid hydrocarbon of citrusy odour as it occurs in nature.

1,8-Cineole is a cyclic ether having an odour of eucalyptus, which occurs in *Eucalyptus globulus* Oil as the main odorous constituent. In the chromatogram it occurs coincidentally with limonene, but is present in Bergamot Oil in only a very small proportion. Cineole, known also as eucalyptol, contributes to the freshness of the odour of Bergamot Oil.

The alcohols alpha-terpineol and linalöl impart mild floral notes and the esters give further florality and a touch of fruitiness to the oil, while terpinenol-4 and the sesquiterpene beta-bisabolene contribute peppery and spicy-balsamic notes which persist almost to the dry-out.

The top note of Bergamot Oil is freshly and sharply citrus in character, for which the citrals neral and geranial, the latter having the same retention time as linalyl acetate, are responsible. Linalyl acetate and linalöl together provide the "lavender-like" body notes of the oil (so far as it can be said to possess body notes) while caryophyllene, the main sesquiterpene of the clove oils, gives a touch of warm, spicy woodiness.

SCRATCH AND SNIFF

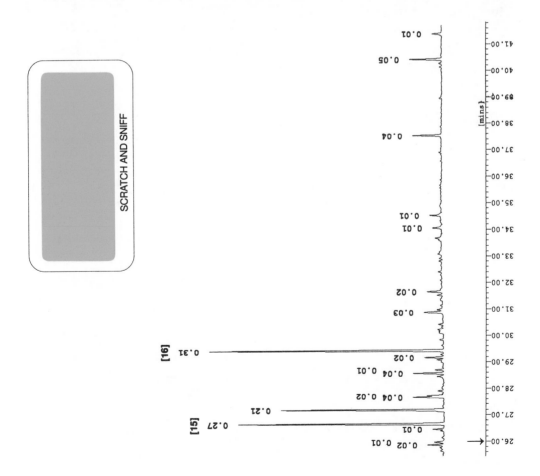

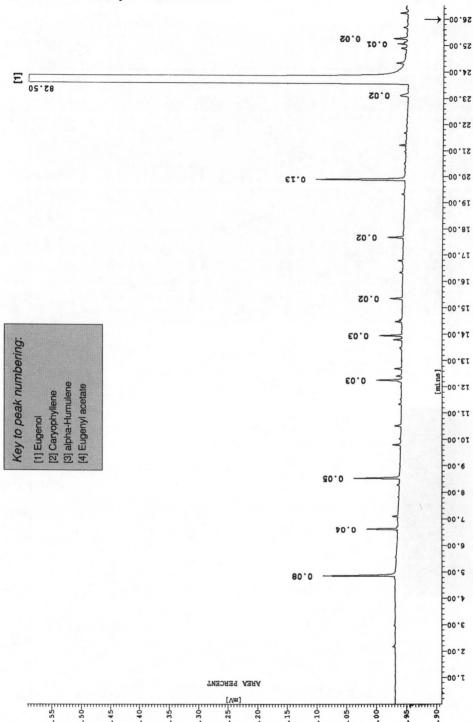

Key to peak numbering:

[1] Eugenol
[2] Caryophyllene
[3] alpha-Humulene
[4] Eugenyl acetate

Fig. 6.8— Chromatogram 2: **Clove Bud Oil**

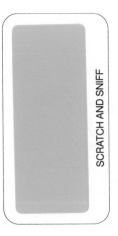

SCRATCH AND SNIFF

Fig. 6.8 (contd.) — Chromatogram 2: **Clove Bud Oil**

The two principal odour-characterizing constituents of Clove Bud Oil are the phenol eugenol, having a warm, spicy and somewhat carnation-like odour typical of sun-dried clove buds, and the sesquiterpene caryo-phyllene, contributing woody and somewhat spicy notes.

alpha-Humulene, an isomer of caryophyllene and possessing a similar, woody–spicy odour, is found also in Hop Oil.

Eugenyl acetate, known also as acetyl eugenol (or acet-eugenol), a crys-talline substance, possessing a sweet, floral, and fruity-balsamic odour, enhances the 'carnation' impression of Clove Bud Oil, especially if the oil is sufficiently diluted with an odourless solvent.

The richness and warmth of the odour of Clove Bud Oil are absent from a correctly proportionate mixture of its major constituents and so these valuable odour effects must be produced by certain of its minor and trace components.

Clove Bud Oil will keep extremely well if properly stored, for the reason that its content of monoterpenes is negligible. In common with other phe-nols, however, eugenol darkens on exposure to air (oxidation) and so do essential oils containing it. This darkening is enormously accelerated in the presence of alkali.

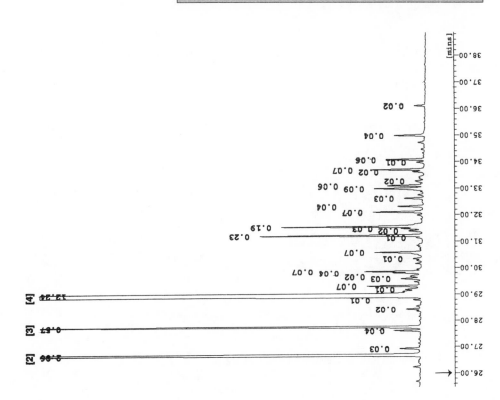

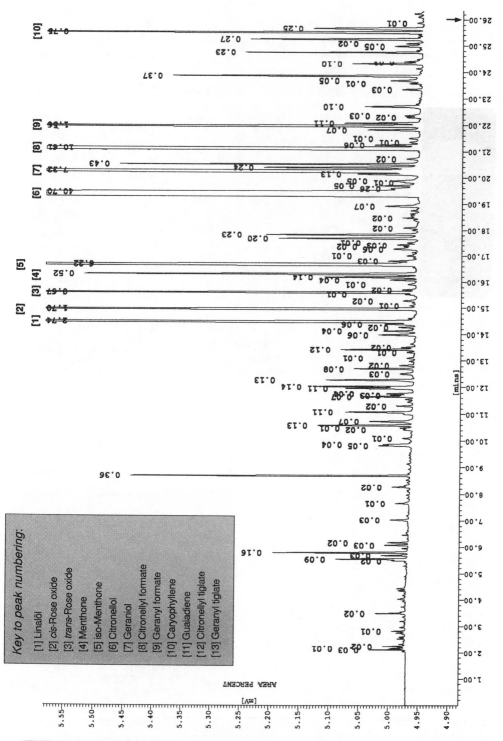

Fig. 6.9— Chromatogram 3: **Geranium Oil, Chinese**

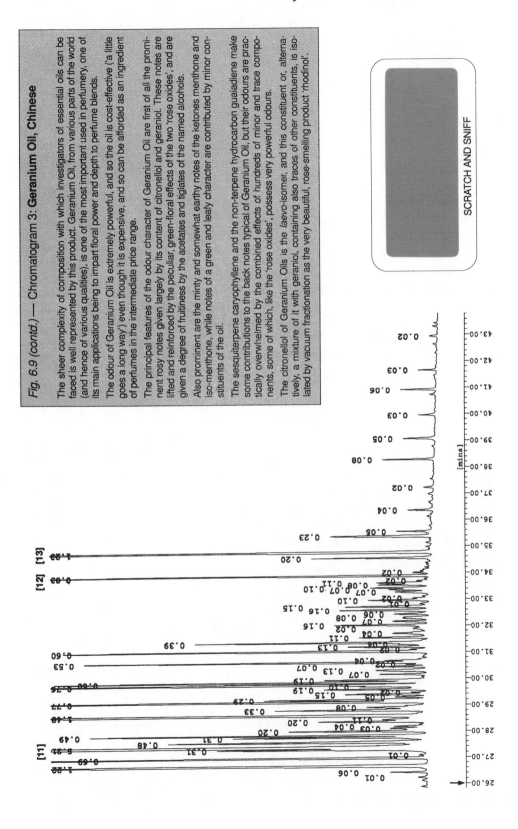

Fig. 6.9 (contd.) — Chromatogram 3: **Geranium Oil, Chinese**

The sheer complexity of composition with which investigators of essential oils can be faced is well represented by this product. Geranium Oil, from various parts of the world (and hence of various qualities), is one of the most important used in perfumery, one of its main applications being to impart floral power and depth to perfume blends.

The odour of Geranium Oil is extremely powerful, and so the oil is cost-effective ('a little goes a long way') even though it is expensive, and so can be afforded as an ingredient of perfumes in the intermediate price range.

The principal features of the odour character of Geranium Oil are first of all the prominent rosy notes given largely by its content of citronellol and geraniol. These notes are lifted and reinforced by the peculiar, green-floral effects of the two 'rose oxides', and are given a degree of fruitiness by the acetates and tiglates of the named alcohols.

Also prominent are the minty and somewhat earthy notes of the ketones menthone and iso-menthone, while notes of a green and leafy character are contributed by minor constituents of the oil.

The sesquiterpene caryophyllene and the non-terpene hydrocarbon guaiadiene make some contributions to the back notes typical of Geranium Oil, but their odours are practically overwhelmed by the combined effects of hundreds of minor and trace components, some of which, like the 'rose oxides', possess very powerful odours.

The citronellol of Geranium Oils is the *laevo*-isomer, and this constituent or, alternatively, a mixture of it with geraniol, containing also traces of other constituents, is isolated by vacuum fractionation as the very beautiful, rose-smelling product 'rhodinol'.

SCRATCH AND SNIFF

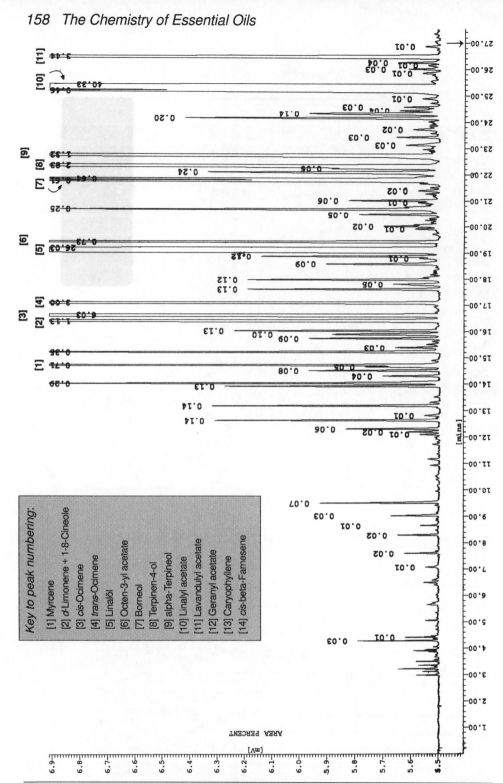

Key to peak numbering:

[1] Myrcene
[2] *d*-Limonene + 1-8-Cineole
[3] *cis*-Ocimene
[4] *trans*-Ocimene
[5] Linalöl
[6] Octen-3-yl acetate
[7] Borneol
[8] Terpinen-4-ol
[9] alpha-Terpineol
[10] Linalyl acetate
[11] Lavandulyl acetate
[12] Geranyl acetate
[13] Caryophyllene
[14] *cis*-beta-Farnesene

Fig. 6.10— Chromatogram 4: **Lavender Oil**

Fig. 6.10 (contd.) — Chromatogram 4: **Lavender Oil**

Lavender is a further example of a complex essential oil of great importance to perfumery. Its high monoterpene content, consisting largely of myrcene, *d*-limonene and the two isomers of ocimene, renders this oil susceptible to oxidation, and so cool storage in tightly sealed containers is an absolute necessity.

Notice that the *d*-limonene peak occurs in the same position on the chromatogram as the peak of 1,8-cineole, which contributes a very moderate, camphoraceous freshness to the odour of the oil. The terpene alcohol borneol also possesses a camphoraceous odour, but of a somewhat 'sweaty' kind. Lavandin Oil is more camphoraceous than either French or English lavender, while Spike Lavender Oil is strongly camphoraceous.

The floral-herbaceous character of the odour of Lavender Oil is based on the major constituents linalöl and linalyl acetate, to which association the ester lavandulyl acetate lends slightly spicy warmth and a degree of fruitiness.

Together with linalöl, floral elements of Lavender Oil include lilac-smelling alpha-terpineol and rosy geranyl acetate, while an additional touch of spiciness is imparted by terpinenol-4 and caryophyllene. *cis*-beta-Farnesene, along with other sesquiterpenes, contributes lingering sweetness and warmth to the latter stages of the evaporation of Lavender Oil.

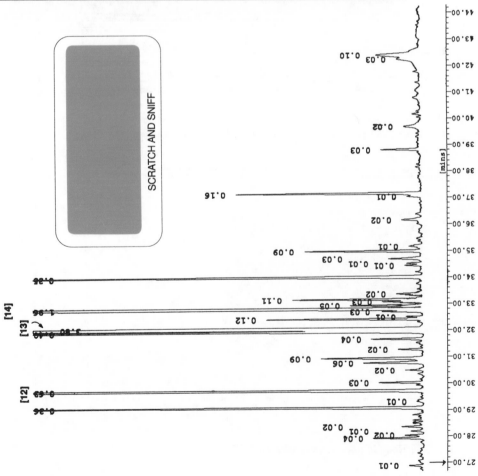

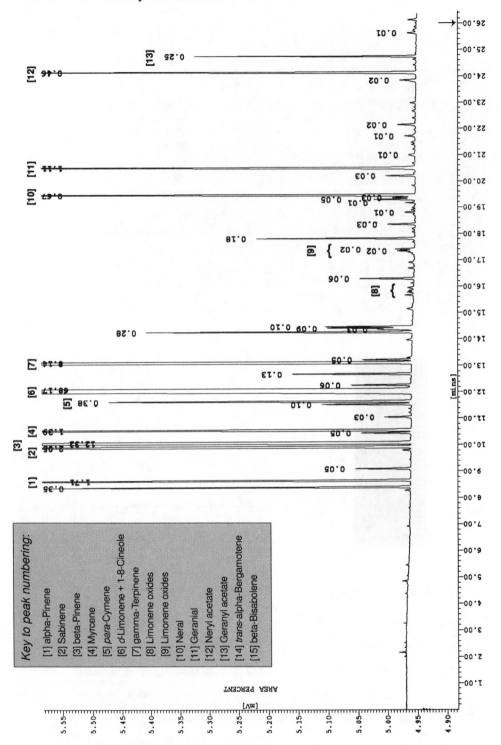

Key to peak numbering:

[1] alpha-Pinene
[2] Sabinene
[3] beta-Pinene
[4] Myrcene
[5] para-Cymene
[6] d-Limonene + 1-8-Cineole
[7] gamma-Terpinene
[8] Limonene oxides
[9] Limonene oxides
[10] Neral
[11] Geranial
[12] Neryl acetate
[13] Geranyl acetate
[14] trans-alpha-Bergamotene
[15] beta-Bisabolene

Fig. 6.11 — Chromatogram 5: **Lemon Oil**

Fig. 6.11 (contd.) — Chromatogram 5: **Lemon Oil**

Lemon Oil is characterized in odour by the combined and very similar odours of the two citrals, neral and geranial, which are given impact and sharpness by the fatty aldehydes C_8 (octanal) and C_9 (nonanal), together with other minor and trace constituents. Chemically, the oil is notable for the very high proportion of *d*-limonene it contains, which is accompanied by the other monoterpenes alpha- and beta-pinenes, sabinene, myrcene and gamma-terpinene. Being readily susceptible to oxidation, these terpenes, together with the fatty aldehydes present, render Lemon Oil capable of rapid deterioration if it is not stored in a cool room or refrigerator, under a minimum headspace of air.

Because it is impractable to express Lemon Oil, and indeed the other citrus oils, from the peel of the fruit in an inert atmosphere (of nitrogen, for example) it inevitably suffers some amount of oxidation, as shown by the peaks corresponding to the limonene oxides in this chromatogram [*see also* Chromatogram 6].

Again we find 1,8-cineole occurring coincidentally with *d*-limonene, but this ether is present in Lemon Oil at such a low level of concentration that any contribution it might make to the freshness of the oil is overwhelmed by the strong odours of the citrals.

The isomers neryl acetate and geranyl acetate have mild, rosy and somewhat fruity odours, but in the small proportions in which these esters occur in Lemon Oil their effects are minimal.

The two sesquiterpenes *trans*-alpha-bergamotene and beta-bisabolene contribute soft, warm and balsamic and mildly spicy notes to the near dryout stage of the evaporation of Lemon Oil.

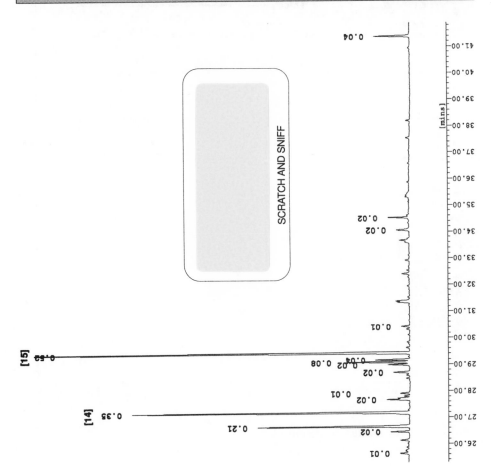

SCRATCH AND SNIFF

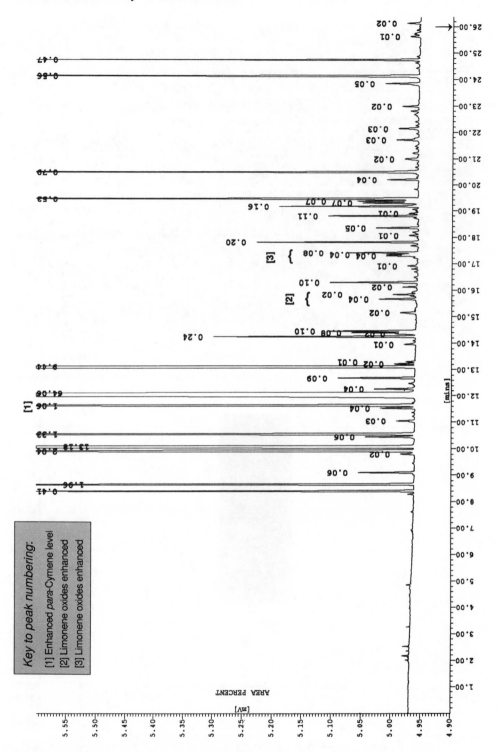

Key to peak numbering:

[1] Enhanced para-Cymene level
[2] Limonene oxides enhanced
[3] Limonene oxides enhanced

Fig. 6.12 — Chromatogram 6: **Lemon Oil, Oxidized**

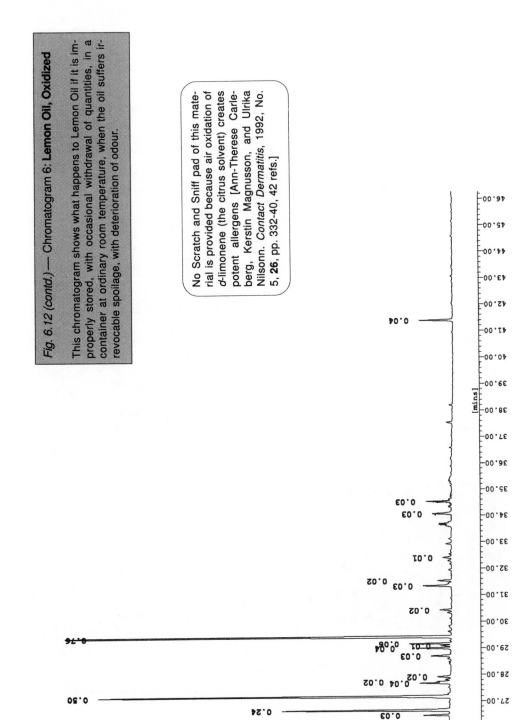

Fig. 6.12 (contd.) — Chromatogram 6: **Lemon Oil, Oxidized**

This chromatogram shows what happens to Lemon Oil if it is improperly stored, with occasional withdrawal of quantities, in a container at ordinary room temperature, when the oil suffers irrevocable spoilage, with deterioration of odour.

No Scratch and Sniff pad of this material is provided because air oxidation of d-limonene (the citrus solvent) creates potent allergens [Ann-Therese Carleberg, Kerstin Magnusson, and Ulrika Nilsonn. *Contact Dermatitis*, 1992, No. 5, **26**, pp. 332-40, 42 refs.]

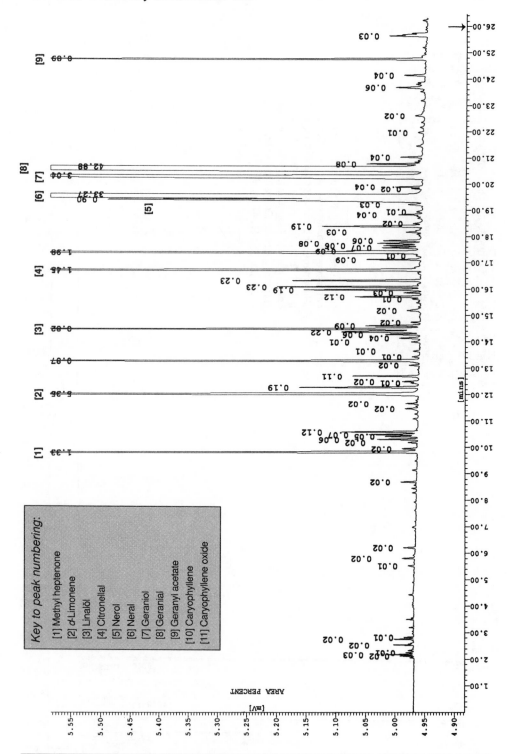

Key to peak numbering:

[1] Methyl heptenone
[2] *d*-Limonene
[3] Linalol
[4] Citronellal
[5] Nerol
[6] Neral
[7] Geraniol
[8] Geranial
[9] Geranyl acetate
[10] Caryophyllene
[11] Caryophyllene oxide

Fig. 6.13 — Chromatogram 7: **Lemongrass Oil**

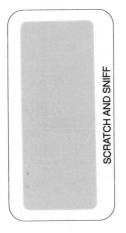

SCRATCH AND SNIFF

Fig. 6.13 (contd.) — Chromatogram 7: **Lemongrass Oil**

In this strongly lemon-smelling essential oil it is not surprising to find a high proportion of citral, in the form of a mixture of neral and geranial. These isomers dominate the odour profile of Lemongrass Oil, but not to completely overwhelm the green, fruity and somewhat oily notes of the ketone methyl heptenone which appear in the top note. The monoterpene content of Lemongrass Oil is small, and the citrals which are present in the oil, are not readily oxidized by atmospheric oxygen, and so the oil keeps well in a tightly closed vessel at ordinary room temperature. It will, however, darken quite rapidly if exposed to light.

Of the other notable constituents of Lemongrass Oil, citronellal adds a rosy-citrus touch to the effect of the citrals, while linalöl and nerol, also geraniol and its acetate, soften to some extent the coarseness of its general odour impression.

Caryophyllene, together with the small proportion of caryo-phyllene oxide present, imparts a perceptibly woody and slightly spicy, tea-like warmth to the odour of Lemongrass Oil in the later stages of its evaporation.

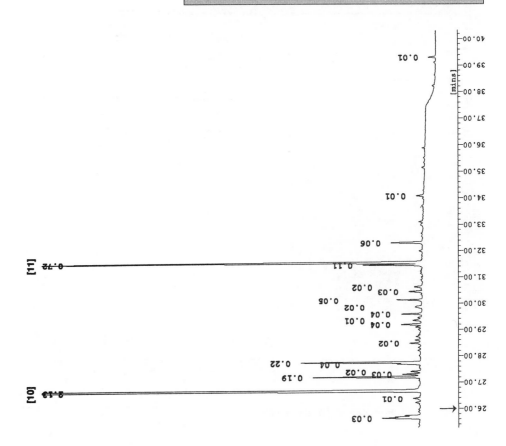

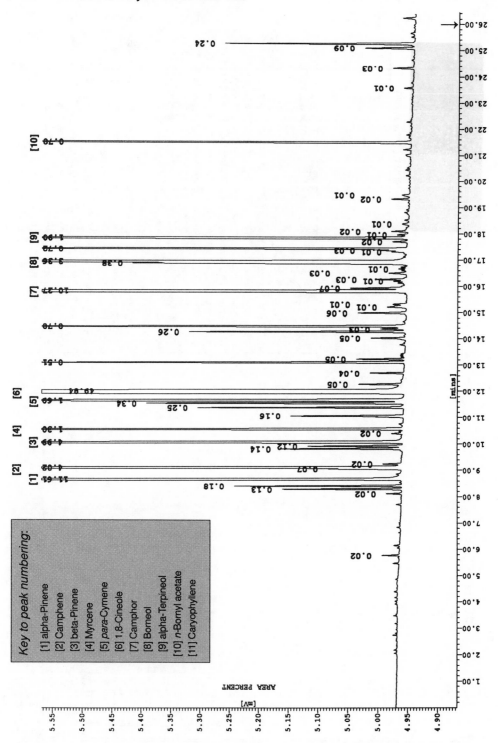

Fig. 6.14 — Chromatogram 8: **Rosemary Oil**

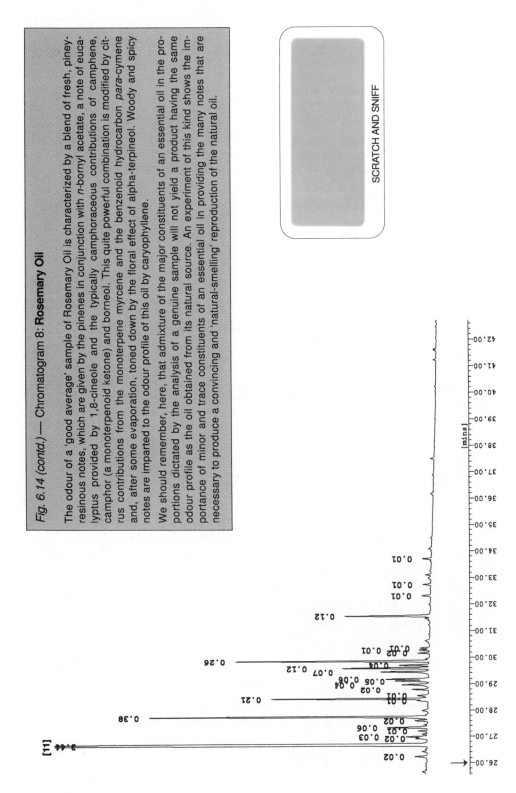

Fig. 6.14 (contd.) — Chromatogram 8: **Rosemary Oil**

The odour of a 'good average' sample of Rosemary Oil is characterized by a blend of fresh, piney-resinous notes, which are given by the pinenes in conjunction with *n*-bornyl acetate, a note of euca-lyptus provided by 1,8-cineole and the typically camphoraceous contributions of camphene, camphor (a monoterpenoid ketone) and borneol. This quite powerful combination is modified by cit-rus contributions from the monoterpene myrcene and the benzenoid hydrocarbon *para*-cymene and, after some evaporation, toned down by the floral effect of alpha-terpineol. Woody and spicy notes are imparted to the odour profile of this oil by caryophyllene.

We should remember, here, that admixture of the major constituents of an essential oil in the pro-portions dictated by the analysis of a genuine sample will not yield a product having the same odour profile as the oil obtained from its natural source. An experiment of this kind shows the im-portance of minor and trace constituents of an essential oil in providing the many notes that are necessary to produce a convincing and 'natural-smelling' reproduction of the natural oil.

SCRATCH AND SNIFF

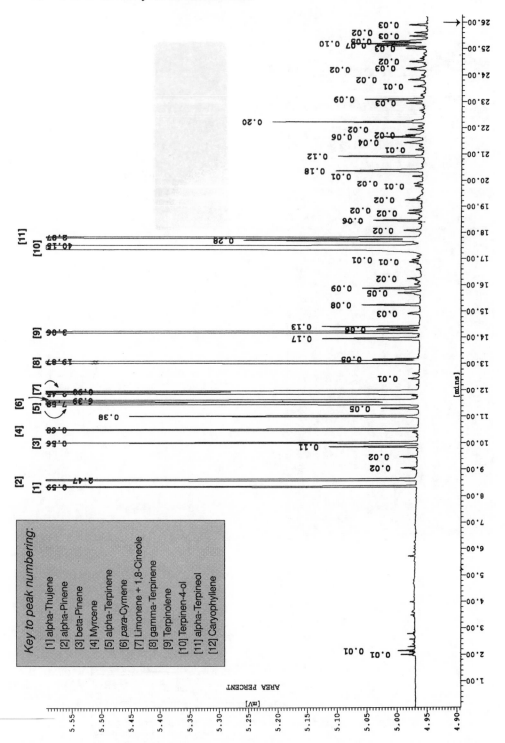

Key to peak numbering:

[1] alpha-Thujene
[2] alpha-Pinene
[3] beta-Pinene
[4] Myrcene
[5] alpha-Terpinene
[6] para-Cymene
[7] Limonene + 1,8-Cineole
[8] gamma-Terpinene
[9] Terpinolene
[10] Terpinen-4-ol
[11] alpha-Terpineol
[12] Caryophyllene

Fig. 6.15 — Chromatogram 9: **Ti-Tree Oil**

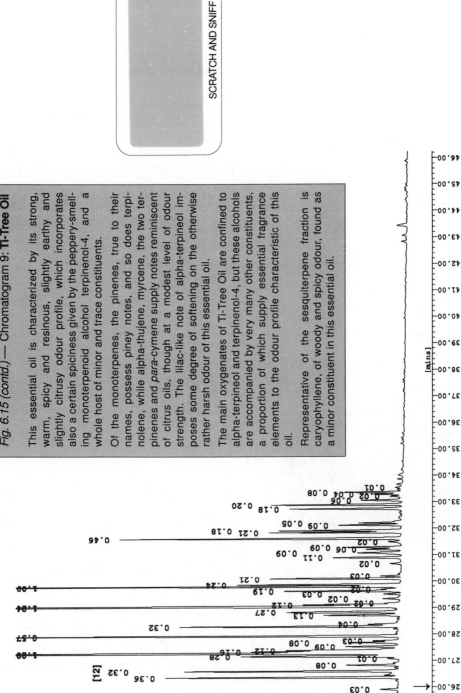

SCRATCH AND SNIFF

Fig. 6.15 (contd.) — Chromatogram 9: **Ti-Tree Oil**

This essential oil is characterized by its strong, warm, spicy and resinous, slightly earthy and slightly citrusy odour profile, which incorporates also a certain spiciness given by the peppery-smelling monoterpenoid alcohol terpinenol-4, and a whole host of minor and trace constituents.

Of the monoterpenes, the pinenes, true to their names, possess piney notes, and so does terpinolene, while alpha-thujiene, myrcene, the two terpinenes and *para*-cymene supply notes reminiscent of citrus oils, though at a modest level of odour strength. The lilac-like note of alpha-terpineol imposes some degree of softening on the otherwise rather harsh odour of this essential oil.

The main oxygenates of Ti-Tree Oil are confined to alpha-terpineol and terpinenol-4, but these alcohols are accompanied by very many other constituents, a proportion of which supply essential fragrance elements to the odour profile characteristic of this oil.

Representative of the sesquiterpene fraction is caryophyllene, of woody and spicy odour, found as a minor constituent in this essential oil.

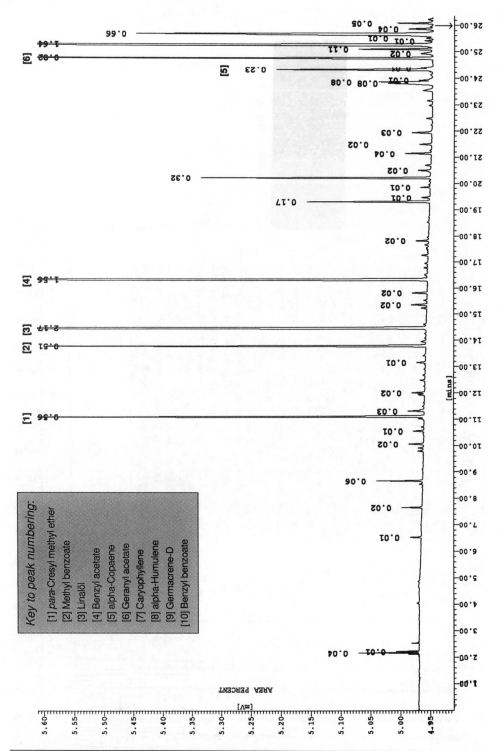

Key to peak numbering:

[1] para-Cresyl methyl ether
[2] Methyl benzoate
[3] Linalôl
[4] Benzyl acetate
[5] alpha-Copaene
[6] Geranyl acetate
[7] Caryophyllene
[8] alpha-Humulene
[9] Germacrene-D
[10] Benzyl benzoate

Fig. 6.16 — Chromatogram 10: **Ylang-Ylang Oil, Extra**

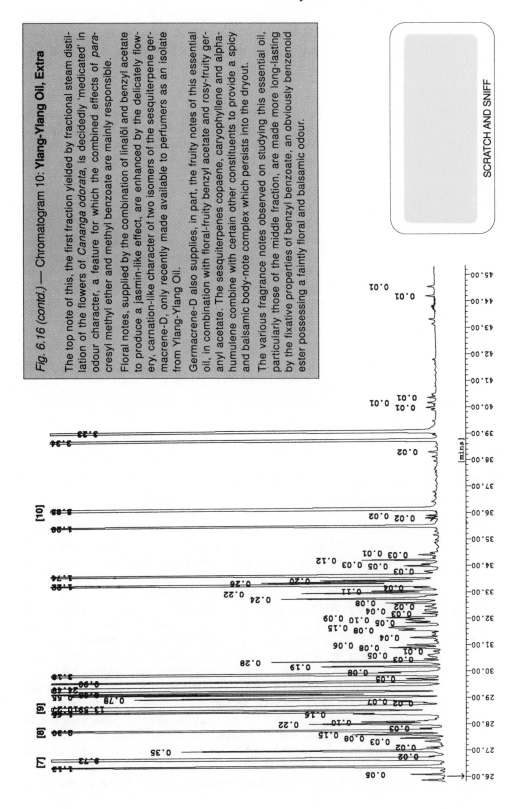

Fig. 6.16 (contd.) — Chromatogram 10: **Ylang-Ylang Oil, Extra**

The top note of this, the first fraction yielded by fractional steam distillation of the flowers of *Cananga odorata*, is decidedly 'medicated' in odour character, a feature for which the combined effects of *para*-cresyl methyl ether and methyl benzoate are mainly responsible.

Floral notes, supplied by the combination of linalôl and benzyl acetate to produce a jasmin-like effect, are enhanced by the delicately flowery, carnation-like character of two isomers of the sesquiterpene germacrene-D, only recently made available to perfumers as an isolate from Ylang-Ylang Oil.

Germacrene-D also supplies, in part, the fruity notes of this essential oil, in combination with floral-fruity benzyl acetate and rosy-fruity geranyl acetate. The sesquiterpenes copaene, caryophyllene and alpha-humulene combine with certain other constituents to provide a spicy and balsamic body-note complex which persists into the dryout.

The various fragrance notes observed on studying this essential oil, particularly those of the middle fraction, are made more long-lasting by the fixative properties of benzyl benzoate, an obviously benzenoid ester possessing a faintly floral and balsamic odour.

SCRATCH AND SNIFF

If positive identification of any peak on a chromatogram is required, several techniques are available, two of which we shall now briefly describe.

6.5.2 Infrared Spectrophotometry (IRS)

The technique of infrared spectrophotometry involves measurement of the energy of different parts of the spectrum of infrared radiation. This lies adjacent to the extreme red part of the visible spectrum and consists of heat rays invisible to the human eye of the kind emitted by an electric fire or heat lamp, which we detect by the increase of temperature they cause when incident upon the skin. The warming effect of infrared radiation is caused by the absorption of its energy, or rather some of it, by the atoms or molecules of any substance upon which it is incident. The result is an increase in the amplitude of their vibration, to which sensory nerve endings lying just beneath the epidermis respond when heat rays fall upon the skin. The basic properties of infrared radiation are noted in figure 6.17.

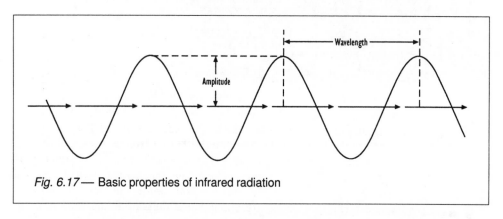

Fig. 6.17— Basic properties of infrared radiation

Heat rays are not absorbed by a molecule in a general, haphazard way, but by causing increased vibration of its different atoms and groups of atoms at their natural frequencies, about the bonds joining them together. With a little stretching of the imagination, this may be likened to the effect of pushing a swing which, if done at just the right moments, increases the height to which the swing rises — i.e. pulses of energy corresponding to the natural frequency of the swing (number of complete, back-and-forth swings per minute) increases the amplitude of the swinging motion: the swing absorbs the energy of the pushes or pulses, provided they are in time with its back-and-forth motions. Now imagine giving the *same number of pushes per minute* to a swing having shorter ropes attached to the seat. The natural frequency of this swing is higher than the one with longer ropes — it swings faster: the pushes do not correspond with the swings and the regular motion of the swing is disrupted; i.e. the energy pulses are out of phase with the frequency of the swing. Similarly, a beam of infrared radiation of any given frequency is absorbed only by those parts of a molecule which vibrate naturally at the same frequency, which depends on the length of the bonds joining them to the rest of the molecule (corresponding to the length of rope of a swing).

There is, however, a further factor involved, which is easily demonstrated by means of two ordinary 30 cm rulers, one wooden and the other of thin, flexible plastic. The object of the experiment is to note the natural frequency of vibration of the *same length* of each of the rulers. Place one of the rulers on a table, so that the 10 cm mark is at the edge of the table with the rest of the ruler, about 21 cm, jutting out beyond the table and at right angles to the edge (*see* fig. 6.18).

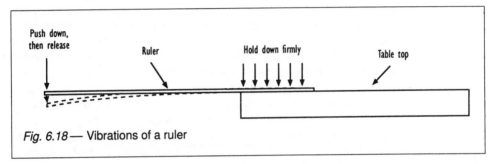

Fig. 6.18 — Vibrations of a ruler

Holding the ruler very firmly on the table, push its outer edge downward, then let go. Note how fast the ruler vibrates. Repeat the experiment with the other ruler. The less flexible of the two rulers vibrates the faster of the two. Similarly, the stronger the bond joining two atoms or groups together, the greater is their natural frequency of vibration. Such analogies between the mechanical world and the world of atoms and molecules are both crude and limited, but provided these limitations are remembered they are better than nothing in aiding our understanding.

Here is a table showing the frequencies of vibration associated with examples of bonds of different length and strength:

Table 6.2 — Frequency of vibration of different bonds

Bond	Bond length (nm)	Relative bond strength (C-C bond = 1)	Frequency (tens of trillions per sec)
C=C	1·34	1·77	4·86 to 5·04
C≡C	1·19	2·42	6·30 to 6·78
C–O	1·43	1·04	3·00 to 3·90
C=O	1·22	2·17	5·10 to 5·25

The frequency range of the vibrations of a molecule lies between about 0·3 and 1·1 hundreds of trillions (3×10^{13} and $1·1 \times 10^{14}$) which latter is the same as 11×10^{13}, per second, or Hertz (Hz.). This frequency range is well within the range of infrared radiation.

To prepare an *infrared spectrogram*, a narrow beam of infrared radiation from a standard source is passed through a sample of the material under investigation, contained in a special cell of the instrument used for this purpose — an *infrared spectrograph or spectrophotometer*. The beam consists of rays of one single frequency, which is slowly decreased from $1·2 \times 10^{14}$ (12×10^{13}) to $1·8 \times 10^{13}$ Hz. Thus the instrument scans the range of vibration frequencies to which molecules of the sample may be able to respond by absorbing radiation at those frequencies. By means of an ingenious device, the instrument makes a pen recording of the percentage of the total infrared radiation transmitted by the sample at the different frequencies scanned. This takes the form of a wavering line, having peaks corresponding to frequencies of least transmittance; that is, of greatest absorption by the sample which, from studies of samples of pure chemicals of known molecular structure, relate to the presence of specific types of bonds and groups of atoms. From the *IR spectrum* of a substance an expert in this technique can deduce valuable information concerning the structure of the molecules of which it is composed.

Applied to an essential oil, IRS gives an overall picture, or fingerprint', of the composition of the oil. The IR spectrograph is very sensitive to small differences of composition, and so is a most useful aid to the comparison of test and standard samples of essential oils, and to the detection of adulteration. The technique has also the advantage of being able to detect and record the presence of nonvolatile as well as volatile constituents of essential oils, and of requiring only a few minutes for the completion of a spectrum.

6.5.3 Mass Spectrometry (MS)

This analytical technique is a powerful aid to the elucidation of the composition and structure of molecules of chemically pure organic compounds. For purposes of the elucidation of the molecular structure of constituents of essential oils, a pure constituent, separated by GLC and represented by a single peak on a chromatogram, is transferred directly to a mass spectrometer. The main features of the working of this instrument will now be described.

Under vacuum conditions, a very small sample of the test compound is bombarded by a stream of electrons. This causes molecules of the test compound to lose one electron, forming positively charged molecular ions of the same molecular weight, the weight of the electron lost being negligible. A proportion of the molecular ions breaks up into positively charged fragments. The positive ions formed by bombardment of the sample and by fragmentation are accelerated by an electrostatic field, then, at high velocity, are made to take sweeping curved pathways in the direction of a detector. Lightest fragments are deflected most, heaviest fragments and molecular ions least, in relation to their masses.[5]

The instrument produces a record of the proportions of the ions of different mass known as a *fragmentation pattern*, from which experts in the technique are able to deduce information on the molecular structure of the compound under investigation. If the molecular ion is registered in the fragmentation pattern, which will not occur if it becomes totally fragmented, its molecular weight is obtained directly. This narrows down considerably the range of possible molecular structures to which the sample corresponds.

6.6 Concepts of Purity

As used in everyday promotional advertising, the word 'pure' is understood to refer to a product which is free from contamination of any kind in relation to its intended purpose: a loaf of bread, a can of soup or an essential oil of high, unadulterated quality, for example. Two other concepts of purity are important in connection with the quality control and assurance of aromatic materials; they are *odour purity* and *chemical purity*.

6.6.1 Odour Purity

Careful odour evaluation at intervals during its evaporation under standardized conditions is, as we have explained, a most important test of the quality of an essential oil. The test is always conducted on commercially available oils by comparison with the odour of a standard sample of the same oil, which is known to be of the quality to which the test sample must conform if it is to be acceptable. Apart from visual inspection, odour evaluation is the only quality control test likely to be available to aromatherapists, beauticians and other nonindustrial users of essntial oils who need to be sure, as far as it is possible to ascertain with the limited resources available, that the oils they use are of the quality required.

The odour purity of an essential oil or other aromatic material may be defined as the extent to which its odour profile matches the odour profile of a standard sample of the same product and grade, when both are allowed to evaporate on smelling strips to final dryout under the same conditions and at the same time.

---

5. A distinction is made between the mass of a body and its weight. A 100 g brass weight contains a certain, fixed and definite *amount* of brass. This *amount* is 100 g, a *quantity* of brass. If the weight is suspended from a spring balance somewhere on the surface of the earth, the balance registers 100 g *weight*. If the same weight were to be suspended from a spring balance on the surface of the moon, the balance would register about 17 g, because the force of the moon's gravitational field at its surface is about ⅙ of the gravitational field at the earth's surface: the *quantity* of brass in the weight *would not have changed*, but its *response* to the much smaller gravitational field of the moon would be correspondingly less.

6.6.2 Chemical Purity

A substance which is chemically pure consists of chemically identical atoms or molecules. The concept of chemical purity applies only to single elements or compounds to which this condition applies. An essential oil, being a mixture of organic compounds, cannot therefore be chemically pure, even though it may be of high odour purity and 'pure' in the sense of being free from contamination.

The chemical composition and odour profile of an essential oil together provide the information from which its purity, in reference to a standard sample, may be ascertained.

6.7 Factors Determining the Quality of Essential Oils

In this section we shall briefly summarize the various factors, discussed in preceding chapters, that are important in determining the chemical composition, and hence the quality, of essential oils.

6.7.1 Genotype of the Source Plant

The genotype of a living organism is its genetic constitution: the composition and order of the genes carried by the chromosomes in the nucleus of every living cell. The genes of a plant determine the composition of the proteins forming the living matter, or *protoplasm*, of the plant. These proteins include the enzymes which control the metabolism of the plant; i.e. all those chemical reactions by which the life of the plant is sustained. In aromatic plants, essential oils are formed in *oil glands* or *cells*; their composition being determined by the enzyme-controlled reaction pathways by which their constituents are synthesized.

6.7.2 Conditions of Growth and Development of the Plant

A green plant obtains the chemical elements that it requires for growth and development to maturity from the surrounding atmosphere and from the soil by which it is supported: carbon from carbon dioxide present in the air, hydrogen from soil water and oxygen from both carbon dioxide and water, all to be used for *photosynthesis*. Mineral salts, absorbed by the root hairs of the plant as ions dissolved in the soil water, are essential for its normal development: nitrates containing nitrogen essential for protein formation, iron and magnesium salts for the formation of chlorophyll, phosphorus, as phosphates, for the formation of cell nuclei and potassium for the control of cell division are but a few examples.

Deficiencies of any of the ions required by a plant causes poor growth and yellowing of leaves and, in aromatic plants, poor yields of inferior quality essential oils. Atmospheric pollution can damage or destroy plant life, as can contaminated soil.

6.7.3 Harvesting and Processing of Aromatic Plant Material

To obtain a high yield of good quality essential oil, the source material must be harvested at the time when its content of oil is at a maximum, using a technique which excludes extraneous matter, such as weeds. Spices and some herbs, iris rhizome and patchouli leaves are examples of source materials needing drying under the correct conditions before distillation; fragrant flowers must be processed as soon as possible following harvesting to minimize loss of essential oil and the onset of fermentation which would introduce unwanted volatiles and spoil the final product.

Assuming harvesting source material in perfect condition, the quality of the essential oil or aromatic extract produced from it will then depend on the conditions of processing and subsequent storage of the product. The design and operation of distillation equipment, for example, must be such as to ensure completion of the process in the shortest possible period of time, but under conditions of temperature and pressure that will not cause any part of the charge in the still to suffer damaging thermal stress. With extraction processes, solvent recovery from aromatic extract solutions under reduced pressure must not allow loss of top notes and must be complete if the resulting concretes, absolutes and resinoids are not to be contaminated with residues of the solvents used for their extraction.

6.7.4 Effects of Moisture on Essential Oils

Resulting from contact with water or hot steam, respectively, essential oils produced by expression or distillation frequently contain proportions of dissolved water. If the storage temperature of the oil is subsequently allowed to fall, the solubility of the water in the oil will be reduced, with the result that some of it may come out of solution. This can cause corrosion in a steel drum, the onset of which is accelerated by the presence of any traces of free acid in the oil. Some essential oils may survive this kind of insult remarkably well —Petitgrain, for example; others, such as Lemongrass or any other oil containing citral or other terpenoid aldehydes, do not. Essential oils should either be dry or, if necessary, be dried by the producer before filling into the final storage containers ready for shipment.

6.7.5 Storage Conditions

In general, essential oils should be stored under the following conditions:

i) in a cool place, at an even temperature;
ii) protected from light;
iii) in tightly sealed containers;
iv) under the smallest feasible headspace of air or under nitrogen;
v) in nonplastic containers, the material of which will not in any way alter their composition.

6.7.6 *Adulteration of Essential Oils*

An essential oil intended for use in aromatherapy must be free from adulteration; that is, it must contain nothing that is not a normal constituent of the oil, as obtained by the process usually adopted for separating it from its natural source.

Adulterants of essential oils of the subtle kind, more typical of today, are not usually detectable by smell, and so in order to set up unadulterated odour standards for the odour evaluation of subsequent supplies, the aromatherapist must make sure to purchase initial and, indeed, all subsequent supplies from a totally reliable source having, or having recourse to, fully equipped facilities for quality control, from which quality certification is readily and willingly available.

6.8 The Safety of Fragrance Materials

The use of aromatic materials as perfume ingredients is the subject of a voluntary code good of practice which is widely accepted in the perfume industry. The code aims to protect users of perfumes and perfumed products from harm resulting from the composition of the perfume compounds used. In the United States of America, the Research Institute for Fragrance Materials (RIFM) has an ongoing programme for the testing of fragrance materials, including essential oils, by independent experts, and gathers information on this subject from other authoritative sources. The data gathered by RIFM is subjected to scrutiny by members of a committee of experts in all aspects of the composition, safety and applications of fragrance materials, from whose deliberations reports are prepared which are transmitted from RIFM to the International Fragrance Association (IFRA), based in Switzerland.

Following careful study of the reports from RIFM, IFRA prepares its own advisory reports on any materials that its experts consider need to be restricted in use as fragrance materials, or banned from this use altogether. These reports, known as 'IFRA updates', are distributed to the members of IFRA, who include the perfumery trade associations, such as the British Fragrance Association. These bodies then forward the reports to their members, who are the individual perfume supply companies. By voluntary adherence to the recommendations of IFRA, the perfume industry in general maintains its enviable reputation as the manufacturer of the safest of all consumer products.

Chapter 7

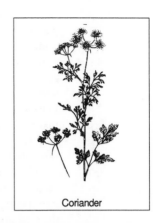

Coriander

Isolated and Synthetic Fragrance Materials

7.1 Inventions and Discoveries

Archaeological evidence in the form of preserved, dated artefacts strongly suggest that the process of distillation was known to an ancient civilization in the region of present-day Pakistan at least as far back as 3000 BC. Stills of this antiquity, and for four millenia afterwards, were crude affairs in comparison with those of today, being heated by a fire lit beneath the distillation vessel and lacking any efficient form of cooling system for condensation of the hot vapours produced, the bulk of which would certainly have escaped into the air.

By the time of the birth of Christ, the Greeks had become skilled in the manufacture of perfumes of many kinds. These included fragrant waters, prepared by treating aromatic plant material with boiling water and passing the vapours produced into the mouth of a receiving vessel — a primitive form of water distillation. By this means, as we now know, they collected in their receivers quantities of water containing dissolved essential oil; but this, the cause of the fragrance of the distillation waters, was unknown to the Greeks. They did, however, observe the presence on the surface of the waters of oily droplets, which they carefully removed and discarded, oblivious of the fact that they were disposing of the very products which would have given them perfumes far stronger than the fragrant waters they so highly prized. In this way the Greeks 'purified' their distillation waters for the next thousand years.

The invention of steam distillation is attributed to the Persian philosopher and physician Ibn Sina (known also as Avicenna) who lived from 980 to 1037 AD. This new and faster process remained, however, as inefficient as water distillation regarding the amounts of distillation waters collected until the invention, by someone unknown, of the water-cooled condenser in Europe, in about 1150. This device, crude at first, involved cooling, by means of flowing cold water, the downward-sloping part of the vapour pipe of the still, so removing enough heat to allow the hot vapours to condense to the corresponding liquids. Using a condenser as part of the still, the resulting reduction in the escape of great volumes of fragrant steam, and increase in the amounts of distillation waters collected, must have been quite dramatic. But the distillers of those days observed that the amounts of 'impurities' accompanying the distillation waters also were greater, necessitating greater effort to make sure that none remained after 'purification'.

Then came the inevitable, revolutionary discovery, again anony-mous — that the oily products of distillation were, far from being impurities, the very source of the fragrance of the distillation waters: the essential oils. This discovery, though marking the earliest origin of the essential oils industry of today, was long in bearing fruit, no doubt because the amounts of oily matter produced by the distillation of most aromatic plants were still too small to suggest their retention and use as perfume ingredients.

The invention of the coil-type condenser, or 'worm', in 1420 pro-vided in compact form the large surface area required for total con-densation of the fast-flowing vapours produced by steam distillation. The commercial distillation of essential oils in Europe commenced at the beginning of the sixteenth century.

Essential oils from citrus fruits were first described in 1560, the same year in which the production of natural aromatic materials for use as perfume ingredients began in Grasse, the Provençal town of southern France which was to become famous for the growing of fragrant flowers for perfumery and known throughout the world for the fine quality of its production. Grasse became and remains today a 'Mecca' of the world of perfumery, attracting visitation by perfumers from far and wide.

Concretes, the waxy extracts produced by solvent extraction, were first introduced by the house of Roure, Bertrand Fils in Grasse, in 1873, and in 1888 Joseph Robert succeeded in developing a large-scale process for the solvent extraction of fragrant plants. This proc-ess was brought into commercial production two years later.

Possibly the very first constituent of an essential oil to be isolated and used was the colourless, crystalline solid, camphor. Isolation in this case involved simply removing the highly odorous crystals from the essential oil distilled from the wood of the camphor tree, from which the crystals separate on allowing the oil to stand in a cool place. Today's Camphor Oil of commerce consists of the residual oil resulting from pressing of the semicrystalline essential oil steam-dis-tilled from the wood of the camphor tree in Taiwan and Japan. Other early examples of constituents isolated from essential oils were the crystals named 'thyme camphor', first observed as a deposit in Thyme Oil by Neumann in 1719, and later rediscovered and renamed thymol by Lallemand in 1853, and the crystals obtained from Peppermint Oil by Gaubius in 1774 and later named menthol, after the botanical source of the oil, *Mentha piperita*. Natural menthol is today isolated from the essential oil distilled from the closely related species, *Mentha arvensis*. Camphor is a ketone, thymol a phenol and menthol an alcohol.

The process of fractional distillation in a vacuum was invented at the end of the eighteenth century and led to the separation of major liquid constituents of certain essential oils. The process involves first pumping most of the air out of a special still containing the essential oil to be treated. The distillation vessel, made of heat-resistant glass or stainless steel, is fitted at the top with a long, wide, vertical pipe called a *fractionating column*, which hot vapours from the distillation vessel must ascend before flowing downward through a curved extension of the vapour pipe to a water-cooled condenser and receiver beneath. In one type of fractionating still the fractionating column is filled with glass or ceramic rings known, after their inventor, as *Raschig rings*. These provide a very large total area for condensation of vapours ascending the column. The entire apparatus is, of course, hermetically sealed to maintain the vacuum conditions required, the reason for which we shall now briefly explain.

At normal atmospheric pressure, pure water boils at a temperature of 100°C; a degree or two higher if the atmospheric pressure is above normal, and a degree or two lower if the pressure is less than normal. Normal atmospheric pressure is that pressure which would support a column of mercury 760 mm in height. Under any conditions of temperature and pressure at which it is distilled, water is perfectly stable; i.e. its molecules remain intact. Essential oils boil, at ordinary atmospheric pressures, at temperatures much higher than the boiling point of water, and at these temperatures the molecules of some of their constituents suffer thermal stress; that is, the vibrations they undergo increase to levels of violence sufficient to risk breaking-up of their structures. Structurally weaker molecules of delicate constituents may be shaken to pieces at the boiling point, the 'pieces' being the simpler molecules of decomposition products having odours quite different from those of the intact constituents. Constituents so affected are said to undergo thermal decomposition under these circumstances, degrading the oil and rendering it useless. Under vacuum conditions, the pressure of the air on the surface of the oil to be distilled is very much reduced, so increasing the rate at which the oil evaporates and reducing the temperature at which it boils. With a good enough vacuum, many oils will boil at temperatures below those at which any of their constituents begin to decompose.

The application of heat to the charged distillation vessel causes the essential oil to boil, whereupon vapour from the oil begins to rise into the fractionating column. The process of boiling occurs when a liquid evaporates throughout its mass, hence the vapour first formed consists of the more volatile constituents of the oil, leaving less volatile constituents in the distillation vessel beneath. The vapour heats the column by the release of latent heat as it condenses back to liquid, and this continues up the column as the vapour rises to the top.

The removal of the most volatile constituents of the essential oil in the distillation vessel raises the boiling point of the remaining mixture of constituents. In this way a temperature gradient is set up, which is highest in the distillation vessel and lowest at the top of the fractionating column. This is the result of the application of heat at the bottom of the still and the cooling effect of the air surrounding the column. Under these conditions, the most volatile constituents of the essential oil (those of lowest boiling point) rise up the column quickly, with minimum condensation once the entire length of the column has been heated, while those of progressively lower volatility (higher boiling point) lag behind down the column in the order of their increasing boiling points (or decreasing volatilities). As the distillation temperature rises, the temperature of the vapours entering the column increases; thus the column temperature at any point up its length slowly rises during the process, reducing the amount of condensation of the vapours of the more volatile constituents in the column and so allowing them to distil over. Thus the distillate obtained consists of constituents of ever-decreasing volatility and ever-increasing boiling point. By periodically changing the receiver for a fresh one, fractions of the essential oil of increasing boiling range and different composition may be obtained.

The vacuum fractionation of an essential oil that is rich in a particular constituent may be controlled to yield that constituent as a fraction known as an *isolate*. By this means, geraniol was isolated from Palmarosa Oil by Jacobsen in 1871, citral from Lemongrass Oil by Dodge in 1890, and phenylethyl alcohol from Rose Otto by Walbaum in 1896.

Vacuum fractionation does not, however, yield isolates of high purity, but products containing portions, usually small, of other constituents of the parent essential oil having boiling points close to those of the main isolate. These confer upon an isolate notes of distinctive character, related to the odour of the parent oil, setting the product apart from the corresponding synthetic chemical as a perfume ingredient in its own right. Thus linalöl isolated from Brazilian Rosewood Oil has a much richer, warmer, more woody-balsamic odour than synthetic linalöl, making it the ingredient of choice for fragrance applications where these qualities are desired. It is, however, considerably more expensive than synthetic linalöl, and so is for this reason of cost-restricted application.

Two very important isolates of modern perfumery separated from Turpentine Oil by vacuum fractionation, are the monoterpenes alpha- and beta-pinene. These products are used in vast quantities for the manufacture of synthetic terpenoid aroma chemicals, including citral. The isolation of citral from Lemongrass or *Litsea cubeba* Oil affords an alternative, though more costly, source of supply of this valuable chemical.

Returning to earlier times, the advances in the science and technology of organic chemistry which took place during the nineteenth century were accompanied by increasing interest in the possibility of preparing constituents of products of natural origin, such as essential oils, by synthesis in the laboratory. Notable successes in this direction were the syntheses of coumarin, the chief constituent of tonka beans, by Perkin and Graebe in 1868, of vanillin, the chief constituent of vanilla, by Haarmann and Tiemann in 1874, and of phenylethyl alcohol, an important constituent of Rose Otto, by Radziewski in 1876 — although in reference to the last example, this synthesis was accomplished before the discovery of phenylethyl alcohol as a constituent of Rose Otto twenty years later. As we shall see, the synthesis and introduction into perfume formulations of naturally occurring chemicals, also chemicals which were at the time of their discovery unknown in nature, was to completely revolutionize the art and technology of perfumery and its application to the fragrancing of products for personal care and care of the home.

The development of the analytical technique of gas–liquid chromatography (GLC) during the years following the end of the Second World War completely changed the outlook of research into the composition of essential oils. Before the introduction of GLC into perfumery, the analysis of essential oils relied on crystallization, vacuum fractionation and sometimes chemical processes to separate constituents and chemical methods to identify them. The procedures used were, however, mostly time-consuming and of very limited usefulness. In contrast, GLC, once sufficiently developed regarding its sensitivity, separating ability and reliability, afforded a means for almost complete separation of the major and minor constituents of an essential oil and of many of its trace constituents as well.

The technique did, and still does, suffer from imperfections, such as the decomposition of certain constituents in the injection block, giving rise to products of decomposition to mislead the analyst when they appear on the chromatogram among the true constituents of an essential oil, the merging of the peaks of constituents emerging from the column at the same time and, in respect of earlier instruments, the very great difficulties encountered in standardizing a chromatograph to give reproducible results. Improvements to the design of GLC instruments have largely eliminated these and other problems associated with their operation, to the extent that modern GLC equipment has opened the door to a veritable wonderland of odorous molecules undreamt of as recently as fifty years ago.

7.2 Isolation of Constituents of Essential Oils

In this section, we shall explore a little further the processes for separating single constituents or bands of constituents from essential oils.

Usable amounts of constituents may be separated from essential oils in a pure or almost pure state by preparative GLC, which is basically different from analytical GLC only in the much larger scale of the equipment used. The process is, however, expensive and too costly to operate on even a moderate (or pilot) scale, let alone on the industrial scale necessary for the production of commercial quantities of aroma chemicals. Hence vacuum fractionation, which we described in section 1 of this chapter, and which is relatively cheap to run, is the process mainly used for liquids, and an equally low-cost process, crystallization, is used for solids that cannot be purified by vacuum fractionation in the liquid state.

When considering the fractionation of an essential oil, it is helpful to visualize the oil as a somewhat eccentric sandwich:

Table 7.1 — Fractions of essential oils as 'layers in a sandwich'

Layer	Representing	Boiling point	Odour/flavour analogy
Upper layer: white bread	Monoterpenes	Low	Pleasant, but not very interesting
Filling: ham, cheese, etc.	Oxygenates	Intermediate	Very interesting: character-determining
Lower layer: brown bread	Sesquiterpenes	High	More interesting than upper layer, but rarely character-determining

With reference to the table above, the first fraction of a typical essential oil, such as Petitgrain Oil, consists largely of monoterpenes, such as *d*- and *l*-limonene. If the receiver is then changed for a fresh one, a second fraction of oxygenated constituents — linalöl, linalyl acetate, geraniol, methyl anthranilate, etc., in the case of Petitgrain — is obtained. Since the separation of constituents by fractionation is never perfect, this fraction will contain also small proportions of monoterpenes and sesquiterpenes, but its production can be controlled so that its terpene content is minimal. Usually the sesquiterpenes (containing some proportion of oxygenates) are obtained as a residue in the distillation vessel. The fraction of oxygenates, known as a terpeneless essential oil, possesses the odour characteristic of the parent oil and finds application as a perfume ingredient where a stronger, less readily oxidized, near-natural note of the parent oil is required. In general, terpeneless essential oils are more soluble in alcohol diluted with water than the corresponding complete oils, a property rendering them useful as substitutes for the latter products in perfume compounds intended for toilet waters and other aqueous-alcoholic products. A terpeneless essential oil may be separated from the parent oil not as a single fraction, but as several successive fractions of closely related composition, from which two or more are then selected and blended together to form the final product, conforming to a prescribed specification.

Using a fractionating column of good separating power, single major constituents of sufficiently high purity for their purpose may be isolated, as noted in section 1 of this chapter. Here is a summary of important examples of these isolates:

Table 7.2 — Examples of isolates from essential oils

Isolate	Essential Oil
Citral	Lemongrass or *Litsea cubeba* Oils
Citronellal	Citronella Oil
Coumarin	Tonka Extracts
Geraniol	Palmarosa or Citronella Oils
Linalöl	Rosewood Oil
l-Menthol	*Mentha arvensis* Oil
alpha- and beta-Pinenes	Turpentine Oil
Thymol	Ajowan Oil
Vetiverol	Vetivert Oil
Vanillin	Vanilla Extracts

7.3 The First 'Synthetics' for Perfumery

Outstanding in the extremely difficult and time-consuming field of early research into the composition of essential oils, which extended over many years, was the French chemist and statesman Jean-Baptiste André Dumas (1800–1884). It was, however, the isolation of coumarin from cured tonka beans by Friedrich Wöhler in 1856 that gave impetus to efforts to synthesize other fragrant chemicals known to occur in nature; a quest having some hope of success since the overthrow of the 'vital force' hypothesis by Hermann Kolbe more than ten years previously.

Crystals of coumarin were first prepared synthetically in 1868 by William Perkin, the great English chemist and father of the British synthetic dyestuffs industry, and the German chemist Carl Graebe. Coumarin was, however, of little interest to the perfumers of the time who, steeped as they were in a tradition of the use of natural materials only as perfume ingredients, were unable to envisage any possible applications of chemicals in artistic creations of such delicacy. But there are, in every walk of life, individuals who think beyond tradition and established fact: visionaries prepared to experiment; adventurers for whom the question, 'What would happen if......?' is demanding of an answer — thinkers and practical people daring to reach out beyond accepted convention to invent, design, construct and create the devices, products and materials of tomorrow. One such was Paul Parquet, who in the early 1880s conceived the idea of a perfume for a toilet soap to be launched by the perfumery house of Houbigant, of which he became owner in 1882. In this perfume, synthetic coumarin was made a key ingredient, and the fragrance quickly gained outstanding popularity among toilet soaps of similar high quality. The soap was named 'Fougère Royale' — Royal Fern — and its perfume became recognized as a great triumph of creative perfumery: a classic of the art of perfume composition. It was the first perfume based on a synthetic chemical to be so recognized and its popularity clearly demonstrated the potential of carefully chosen, synthetic chemicals as perfume ingredients. 'Fougère Royale' was launched in 1882, and from the mid-nineteenth century, once its popularity had become established and the secret of its composition generally known, the necessities of commercial competition slowly began to erode the prejudices of perfumers against chemicals as perfume ingredients, eventually to the extent of their use to generate the novel and very beautiful notes of the great fragrance classics of the twentieth century.

The invention of improvements to the techniques of organic synthesis which occurred during the latter half of the nineteenth century and into the twentieth, presented chemists with ever-widening opportunities for the synthetic reproduction of naturally occurring chemicals having fairly simply molecules. There were aldehydes, such as vanillin and citral, a range of fatty aldehydes, alcohols, such as menthol, alpha-terpineol, citronellol, linalöl and geraniol, and their esters with acetic (acetates) and other organic acids. Also of the greatest importance were ketones such as the wonderfully fragrant ionones, and chemicals as yet unknown in nature (some even to the present day) — the ethers diphenyl oxide and beta-naphthyl methyl ether, the aldehyde heliotropine, ethyl vanillin, an aldehyde twice as powerful in its powdery, vanilla-like odour as vanillin, and an increasing range of musk-smelling synthetics — musc Baur, named after the discoverer of the first synthetic musk, musk ketone, musk xylol and many more.

The gradual acceptance of aromatic chemicals. (later to become known as aroma chemicals) by the more progressive of perfumers did not displace their conviction of the absolute necessity of natural materials for the creation of the finest quality of fragrance. In more recent times it was discovered that the reason for this belief was indeed well founded, as perfumes of entirely synthetic composition lacked the bouquet of minor and trace constituents present in natural materials which were found to be essential to the 'naturalness' of high-quality perfumes. Even today, with more than 5,000 aroma chemicals available to the perfumer, natural materials are used alongside aroma chemicals for this same purpose and to introduce fragrance notes and qualities, such as those of Patchouli Oil, which are simply impossible to produce synthetically.

Certain aromatic chemicals were first synthesized long before they were discovered in nature. Examples are benzyl acetate, first prepared by Cannizzaro in 1855 and discovered as a major constituent (65 per cent!) of Jasmin Absolute in 1895 by Hesse and Muller, and phenylethyl alcohol first synthesized, as we have noted, by Radzizewski in 1876 and found in Rose Otto and Rose Absolute by Walbaum in 1896. Only after their discovery as constituents of aromatic materials of natural origin were such chemicals generally accepted for use in perfumery.

The odours of aromatic chemicals as they were first produced a century ago are today known only from surviving descriptions written by perfumers who used them. Sufficient documentary evidence of this kind exists to convince us that the odours of the same chemicals, as manufactured for use in perfumery today, are in many cases different from those they once possessed, many years ago. Since the same chemical always consists of the same molecules, wherever, however and whenever it is made (law of constant composition) then it should always have the same odour. This apparent paradox may be investigated by questioning the purity of the different samples, and from published literature finding that a) these chemicals are now synthesized by methods different from those originally used, and b) aroma chemicals are today purified to much higher standards than when they were first produced. Different methods of synthesis of the same organic chemical give rise to different side reactions; that is, reactions which take place at the same time as the main reaction producing the required chemical, and these give rise to different impurities having different odours, the extent of the removal of which has a marked effect on the odour of the final product. Certain aroma chemicals in use today, geraniol, for example, are remembered by perfumers of senior years to have been much inferior in odour quality even as recently as the 1960s, so great have been the advances in synthetic and purification techniques in the intervening period of time.

Many aroma chemicals in regular use in perfumery are available in several different grades — highly purified for fine fragrance use, less highly purified for purposes of general perfumery, and still less purified for the creation of industrial perfumes for use as odour-masking agents. The progressive purification of an aroma chemical frequently results in a weakening of its odour, sometimes almost to vanishing point, a phenomenon showing how profound the effect of the presence of impurities can be on the odour of a chemical. Manufacturers of speciality grades of aroma chemicals sometimes 'bouquet' the purest grades of certain aroma chemicals by the addition of small amounts of other materials, carefully selected to beautify to a maximum their odours without significant change to their basic character. Naturally, the purest grades of 'unbouquetted' chemicals command high prices, with speciality grades being even more costly.

7.4 Aroma Chemicals as Odour Notes

The introduction of aromatic chemicals worthy of the name into perfumery began, as we have seen, with coumarin around 1880. By the turn of the century, the trickle of new aromatic chemicals to appear in manufacturers' catalogues had become an ever-increasing flow, and by mid-twentieth century amounted to a veritable tide. Few of these materials, however, offered perfumers anything completely revolutionary by way of creative opportunity until, some 15 to 20 years later, refinements of analytical techniques made possible the discovery and identification of constituents of essential oils which hitherto had appeared as the slightest perturbations on the GLC trace. The often dauntingly difficult synthesis of these constituents fell to the lot of specialist researchers, who were mostly young chemists fresh from university success and seeking higher degrees as foundation stones for their careers. Spurred on by fascination with organic chemistry, by the goal of personal achievement and by the promise of the career progress which would follow fulfilment of the task in hand, they not infrequently brought to the light of day chemicals new to science which were subsequently subjected to rigorous programmes of testing to determine their suitability as perfume ingredients.

Occasionally, a chemical having an exciting new kind of odour would be discovered, only to be later rejected on grounds of some deficiency rendering it useless as a fragrance material — a disappointment of the kind typical of scientific and technological research. Only the most outstanding of those precious few new chemicals of undisputed merit, which also satisfied the exacting demands of the technologist, went on to become the 'secret ingredients' of great perfume creations, so to earn fame and fortune for their originators and permanent places on the perfumers' shelves.

The introduction of new aroma chemicals continues today, though in recent years abated by the mounting costs of the research and development necessary to discover them and find cheap synthetic pathways for their commercial production. Customers for perfume compounds set strict limits on the amounts of money they are prepared to pay for them, and these cost restrictions filter through to manufacturers of perfume ingredients. In costing a new chemical of promising commercial potential, the costs of safety testing and product licensing have also to be taken into account, in addition to costs incurred in providing facilities for production, purification, promotion, marketing and further product development. It is little wonder that the introduction of a novel molecular structure into the world of aroma chemicals is now quite a rare event.

To summarize, among the thousands of aroma chemicals introduced by enterprising manufacturers over the past century, relatively few have survived the test of time, having presented little in the way of special odour properties to excite the imagination of the perfumer. We shall now aim to gain a perspective of how these materials changed the course of the development of perfumery, bringing creative and commercial opportunities to perfumers and benefits to users of personal-care and household products undreamt of at the time of their introduction many years ago.

There are certain analogies between perfumery and music which are useful in comparing the odour properties of aroma chemicals with those of natural aromatic materials. The simplest kind of musical tone is one lacking in harmonics, possessing a wave form consisting of uniform undulations. The flute pipes of an organ give sounds of this kind consisting of pressure waves propagated in the air; they may be represented as shown in figure 7.1.

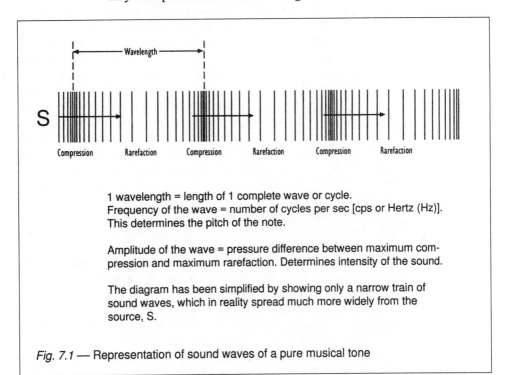

1 wavelength = length of 1 complete wave or cycle.
Frequency of the wave = number of cycles per sec [cps or Hertz (Hz)]. This determines the pitch of the note.

Amplitude of the wave = pressure difference between maximum compression and maximum rarefaction. Determines intensity of the sound.

The diagram has been simplified by showing only a narrow train of sound waves, which in reality spread much more widely from the source, S.

Fig. 7.1 — Representation of sound waves of a pure musical tone

As the diagram shows, these waves are alternating regions of compression and rarefaction of the air but, unlike light waves, they are longitudinal. However, like light waves, sound waves possess the properties of wavelength, amplitude and frequency. The shorter the wavelength of a sound wave the higher is its frequency and the higher is the pitch of the sound it produces; the greater its amplitude, the louder is the sound.

In music, a pure tone is given by a sound wave of one single frequency; the sound to which it gives rise has both pitch and loudness, but no quality. The Greenwich time signal is an example of a sound of this kind. The distinctive tones of different musical instruments are given by sound waves consisting of mixtures of many different frequencies, harmonically related to the frequency of the fundamental, or principal, frequency which usually gives the pitch of any note played.

As far as is at present definitely known, there are no 'pure odour tones' from which all other odours can be produced by correct proportional blending. There do, however, appear to be certain odours which cannot be accurately reproduced by blending together other odours of essentially different kinds. An example, here, is the odour we know as 'bitter almond', as represented by benzaldehyde. There are several other chemicals having this kind of smell, but none of their odours is precisely the same as any of the others, although they are of the same odour type. It is found to be impossible to reproduce the odours of any of these chemicals by blending together others which do not themselves possess the bitter almond smell.

Analogies between musical sounds and odours are more useful when applied to perfumes, and we shall return to this theme in Chapter 8 when discussing the art of perfume creation.

Quite probably, the first feature of the odour of coumarin to be observed by the perfumer Paul Parquet (*see* p. 186) was the soft, sweet hay-like aspect of its profile, which is similar in odour type to, though greatly different in richness of odour character from, the absolute of the natural source of coumarin, namely, dried and cured tonka beans; differences between the odours of the two products no doubt led Parquet to use synthetic coumarin in preference to Tonka Absolute in the creation of 'Fougère Royale'.

A very important difference between the odour character of a typical aroma chemical, linalyl acetate for example, and an essential oil or aromatic extract, such as Lavender Oil, containing the chemical as a major constituent, is that while both are perceived as being of complex odour in possessing a number of different, recognizable odour features, the odour of the chemical is, during its evaporation from a smelling strip, relatively static in character, while that of the essential oil, evaporating under the same conditions, undergoes gradual but readily observable changes to final dryout. A natural product is for this reason more interesting to smell and easier to use as a perfume ingredient than an aroma chemical, and is parallelled in its behaviour on evaporation by a skin perfume of the traditional kind which is structured to display a top note of brief duration as a contrasting introduction to a long-lasting main fragrance theme.

An aroma chemical may therefore be regarded as a means for the production of an odour complex of a certain kind, as a violin gives sound of a certain character. We may take the analogy a step further in recognizing that while the *characteristic* tone of a violin is the same for all makes of the instrument, the different makes display differences of tonal quality by reason of differences in the detail of their construction. Analogously, while the *characteristic* odour note of an aroma chemical is the same for all pure grades of the product, lower grades display differences of odour quality by reason of differences in the nature and levels of the impurities that they contain. Furthermore, just as a very cheap violin may produce sounds of inferior character, yet inspire a child to take up the instrument (albeit to the initial devastation of the child's parents) so a very cheap grade of aroma chemical may be of coarse, crude odour, yet provide just the note and odour impact required to render it effective as an active odorous ingredient of an air freshener, for example.

If an aroma chemical is regarded, by analogy, as comparable to an orchestral instrument of a particular kind, a typical essential oil represents to the human sense of smell a naturally harmonized combination of many instruments.

How then may we regard a perfume? We will address this question in Chapter 8.

7.5 Aroma Chemicals and Classical Perfumery

Using aroma chemicals, a perfumer is able to create blends having odours of character very different from the odours of combinations of essential oils. This was not, however, the way in which aroma chemicals were first used to produce perfumes, probably because those that became available up to the end of the nineteenth century and which were regarded as suitable for use in perfumery were so few in number and so contrasting in odour that most perfumers regarded their experimental combination as a waste of time.

The technique adopted by the more adventurous of perfumers to investigate the fragrance properties of the new materials was extremely cautious, consisting of replacing one or more of the natural ingredients of an existing perfume by carefully selected chemicals, or by simply adding a chemical in graduated steps to a prepared blend of natural ingredients, to see what the result would be. Either of these procedures was, on the basis of trial and error experimentation, frequently found to produce interesting and sometimes very beautiful fragrances of novel character. The really big surprises, however, came with aromatic chemicals unknown in nature; chemicals such as methyl ionone, amyl salicylate, anisaldehyde and hydroxycitronellal, with the aid of which the first great classics of perfumery were created by perfumers who became recognized as masters of their difficult and exacting art.

The main fragrance themes of the great perfumes of the turn of the twentieth century, such as Piver's 'Trèfle Incarnat' (1896), François Coty's 'L'Origan' (1905), Guerlain's 'Après l'Ondée' (1906) and the 'Narcisse Noir' of Caron, were not determined by the notes of aroma chemicals but, just as blue is necessary for the production of crimson from red, certain chemicals were instrumental to the realization of the novel fragrance appeal and beauty of these perfumes.

In 1921 came the launch of the renowned 'No. 5' of Chanel, in which the master perfumer Ernest Beaux had used certain fatty aldehydes at dosage levels which the very unpleasant and powerful character of their odours suggested would be unacceptable. Set upon a rich, floral, woody and balsamic base, however, the effect of this emphasis on the aldehydes was to produce a diffusive and highly original perfume which very quickly gained lasting popularity. 'No. 5' was the first perfume to be characterized by notes of synthetic chemicals, and its phenomenal and continuing success invalidates the view, frequently expressed or implied, that because a material is a chemical it must necessarily be of inferior quality in comparison with natural products. Fatty aldehydes are not expensive chemicals, and their odours in the pure state are highly objectionable but, like common clay, in the hands of the inspired creative artist they can become media for the expression of great beauty. 'Chanel No. 5' was also the first perfume to be launched by a dressmaker, and was followed in this context by others of equal elegance and distinction, such as 'Joy' (Patou, 1935), 'Shocking' (Schiaparelli, 1937), 'Bandit' (Piguet, 1944), 'Ma Griffe' (Carven, 1946) and 'Miss Dior' (Dior, 1947).

7.6 The Consumer Revolution

By the time of the outbreak of the Second World War, the dimension of fragrance was becoming firmly established as an attractive feature of a growing variety of perfumed toilet preparations and beauty aids. Among perfumes sold at almost every pharmacy and department store were the following, in respect of which we quote the prices for which the smallest sizes were sold in the monetary system then in use: 12 pence (d.) = 1 shilling (s.), which today is equal to 5p. In the late 1930s, when a Ford 8 family saloon (the equivalent of the present-day Mini) could be bought for £100 and a good bicycle (with mudguards) for less than £5, the purchasing power of money was very much greater than it is today.

Table 7.3 — Cost of some popular perfumes in the late 1930s

		s.	d.
'Californian Poppy'	Atkinson	1	$4^{1}/_{2}$
'Ashes of Roses'	Bourjois	1	0
'Ashes of Violets'	Bourjois	1	0
'Eau de Cologne'	4711	2	6
'Phul Nana'	Grossmith	1	3
'Shem el Nessim'	Grossmith	1	3
'Lavender Water'	Potter & Moore	1	0
'June'	Saville	1	3
'Lavender Water'	Yardley	2	6

The above-named perfumes were, and those of them remaining today are, of excellent quality, and in most cases displayed the skill of the perfumer in replacing costly natural materials by bases of largely synthetic composition without greatly sacrificing 'natural-ness' of fragrance character. By this time, the prices of regularly used aroma chemicals had in real terms fallen drastically since they were first manufactured. This arose as a result of increasing demand, setting a trend that was to resume after the War with the need to perfume a completely new kind of product — the synthetic detergent.

In France before the First World War and in Germany between the Wars, synthetic chemicals were discovered which possessed the cleansing and foaming properties of soaps, but to a much greater degree and which were, unlike soaps, just as effective in hard water as in soft. During the Second World War, the shortage which arose of vegetable oils for soap-making gave impetus to the development of the manufacture of soap substitutes, using soapless detergents as the active ingredients. Later, following the cessation of hostilities, syn-thetic detergents ('syndets') were discovered which were far superior to soap in their detergent power, as well as in their emulsifying prop-erties for the manufacture of products for personal care and care of the home; products such as hair shampoos and conditioners, skin creams and lotions, dishwashing detergents, domestic laundry deter-gents and furniture polishes.

At the same time, traditional techniques of selling were undergo-ing profound change with the development of the theory and practice of mass-marketing. The customer, whose value was enshrined in the maxim 'the customer is always right' and recognized in the better shops by a high level of personal service, became the consumer, an entity to be tempted into sprees of self-selection by the sheer ease with which a wire trolley could be filled with groceries to the point of collapse. Once the advantages of self-selection became apparent, this form of selling spread to all but the most conservative of retail-ing establishments. Shops became known as 'retail outlets', and in the jargon of today they are called simply 'doors' — portals through which consumers rush to avail themselves of the necessities of civi-lized living and out through which they later rush in the opposite direction to get down to the business of consuming them.

By the 1950s, the unceasing quest of shoppers for preferred exist-ing products and for new ones that they had never before realized they needed, was firmly established as 'consumer demand'. The race by consumer product manufacturers to 'beat the competition' by im-proving their products already on the market and by inventing new ones that their competitors had not (yet) thought of was on, and flourishes today with unremitting zeal. It was in this era of burgeon-ing consumerism that the subject of fragrance came under the spot-light of marketing experts, in relation to the role it played in the sales promotion of non-food consumer products, which had already long been expressed by the affirmation that the 'the perfume sells the product' within the perfume and perfumed-product industries. The fact was well established that the comparative merits of different products having the same purpose and sold at about the same price were judged by consumers by opening the containers and taking a sniff at the contents thereof.

Perfume thus became all-important as a sales promoter and it was, in fact, discovered that consumers regarded the fragrance of a perfumed product as an inseparable part of that product, having much to do with the efficiency of the product in doing the job for which it was intended, rather than the completely nonfunctional additive that in fact it is. Tests were carried out in which two separate and identical lots of domestic laundry were machine-washed under the same conditions with the same washing powder, divided into two equal amounts, the only difference between the two lots of powder being that one was perfumed and the other unperfumed. Almost invariably, the perfumed powder was judged to have washed the laundry cleaner than the unperfumed powder. The perfume, therefore, had improved the *perceived* functional performance of the powder, even though it could not possibly have made any difference to its actual performance.

From the time in the 1950s when the commercial importance of perfume in functional consumer products was fully realized, and with the growth of the manufacturing industry that took place, the demand for perfume compounds, with respect to both quantity and variety, increased and consequently so did the demand for the requisite raw materials for their manufacture. The price levels at which it was necessary to sell functional products to be competitive in the market place had to be kept as low as possible, consistent with the value judgements of consumers (too low — 'inferior quality'; too high — 'find something cheaper!'). Since the perfume in such products was always the most expensive ingredient, its cost had to be kept as low as possible consistent with the need to convey to consumers through the medium of its fragrance clear impressions of high quality and functional superiority. To fulfil these requirements, many of the natural materials used in fine fragrance compositions were too costly, or unstable in functional product bases, or both, and had to be replaced by aroma chemicals.

The increased demand for aroma chemicals thereby generated resulted in the scaling-up of the processes for their manufacture, so reducing production costs per kilo and hence making possible reductions in selling prices to perfume manfacturers. The general upsurge of trade in aroma chemicals which took place in the late 1950s and the 1960s and 1970s financed not only improved production but also the research to discover new chemicals for the perfumer. This research yielded a veritable bonanza of success until the recent world recession of trade caused massive redirection of funds earmarked for research to more essential and immediately profitable purposes.

7.7 Imitating Nature

One of the most interesting and economically important applications of aroma chemicals is in the synthetic reproduction of the fragrances of flowers and other natural aromas. This commenced in France in the early years of the twentieth century. At this time, perfumers had perforce to rely on sensory evaluation and laborious procedures of chemical analysis for gaining information on the composition of natural sources of odour, such as essential oils.

Of the many different floral oils, the absolutes of the flowers of Rose, Jasmin and Violet (of which the last has long disappeared from the perfumer's shelves) together with the essential oil distilled from orange blossom, Neroli Oil, were known to produce highly appreciated perfumes when blended together in various proportions. Violet Flower Absolute was eventually replaced by Orris Oil, a solid essential oil having a fine violet-like odour, produced by the distillation of dried iris rhizome reduced to a fine powder, and the odours of Rose, Jasmin, Neroli and Orris became known as the 'big four' fragrance notes of perfumery. A fifth and greatly loved odour note was that of Lily-of-the-Valley, or Muguet, but for technical reasons it was found impossible to produce either an essential oil or an absolute from the flowers. The nearest approach to a Lily-of-the-Valley fragrance before the advent of aroma chemicals was produced by blending *extraits* (alcoholic solutions prepared from flowers) of Rose and Lilac. The synthesis in Germany of the fragrant chemical hydroxycitronellal and its commercial availability as a perfume ingredient in 1905 was a great forward step in the realization of 'true-to-nature' Lily-of-the-Valley fragrances. 'Hydroxy', as this chemical came to be called, with its note of lilies and lime blossom, was for about twenty years the only synthetic fragrance of its type and was eventually manufactured in tonnage quantities as a most versatile ingredient of countless perfumes.

Using 'hydroxy' and other fragrant chemicals discovered in the early years of the twentieth century, perfumers found possible the reproduction of an ever-widening range of natural scents, although for really convincing results proportions of carefully selected natural products were essential. Once GLC analysis had revealed the true complexity of natural perfumery materials, and the identity of some of their important minor and trace constituents had become known, it was realized that the 'naturalness' conferred upon a perfume by the skilled use of appropriate essential oils and absolutes was due to the contributions to the fragrance profile of these same constituents, many of which were of extremely powerful odour. Imagine trying to duplicate the special, 'naturalizing' bouquet of an essential oil of upwards of three hundred constituents using aroma chemicals, many of which had yet to be synthesized — an impossible task! This kind of 'creative enhancement' of blends of aroma chemicals remains necessary even today, when so many more naturally occurring minor and trace constituents of essential oils are available as aroma chemicals than were at the beginning of this century. It is simply impracticable to attempt a total reproduction of, for example, the composition of a variety of rose from an analysis of its scent; nor, fortunately, is it necessary to attempt to do so, for it has been found that by no means all constituents of a natural product make essential contributions to the character and 'naturalness' of its fragrance profile.

The first synthetic reproductions of flower fragrances to be widely accepted and used as perfume ingredients were remarkable for their time — beautiful in concept and effective in their application to the creation of quality fragrances; some remain in use today, as highly regarded as ever they were. Such products, which aim to simulate the fragrances of the natural sources of odour that they represent, rather than duplicating the composition and odours of the essential oils and other perfume ingredients obtained from them, are known as *bases*; they save the creative perfumer much time and trouble, and among them are today numbered products representing not only the scents of nature, but also abstract fragrance ideas; brilliant, imaginative odour effects to inspire the perfumer to new heights of creativity.

7.8 Simulating Natural Products

As we have noted, the odour of a distilled essential oil differs from that of its source because the harsh conditions of its production alter the compostition of the oil by chemical changes such as hydrolysis. Essential oils are most valuable ingredients of high quality perfumes; but the best suffer from natural variations in their odour profiles and relatively high cost. For both reasons a preoccupation of perfumers of technical inclination has always been their synthetic reproduction, particularly in the case of the more costly of regularly used oils, such as Bergamot, Ylang-Ylang and Geranium, and the very expensive absolutes of Jasmin, Rose, Hyacinth, Tuberose and other flowers. Technical artistry of this kind has been brought to a high level of perfection over the past thirty years and has resulted in the production of the so-called 'reconstitutions', or synthetic equivalents, of many natural perfumery materials at fractions of the costs of their natural counterparts. Thus, in a perfume formulation, a high-cost natural material may be partially or even totally replaced by a corresponding reconstitution of good quality without noticeably (at any rate to the untrained nose) compromising on fragrance quality, but with considerable saving on cost. Cost-cutting is an exercise frequently demanded by product manufacturers trying to maintain competitive price levels against inflation.

The demand for perfume compounds of all kinds could not possibly be met today by the world's total production of natural materials alone, a situation which underlines the importance of aroma chemicals as perfume ingredients. Their bulk manufacture and purification to high levels of safety and fragrance quality have been instrumental in promoting the growth of the perfume industry to its present-day level of creative and technological capability and have enormously benefitted the consumer, whose choice of expertly fragranced products is now wider than ever before.

7.9 Exploring the Scents of Living Flowers

Perfumery without flowers is almost unthinkable. We have already noted the importance of the 'big five' fragrance notes Rose, Jasmin, Neroli, Violet/Orris and Muguet, and it is significant that of all of the great classic perfumes for women embody these notes, either as the complete fragrance entities or as representative ingredients. Fragrances for men — shaving lotions, antiperspirants, colognes, etc. — generally employ floral elements at lower levels of concentration in favour of the accentuation of citrus, herbaceous, woody and musky–ambergris notes, yet notes of flowers remain important.

By the 1970s, GLC analysis coupled with mass spectrometry for determining the composition of essential oils and aromatic extracts, had become so revealing a research tool that detailed knowledge in this area was rapidly accumulating. Very little of a definite nature had, however, been discovered of the composition of the truly natural fragrances exhaled by living flowers until, in 1980, a programme of investigation to this end was launched by one of the international perfume and flavour companies. Something of the difficulty of work of this nature can be imagined when it is realized that the weight of the volatiles per litre of air entering the nose on smelling a flower is of the order of no more than a few billionths of a gram — about a thousand times less, at the time, than the least amount required for the most sensitive technique of GLC analysis available. Concentration of the volatiles was therefore necessary, and this was achieved by the capture of natural fragrances, using either a very efficient condenser, called a *cold trap*, or by adsorption onto the surface of a specially prepared, chemically inert, granular solid.

The technique developed is known as the *capture of headspace volatiles*. A single fragrant blossom or inflorescence is enclosed in a perfectly clean and odour-free glass bulb fitted with two side-arms, through one of which purified and odour-free air is slowly pumped into the bulb. The air carries the volatiles responsible for the scent of the flower out of the bulb via the other side-arm to a narrow glass tube, called a *microfilter*, containing a few milligrams of a finely granular adsorbent, onto the surface of which molecules of the volatiles stick as the air carrying them flows over it. Once the adsorbent has trapped sufficient of the volatiles for analysis, the pump is turned off and the microfilter detached. The trapped volatiles are then desorbed from the adsorbent by gentle heat or by using specially purified organic solvents, and their composition is determined by capillary GLC and mass spectrometry (fig. 7.2).

This ingenious technique has yielded most interesting and sometimes surprising information. Constituents of totally unexpected

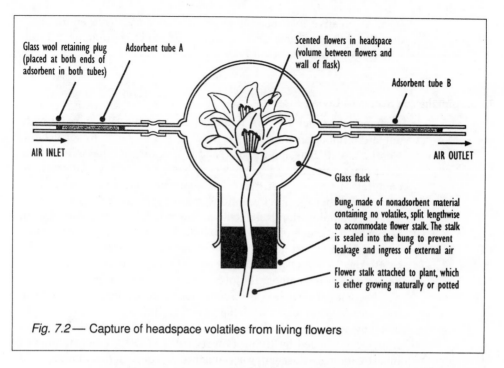

Glass wool retaining plug
(placed at both ends of
adsorbent in both tubes)

Adsorbent tube A

Scented flowers in headspace
(volume between flowers and
wall of flask)

Adsorbent tube B

AIR INLET

AIR OUTLET

Glass flask

Bung, made of nonadsorbent material
containing no volatiles, split lengthwise
to accommodate flower stalk. The stalk
is sealed into the bung to prevent
leakage and ingress of external air

Flower stalk attached to plant, which
is either growing naturally or potted

Fig. 7.2 — Capture of headspace volatiles from living flowers

composition have been identified and molecules of novel structure discovered. In recent years, the data obtained by headspace capture has been applied to the development of fragrance compositions of greatly enhanced natural quality to intrigue the nose of the consumer.

Of more academic interest are the discoveries of differences, in some cases very marked, between the composition of the fragrance from the same flower before and after detachment from its stalk, from different flowers on the same plant at the same time of day or night, and from the same flower as daytime yields to nightfall.

We should finally note that only in a computerized world is it possible to store, correlate and make readily available for future use the mass of data on the composition and odours given by headspace analysis coupled with sensory evaluation. The practical value of this information lies in identifying constituents which, if of truly novel and supremely useful character, may be synthesized as the aroma chemicals of tomorrow, to be woven into sparkling new fragrance ideas by the fertile, creative mind and technical skill of the artist in fragrance.

Chapter 8

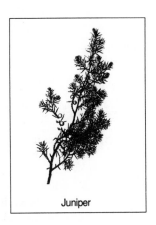

Juniper

Perfumery — The Fragrant Art

8.1 Origins of Perfumery

Perfumery is believed to have originated at the dawn of civilization, when it was first observed by early man that certain woods, twigs, barks, leaves and resinous matter from plants gave forth pleasing aromas when left smouldering on a fire. Much later, with the development of nomadic, tribal societies, there arose notions of omnipotent beings who possessed supernatural powers to control parts of the natural world, and the sometimes violent and frightening phenomena of tempest, earthquake and volcanic eruption. These were the gods of primitive civilizations, who were to be believed in, worshipped and placated for the good of the tribe and to dispel evil spirits.

One form of symbolic representation adopted in antiquity was provided by the burning of aromatic plant matter, the ascending smoke lending visible reality to the supplications of believers and providing atmospheres conducive to worship. This form of religious symbolism has, as we know, persisted through the ages of mankind to the present day, passing from pagan ceremonial into the great religions of the world, the means for its expression developing from the use of fragments of plant matter to that of various forms of manufactured incense composed of much the same materials, granulated or ground to powder in proportions prescribed by ancient recipes. Today, in traditional high church ceremonial worship, granules of frankincense are heated in a censer, or thurible, by means of glowing charcoal kept burning by a gentle flow of air. The incense is not burned in the thurible, but is vaporized, with some decomposition, to produce the smoke and characteristic, sombre fragrance. The smoke from incense is composed of a complex mixture of volatiles, some of which are of very low volatility and so readily condense on surfaces with which the smoke comes into contact. Hence the 'smell of incense' one notices on entering a place of worship where incense is used. The smell of frankincense granules is quite different from that of the vapours they produce on heating, since only the more volatile constituents of the material are released at room temperature and because much of the essential oil it contains is trapped by its high content of odourless resin.

A more long-lasting offering to the deity took the form of vegetable oil in which had been soaked aromatic herbs, flowers or other scented parts of plants which, it had been discovered, would impart their fragrance to the oil if the two were left in contact over a sufficient period of time. In this way, the first liquid perfumes were produced, at first exclusively as gifts of rarity to the gods, and then later to God by His earthly representatives, the priests.

In course of time, the oily perfumes made by the priests of old became appropriated by ruling monarchs for their own use, then by the dignitaries of their households and eventually by the priests themselves. The ultimate step in the secularization of perfumes came when the priests who made them found a ready market for their sale among the general population, so that they could make their own offerings to the 'Gods of the Hearth', who were believed to protect the household from harm, and for use as gifts to the rich and powerful and to the nobility, and also as personal fragrances. In this way there arose the tradition of the giving of perfume as something precious and personal to honour the recipient, as exemplified at the Nativity, which we maintain today. The modern perfumer is the direct professional descendent of the priests of antiquity, whose tradition of closely guarded secrecy is perpetuated in the computerized security systems of every creative perfume laboratory.

8.2 What is an Art?

We may attempt to answer this question by reflecting on what is involved in painting a picture — the activity which usually springs to mind whenever the subject of art is mentioned.

First, there has to be some form of desire to represent something or to communicate an idea, by means of shapes, forms and colours, on paper, canvas or other suitable surface. Inseparably from a general urge to paint, the artist must have at least the germ of an idea of what to paint — a vision which at the most sublime level comes to mind through inspiration — a kind of synthesis of the elements of a mental construct arising from an immediate experience involving visual, aural, tactile, olfactory or gustatory sensations, either singly or in combination, or from memory of an experience of the past. Such inspiration may cause the artist to form trains of thought, to be brought together, arranged, rearranged, perhaps given expression in the form of sketches, and finally lodged in the mind, there to await expression as the visual image of a painting. More dramatically, an inspiration can be quite sudden and physically breathtaking, the pieces falling together as though directed by some external agency, quite independently of any effort on the part of the artist. Imagery so synthe-sized can be demanding of immediate expression, and may be lost *forever* if not recorded in some way at the time of inspiration. For this reason, a poet or author is well advised to carry a voice recorder at all times.

In the context of commercial art, the subject to be represented arises from a need to communicate the virtues of something in order to attract sales, whether that 'something' is a product of some kind, a theatrical performance or the Cup Final. Cleverly designed commer-cial artistry, extending through to the vocal art of the salesperson, is *the* positive catalyst for sales, and since sales, and ultimately sales alone, keep us all in the land of the living, all forms of commercial art are of the greatest importance to the perpetuation of our civiliza-tion.

A concept to be expressed by an artist may be concrete — an object or collection of objects — or abstract, arising from the imagi-nation and not directly representative of anything of material nature. Whatever the subject may be, its artistic representation requires some kind of interpretation, if only translation from three dimensions into two. In commercial art, review of past successes and failures and research into the work of other artists may be helpful in achieving the desired goal. Drawings, sketches and models can all help towards bringing the subject to life until, one morning, all is ready. Brushes, paints and canvas are to hand, the studio illumination is adjusted, and the artist sets to work.

The extent to which a work of art is fully communicative of the subject given expression depends on the technique employed by the artist for its realization and his skill in using it. The word 'creativ-ity', a term often associated with the arts, implies the bringing into existence of something having no prior existence; in reference to an art, it refers to the bringing together, or arrangement, of the elements of the art — colours, musical notes, contours, mathematical symbols, fragrance notes — in sequences, patterns or combinations which are *original*. In painting, this amounts to the making of an original ar-rangement of forms and colours, which together give expression to the artist's interpretation of what he or she sees, feels or imagines.

Thus far, then, we can propose that an art is a means for creative self-expression arising from some form of inspiration, employing a medium of some kind for the purpose of communicating the ideas of the artist and demanding a skilled technique for their representation.

Much of art is concerned with the expression of beauty, though this is by no means necessarily so, as a visit to an art gallery will soon reveal. For a painting or other art-form to be accorded the dis-tinction of being regarded as a work of art, however, it must have aesthetic appeal, and here we encounter very strong elements of sub-jectivity, for that which is beautiful to one observer may not be beau-tiful to another. It is, furthermore, possible for someone to find beauty expressed in artistic representation of scenes of the most terrible violence and carnage, perhaps because of the artist's sensitivity in creating the portrayal, or skill in using dramatic cloudscape to impart living impact to the awful scene that we behold. All of this, and more, is embodied in our appreciation of a work of art, which is always a highly subjective assessment of its merits — a matter of individual opinion and judgement. The same elements of subjectivity are involved in our response to the other visual arts, and to music. Mathematics is essentially impersonal, but can be wondrously beautiful in the insights that it gives us into the nature of the physical world and in the ways in which great mathematicians explore its pathways for enlightenment or for the solution of problems. Perfumery is different.

Whereas perfumers of former generations found time for the contemplation of fragrance for its own sake and for reflection, almost at leisure, on ways in which natural fragrances might be represented, interpreted or combined, albeit ultimately to achieve a commercial purpose, the thoughts of modern perfumers are very much concerned with the achievement of fragrant commercial goals within tight time schedules and sometimes severe limitations of cost. Practice of the arts associated with the sales promotion of perfumes and other fragranced products, involving as they do the design of containers, packaging, advertisements and promotional presentations, demands for success detailed knowledge of the various forms of social grouping (age, sex, ethnic origin, income, fragrance preferences, etc.) in order to establish as closely as possible which designs will be most likely to attract consumers in the market for which the product is intended. This involves detailed studies of currently successful products of the same kind, coupled with an estimation of their likely future progress in the market place. A further, unique aspect of perfumery is that it is almost entirely concerned with the production of odours which are pleasing to the human sense of smell, and with odours which cover or eliminate unpleasant odours. Finally, we should note the powerful influence on sales of a fragranced product of a promotional association between the product and a currently popular personality of sport or entertainment. Recommendations of this kind, entering the home via fashion magazine or television, suggest worlds of glamour which no-one really believes are attainable through the use of any product, but which may in the imagination be contemplated for a while through the magic of an artist in fragrance.

8.3 A Perfumer's Training

Throughout its history, from beginnings in the ancient world, development in Greece and Rome, during its spread throughout Europe and into the Americas and in modern practice, perfumery has been and remains a secret art. Formulae for successful perfumes constitute a perfume company's greatest asset and are protected by some of the tightest security systems available. Using instrumental analytical procedures in combination with sensory evaluation, it is nevertheless usually possible for a rival perfume company to produce a good match of an originator's perfume for almost any given product with a little expenditure of time and trouble, provided that the necessary sensory and analytical skills are available, and it is this proviso which acts as a brake to the wholesale copying of perfumes by any-one and everyone. Good noses command good salaries, and not only is the analytical equipment also required costly, but so are the spe-cialists needed to operate it and to interpret correctly the results it yields. It is, of course, the perfumer whose responsibility it is to pass judgement on a perfume put together as the result of an analysis, and to know how to adjust its composition to match the original in the product for which the match is required, so that it will be safe and compatible with the product base under all anticipated conditions of storage and use.

In every form of art there are practitioners who never undergo a day's formal training throughout their lives. Some of these excep-tionally gifted people display extraordinary degrees of creativity and perfection of technique. In perfumery, the existence of such natural proficiency is usually discovered in adulthood, mainly for the reason that, apart from a small number of them, aromatic materials are un-available beyond the confines of the perfume or flavour laboratory and those few institutions offering courses in perfumery. Thus, in contrast to the practice in other arts, only relatives of perfumers are ever likely to find opportunities to 'dabble' in the fragrant art. How, then, did people working in the perfume industry ever find their way into it? The simple answer is, with the exception of those having family connections in perfumery, mostly by chance. For example, a school leaver seeks temporary work for a few weeks after sitting 'A' levels before going on to university or taking up a chosen career, and finds a job washing bottles in a factory making perfumes. Becoming interested in the multitude of smells and noticing that some of their names are similar to the names of chemicals used in 'A' Level chem-istry, the student begins to haunt the perfume laboratory during the lunch-break. This interest is noticed by the perfumers, and the bottle-washer is given a trial as a perfumer's assistant. The important step has been taken; the candidate is accepted for training within the com-pany, works hard, studies the books and papers diligently, takes every opportunity to learn and experiment and is eventually pro-moted to Junior Perfumer: a perfumer at last! But this achievement, the result of complete dedication to the task in hand over several years, is but a beginning, for full professional status as yet lies sev-eral more years in the future.

The one essential qualification a candidate for training as a per-fumer must have is a normal sense of smell. Sensitivity to odours does vary among individuals, though rarely much beyond the norm. Professional training in perfumery has no effect on the sensitivity of the olfactory organ, but acts to develop the mind, tuning it in to the world of smells, developing the memory for odours and combinations and sequences of odours and their perceived relationships with other forms of sensory input to the mind — visual, aural, tactile and gustatory — while all the time enhancing the perception of the trainee of finer and finer differences between odours which to the layman seem identical. All this is achieved through a structured programme of sensory experience of individual aromatic materials, experiments to discover the odour effects of materials in combination — the *accords* of perfumery, which are analogous to chords of musical notes — and, early on in the programme, 'deep-end' exercises in which the candidate is given commercial perfumes to match — with no analytical aid other than his or her own nose. Practical sessions are interspersed with lectures on the history, art, technology and commercial aspects of perfumery, and include the vital subjects of applications of perfumes, product safety and legality and quality management, control and assurance. Most candidates take a course in cosmetic science, usually before entry to professional training, while some complete a correspondence course in perfumery either before or soon after entry into the industry to prepare for their careers. Commercially orientated candidates may opt for a degree course in the business of perfumery.

Since perfumery is fundamentally an art, proficiency can be gained only through unflagging interest, patience and experience, sustained by a clearly defined future goal and pursued with dedication. Underlying the art of perfumery is a technology, by the application of which the materials of the perfumer's palette are manufactured and the production of fully effective and otherwise totally acceptable perfume compounds made possible. In the practice of perfumery, art and technology merge, for the perfumer must be as familiar with the physicochemical properties of his materials as he is with their behaviour as elements of fragrance creation. Perfumes are made to be sold, and it is on his ability to produce successful perfumes that a perfumer's worth is judged. This will frequently involve the subjugation of a perfumer's standards of aesthetic excellence to those of his customers, in consideration of current fragrance trends in the market place for the various categories of consumer products. Thus do consumer preferences determine, to a very large extent, the nature of products offered for sale in the market-place and, in respect of perfumed products, the nature of the fragrances which proclaim the excellence of their performance. The training of a perfumer, through the matching of successful perfumes and modification of the resulting formulae for any desired application, provides the essentials of composition and technique upon which he or she can build successful personal approaches to the commercial and creative challenges to be faced on every working day.

Creativity in perfumery cannot be taught, but is either innate or develops in one way or another during training. Typical signs of latent creative originality are the ability to combine materials in just the right proportions to produce a desired fragrance effect, apparently with little difficulty, and the desire to wander from the beaten tracks of formulation to produce promising and sometimes intriguing and unconventional results. In the next section we shall discuss the matching and creation of perfumes in a little more detail.

8.4 The Fragrant Art

The perfume for a product, such as a toilet soap, hair shampoo, household detergent or pot-pourri, is normally selected from a number of samples submitted for the approval of the product manufacturer by several different perfume supply companies. Some weeks or months previously, a finished-product company will have determined the nature of a product to be launched and the kind of fragrance or fragrances believed best suited to its promotion, and will have prepared a document, known as a perfume brief, in which all the fragrance, technical, commercial and promotional information required by a perfumer in order to create a suitable perfume appears. The brief will also supply other important data, such as the final date for submission of perfume samples, how the samples are to be presented and the maximum price the manufacturer is prepared to pay for the perfume. This is the specification to which the several perfume companies normally briefed will work to produce what each one hopes will be the winning perfume. Ideally, the product manufacturer supplies a sample of the unperfumed product base, so that perfumes proposed for submission can be tested for compatibility with the base. Following discussion between the perfumer and representatives of the product company to clarify the terms of the brief, the perfumer secures the collaboration of an odour evaluator to select possible candidates for submission from the perfume company's fragrance library, which contains samples of both successful and failed perfume submissions of the past. One or more of these perfumes may be suitable for submission, though perusal of the formula and cost will usually indicate the need for adjustments to be made to the formula to comply with the terms of the brief in hand, and satisfy the perfumer that the fragrance is right for the product.

If the terms of the brief require the perfume to relate in its fragrance to an established, commercial perfume, then if not already available as a match sample in the fragrance library, a match of this perfume will have to be made. This involves, first of all, analysis of the perfume by gas–liquid chromatography (GLC) and, where interpretation of the results reveals the presence of unidentified ingredients, the use of other techniques to establish their composition. While this work is in progress, the perfumer, frequently with the collaboration of colleagues, makes a close sensory examination of the original perfume to determine, as far as possible, the patterns of composition which form its fragrance profile, from top note through to final dryout. The perfumer's training, in being required to match perfumes without the aid of analytical instruments, is here invaluable.

From the results of analysis, a formula is written from which a 'GLC match' of the perfume is prepared. Depending on the amount of analytical information obtained, this may or may not resemble the original perfume. Using his creative and technical skills, the perfumer then sets about the task of making as close a match of the perfume as is necessary for the completion of this stage of the work. Usually, a brief will not demand an exact copy of an existing perfume, but either a match sufficiently close to be familiar to consumers in some way, but distinguished from the original by a creative 'twist of originality' that will set the product apart from others of a similar kind, or some lesser resemblance to the original, to be incorporated, perhaps, as just one element of the fragrance profile. To test the correspondence of the fragrance of a match sample of a perfume to the original, a perfumer frequently uses the *triangle test*, in which two smelling strips are impregnated with the original perfume or with the match sample and a third strip with the other. The strips are coded for easy identification and then smelled in turn, with the identification marks concealed. If, then, the sample that is different from the other two can be identified without difficulty, the match sample is not close to the original and may need further work in order to make it so. If a test of this kind is carried out formally, by an odour evaluation panel, results are recorded by the members on an equilateral triangle, the apexes of which are marked with the codes inscribed on the smelling strips, either by means of an 'equals' sign placed between the code markings of the identical samples and crosses between the different ones, or by ringing the code marking of the 'odd man out'. The triangle test is repeated at predetermined intervals of time in order to assess the correspondence of the match sample and original at different stages during their evaporation.

Fortunately for the progress of perfumery, the present-day emphasis on fragrance matching has not resulted in the complete demise of creativity. Consumers do, however, tend to reject a totally novel fragrance that does not relate to anything with which they are already familiar. Thus perfumers tend to produce perfumes which relate to the highly appreciated fragrances of successful consumer products that have made names for themselves in the market-place. This greatly reduces the possibility of the commercial failure of a perfumed product and loss of its development, promotion and launch costs, which can today amount to a seven-figure sum.

Many of the perfumes used for fragrancing functional consumer products are based on more or less original ideas conceived in the fine-fragrance sector of perfumery, where cost restrictions are not so stringent and where, therefore, high-quality ingredients can be used which these restrictions would prohibit in more general applications, such as in perfumes for personal-care and domestic products. Fine fragrances are so called for the excellence of their fragrance qualities; they are created for use as personal perfumes and for the highest quality toilet preparations. When speaking of the 'quality' of a perfume we enter further realms of subjectivity, for not only are there many standpoints from which quality may be judged, but also the very act of passing judgement is subject to the vagaries of human opinion. A reasonable and practical approach to the assessment of fragrance quality is to follow the practice of the wine-taster and gain the required basis of knowledge through experience and practice. A period of employment at the perfumery counter of an establishment selling perfumes would be excellent for this purpose.

Until the early 1960s the 'quality' element of a fine fragrance was impossible to reproduce without the use of expensive, natural ingredients; thus a match of such a perfume could be made for, say, a toilet soap to be sold in the middle price range, and the soap would smell like the perfume — but that would be all; the 'luxury' aspect of the fragrance would be missing. 'If only', a perfumer would think, '....if only I could find something to give this perfume the *quality* of a fine fragrance without going over the top with the cost'. But every perfumer knew this to be impossible — every perfumer, that is, excepting one, who, like Parquet of Houbigant, was prepared to question the pontifications of convention and experiment with a newly synthesized aroma chemical, again as it happened, as an ingredient of a perfume for a toilet soap. The result was little short of a miracle, in the form of a perfume of modest cost which clearly displayed impressions of the high quality associated with the best of fashion fragrances. Using newly developed techniques of analysis, the secret of this remarkable achievment was ultimately revealed, but by that time effective sales promotion, coupled with the truly revolutionary fragrance breakthrough that it supported, was well on the way to establishing for the product a name which would become a household word, as it is today.

We have discussed something of the nature of creativity in perfumery, but how does a perfumer translate his ideas into a perfume? Whatever the creative technique he adopts, the ingredients for the perfume are combined in consideration of their properties of odour profile, odour strength and odour persistence or lasting power, diffusiveness, etc., always with reference to other important data, such as physicochemical behaviour, safety in use, legality in the country of import, and so on. The great French perfumer Jean Carles, among whose creations was the perfume 'Ma Griffe' (meaning 'My Signature') launched by Carven in 1944, advocated a simple method, based on the concept of fragrance 'accords'. If, for example, in following the recommendations of Carles, a perfumer first makes a mental or written sketch of the perfume to be created, this becomes a goal towards which to work. The fundamental note of the main fragrance theme of the perfume is then identified, and a suitable ingredient having this note is chosen, together with a second ingredient representing a further important note. In the case of a fine fragrance, let the first ingredient be Sandalwood Oil and the second a skin-safe Oakmoss Base. The ingredients are mixed in the following proportions by counting drops (preferably with the sample container tared on an electronic balance so that the actual weights of all ingredients will be known):

	A	B	C	D	E
Sandalwood Oil, East Indian	9	8	7	6	5
Oakmoss Base	1	2	3	4	5

The accord to be created is based on sandalwood and not on oakmoss, and so, according to Carles, the proportion of Sandalwood Oil must not be less than that of the Oakmoss Base.

The five accords are carefully smelled, and that which most closely represents the desired approach to the base of the perfume (C, say) is selected for further experiment. A third important ingredient is, let us say, a synthetic musk base which, because of its strength, may have to be used as a 10 per cent solution:

	F	G	H	I	J
Accord C	9	8	7	6	5
Musk Base, 10%	1	2	3	4	5

The best of this second series of accords, F to J, is now chosen, and as many further experiments are completed as are necessary to produce the main theme of the perfume, using the same technique. Modifiers of the fragrance may now be incorporated to complete the main theme in accordance with the original plan. These will certainly include floral elements in some proportions — higher for a feminine fragrance and lower in the case of a perfume for a masculine toilet water — also other notes, such as herbaceous, green, spicy, fruity, etc., as necessary for achievement of the desired fragrance profile. The completed 'main theme complex' consists of both middle and basic notes in terms of volatility and may already be sufficiently well blended, so that individual notes merge to form a single, complex fragrance impression, which may be long-lasting if required, in the product under in-use conditions (on the skin, for example). If it is not sufficiently well blended, then appropriate adjustments are made to the formula. The top note accord or complex is then created using the same procedure and is then blended with the base in the most effective proportions. Further adjustment may finally be necessary in respect of the proportions of basic, middle and top notes, also to provide sufficient 'lift' of lower notes into the top, for which Ylang-Ylang Oil, Extra, is one of the best-known agents. Jean Carles' technique may be used for the construction of perfumes at all levels of cost, the only drawback being that it is time-consuming. It is, however, time-saving in research to find suitable applications for newly discovered aroma chemicals, in comparison with the 'trial and error' approach so often adopted in everyday perfumery. This usually yields acceptable and sometimes good results, though probably not the best that could be achieved, given sufficient time.

We should note that for some products — dishwashing detergents, for example — a fragrance must have impact when the product is used, but no lasting power, while, conversely, certain fragrance elements of perfumes for domestic laundry products are required to be substantive to textiles; that is, they must cling to the fibres, surviving the washing, rinsing and drying cycle to give a lingering odour impression of clean freshness.

A recent invention of considerable interest to perfumers is that of the 'artificial nose', which depends for the detection of odorous molecules on their adsorption onto specially prepared surfaces. This causes energy changes which when amplified are used to record graphically a profile related to the odour of the stimulant molecules. If the current rate of the advance of technology is any yardstick, it would seem likely that the electronic 'sniffers' currently in use in perfumery, brewing and other industries where odour or flavour quality is an all-important feature of product appeal, will quickly be superseded by others of far greater versatility and sensitivity, making possible the preparation of detailed and reliable 'olfactograms' of all commercial perfumes. Such a development might well open up opportunities for the patenting of a *fragrance* (as distinct from its formula) as intellectual property, rendering its matching or the creation of a similar fragrance (whatever the formula) illegal.

As in all spheres of human activity, the wonders of today become unremarkable features of everyday life tomorrow. Thus today we find the brightest stars among recently discovered aroma chemicals sitting on the shelves of the perfume laboratory alongside those of fifty years ago — all nevertheless capable of renewed brilliance in the hands of the artist in fragrance.

8.5 Perfume Manufacture

Whether conducted on a small or large scale, the operations of perfume manufacture are in principle very simple. The ingredients, always double-checked for their identity by odour and by container label, are weighed into a mixing vessel of glass or stainless steel, and stirred, each item being marked off on a formula sheet as the work progresses. Minimum heat is, if necessary, applied to effect solution of solid or semi-solid ingredients and following thorough final mixing, the resulting compound (known also as perfume oil or 'juice') is filtered into a suitable container for transport to the customer, who incorporates it into an unperfumed product base to form the product to be launched into the market.

The ingredients of a perfume oil are weighed and mixed according to a formula prepared for bulk manufacture and in the predetermined order specified on the formula sheet, which today usually takes the form of a computer printout. In general, large quantities of stable ingredients of low viscosity and moderate to low volatility go in first, and in this preliminary mixture are dissolved any solids and semi-solids included in the formula. Stirring is continuous and any heat applied is kept to a minimum consistent with rapid dissolution. Any other ingredients of low volatility (basic notes) are then incorporated. If heating has been employed, the mixture is then cooled before adding readily oxidizable ingredients, such as fatty aldehydes, delicate essential oils, for example Bergamot Oil, and finally, any other top notes which have not already been added. The finished perfume compound is then further stirred, but not so rapidly that air is pulled in by a 'whirlpool' or vortex effect, and is then filled into storage containers via an on-line cartridge filter. The logic of this compounding sequence is fully justifiable on grounds of preservation of the integrity of the ingredients. In some large perfume manufacturing installations the compounding operations are fully automated under computerized control, so almost completely eliminating the possibility of error.

Ideally, perfume compounds should be allowed to age at a cool temperature for at least one month following compounding, to allow time for reactive ingredients to interact. Certain alcohols, for example, present in a perfume as constituents of one or more essential oils, or as aroma chemicals, are capable of reacting with esters or with aldehydes, and also with the traces of free organic acids frequently found in essential oils. Many other odour-changing reactions are also possible. All this chemical activity takes time to reach a state of equilibrium, and when it does so the compound may be said to have reached a metastable state, meaning that further change of composition, and hence of odour, will normally be very slight if the compound is left alone, but that they could be rapid if it is exposed to the air or incorporated into a product base. The purpose of ageing a perfume compound is in most cases immediately obvious on comparing the odour of a fully aged compound with that of the same compound freshly prepared. Ageing noticeably improves the blending of the different fragrance notes of the ingredients into a coherent, complex odour impression, within which it is difficult to identify any one component. Conversely, in experimental work, ageing can reveal formulation errors by the appearance of harsh, sickly sweet or other unfortunate odour effects.

The object of perfuming a product is first of all to mask or eliminate any objectionable odour present in the unperfumed product base, such as may occur, for example, in toilet soap noodles or in shampoo, hair conditioner or detergent base formulations. In alcoholic perfumery, ethanol of perfumery quality presents no problems in this respect, but alcohol does possess an alcoholic or vinous smell which slowly softens if the final product is, like a wine, allowed to mature.

The primary purpose of perfume is to impart pleasing fragrance to persons or products, or to the air. A personal fragrance should help to enhance the image the user wishes to present to the world at large and this fact needs to be considered when a perfume or toilet water is bought as a gift. In a functional consumer product the mission of the fragrance is, as we have seen, to promote sales of the product, to which end it is designed to convince the user of the excellence of the product for its purpose. Here, the psychological skills of the perfumer, working in collaboration with marketing personnel, are combined with a high degree of aesthetic sensitivity and creative flair in an all-out effort to make the product a commercial success. The product base must, of course, fulfil the promise of the fragrance and all other aspects of the promotion of the product regarding the excellence of its functional performance, otherwise nothing the perfumer can do will prevent its failure in the market place.

Almost all product bases are chemically or physically reactive in one or more ways, and so a perfume must be composed with regard to its mutual compatibility with the product base. The essential requirement of perfume/product base stability during the anticipated period and under the anticipated conditions of the storage and use of the product, is investigated by testing the finished, perfumed product in its container and packaging under conditions far more severe than it is ever likely to have to withstand in the hands of the retailer and user.

Since product bases vary widely in composition and hence in the nature of their physicochemical reactivity, a perfume compound which is fully compatible with a given product base may not be compatible with another. Hence for a line of products — perfume, toilet water, talcum powder, toilet soap, etc. — required to display the *same* fragrance, a perfume compound of somewhat different composition from all the others will be likely to be required for each of them.

The most popular kind of perfume for personal use has traditionally taken the form of a solution of a perfume compound in alcohol, or aqueous alcohol in the case of toilet waters, such as eau de parfum, eau de toilette, aftershave lotion, etc. A product of this kind is made by dissolving the compound in ethanol of the required strength to make a solution containing upwards of 10 per cent compound for extrait and below 10 per cent for toilet water. Traces of an antioxidant and a sunscreen may be added to combat the worst ravages of improper storage as, for example, in a shop window or on a dressing table in full sunlight, or misuse, such as the common but destructive practice of upending an opened bottle of perfume on the skin, while in toilet waters a small proportion of an emollient may be added to prevent dehydration of the skin. A trace of a harmless dye is sometimes used to impart to a watery-looking creation the appearance of richness it fully deserves or to transform a special but quite ordinary-looking perfume into something mysterious and exciting. Many essential oils, the chamomiles and untreated citrus oils, for example, also a few aroma chemicals, exist as coloured products, and so by no means do all coloured perfumes contain added colour.

Once upon a time all extrait perfumes and toilet waters were allowed to mature before being filled into their containers ready for sale. Some still are, but not usually for the long periods of time that were once the rule; a reflection of the urgency of commercial activity characteristic of our time.

8.6 Quality Control of Perfume Compounds

The quality of perfume compounds is controlled and checked by procedures similar to those employed for essential oils, described in Chapter 6. Most important are the evaluation of fragrance profile and of the results of gas–liquid chromatography and infrared spectrophotometry, all of which are made comparatively, with reference to samples of previous batches of the same perfume or, better, to standard samples, accurately prepared in the laboratory using ingredients drawn from current factory stocks.

Compounding deficiencies, i.e. ingredients short-weighed or omitted altogether, are serious enough, reflecting unfavourably on vigilance during compounding. Errors of this nature can, however, be easily remedied, as bulk compounds are held in mixing vessels until cleared by the quality control laboratory. This is not, however, the case where an ingredient is found to be in excess of the quantity required or where a wrong ingredient has been accidentally substituted for the right one, the outcome of which, once the ensuing ructions have subsided, will depend on several factors, not the least of which will be the quantity of perfume compounded. For example, an excess of 5 per cent of Geranium Oil in a 50 kg batch would be a nuisance to correct by proportional addition of all the other ingredients, to produce a 100 kg quantity of the perfume, 50 kg of which could be consigned to cold storage in the hope that it could be sold to the same customer in fulfilment of the next order. More life-threatening would be, for instance, the mistaken use of the prescribed quantity of a 100 per cent fatty aldehyde in place of the required 10 per cent solution in a 1000 kg batch. If all resources of ingenuity fail to solve a problem of this kind, efforts are made to salvage at least something from the disaster by first attempting to render the odour of the product acceptable for some purpose or other — in this case as a perfume for a disinfectant, for example, by loading it with, say, isobornyl acetate, a pine-smelling aroma chemical, and then selling it as a 'one-off' supply at an attractive price.

The work of a perfume compounder is comparable, with respect to the vigilance and accuracy required, with the dispensing of medicines by the pharmacist of a decade or so ago, with the difference that the consequences of a compounding error are more likely to be financially disastrous than physically harmful.

As in the sensory evaluation of essential oils, careful smelling by trained and experienced odour evaluators can reveal odour differences between freshly prepared and stored standard samples of the same perfume that are impossible to correlate with any difference of composition revealed by chromatography, the differences being so small as not to show up on comparison of the respective chromatograms. There are many possible causes of such differences, the most common being variations in the composition of any essential oils present in the perfume — variations that have not been sufficiently evident for their rejection following delivery — and the quality differences almost always found on comparing a fully aged perfume compound with a freshly prepared sample of the same perfume. A further possibility is the presence of lingering 'still notes' in one or more of the essential oils in the perfume, which will have long vanished from the sample kept as an odour standard and which will disappear from the batch sample of perfume before it is used by the customer. Notes of this kind are produced when culinary vegetables, such as cabbage, are cooked by treatment with boiling water.

Ideally, to maximize the uniformity of fragrance quality of a perfume compound and the product for which it is intended, all batches of the compound should be allowed to age over the same period of time before being incorporated into the product in exactly the same way. In the case of an alcoholic perfume, all batches of the bulk finished product should be allowed to mature under the same conditions before chilling, cold filtration and filling.

8.7 Fragrance Experiments with Essential Oils

Perfumes of today contain appreciable and frequently high proportions of aroma chemicals, none of which are generally available except to the perfume, food flavour and other industries needing them. These industries purchase bulk supplies of aroma chemicals, 50 kg of some of them representing a very small order indeed. Thus, many extremely useful fragrance notes are simply unavailable to the intending experimenter not employed in one or other of the user-industries. Arising mainly from the practice of aromatherapy, however, is the availability of quite a wide range of essential oils for professional application, while a smaller range is found on open sale in the pharmacy (where once many of them were in regular medicinal use), beauty salon or department store for domestic aromatherapeutic treatments and the making of room fragrances. These oils may usefully be employed for experimental work on fragrance composition within the limitations of what is available.

Essential oils are expensive if purchased in small quantities, and so for the purpose of blending experiments it is advantageous to use them in the form of solutions in an odourless solvent. In industry, several solvents, including perfumery-grade ethanol, are to hand for this purpose, but none are generally available in small quantities. An acceptable alternative is to be found in refined Jojoba Oil, which in this quality grade, beside being a good solvent for essential oils, is a colourless, almost odourless, mobile liquid which remains liquid down to about 12°C, below which temperature it freezes to a waxy, semi-crystalline mass. Solutions of essential oils in Jojoba Oil freeze at lower temperatures. Grades of Jojoba Oil that do not conform to the above specification are unsuitable for the purpose under discussion because they carry a not unpleasant, but oily odour.

The equipment needed for making up solutions for blending experiments, and for the experiments themselves, is very simple, consisting of supplies of the following items:

> Amber glass, screw-capped, 10 ml dropper bottles for solutions
> Amber glass, screw-capped, 10 ml sample bottles for experiments
> Labels for the solution and sample bottles
> Glass teat-pipettes, all of the same kind, if required
> Smelling strips
> *Refined* Jojoba Oil
> Essential oils

Regarding the pipettes or droppers, these must be cleaned and rendered odour-free after a session of experiments (with their teats removed, of course). Alternatively, disposable, polythene pipettes may be used; these cannot, however, be rendered odour-free for reuse. *With teated glass droppers, care must be taken not to allow solutions to be sucked up into the teats.*

An old tray is useful as a working space for experiments to prevent contact between oils and solutions with clothing, and the surfaces of household furnishings.

Certain essential oils can ruin polished surfaces and plastics.

During experimental work of any kind, including sensory evaluations, eye protection should be worn.

This may seem fussy, but the unexpected is always waiting to happen and sooner or later will do so. Essential oils and their dilutions in Jojoba Oil in quantities of a few millilitres do not present a serious fire hazard if carefully and thoughtfully stored and used, but it is better to be safe than sorry. Keep them always away from naked flames and do not permit smoking where they are stored or being used. Dispose of used, unwanted smelling strips and any mopped-up spillages of essential oils or solutions in an external waste bin. Unwanted experiments should be stored in an appropriately labelled container, for eventual disposal in the approved, environmentally safe manner at your local waste-disposal facility.

The author of this book recommends that experimental blends of all kinds containing essential oils should not be applied to the skin, because it will not normally be possible for them to be independently tested for skin safety as commercial fragranced products are so tested. Experimental blends may be used as room fragrances, by evaporation from a suitable vaporizing ring, but do not allow drops of essential oil or of an experimental blend to come into contact with the hot surface of an electric lamp bulb, for it might then shatter.

For the experiments suggested in this book, Jojoba Oil, though acceptable as an essential oil solvent, suffers from the same disadvantage as do other vegetable oils used for the same purpose, which is that, unlike alcohol, which imparts excellent 'lift' to fragrance compositions, it greatly reduces the fragrance impact of dissolved essential oils. This effect is not, however, a great drawback in respect of room fragrance work; the presence of a large proportion of a vegetable oil helps to prolong the in-use odour persistence of the product. The Jojoba Oil content will not evaporate from a heated diffusion ring containing an experimental blend, *and so presents a hazard if the ring is not allowed to cool* before disposal.

Suitable dilutions of essential oils for perfume experiments are given in table 8.1. These may be prepared by counting drops, of which 200 will comfortably go into a 10 ml sample bottle. Although a somewhat onerous task, it is best to prepare all the solutions before commencing experimental work so that their odours may be studied, and to provide a resourceful fragrance palette for extended work on fragrance blends. Keep the solutions in a cool place.

In the following table (table 8.1) the relative volatilities of the essential oils (not their solutions) are noted as T (Top note), M (Middle note) or B (Basic note). The Jojoba Oil in the solutions reduces the rate of evaporation of the essential oils, but not equally in respect of solutions of different oils of the same strength.

Note that the list includes essential oils which are either the subject of recommended restrictions in respect of use in aromatherapy, or which are not recommended for use in aromatherapy.[1] The prepared solutions should be clearly labelled NOT FOR AROMATHERAPY and kept away from aromatherapy oils and from access by children.

Experiment 1

For this first experiment, a simple representation of a well-known fragrance type, Eau de Cologne, may be attempted, commencing with 30 drops of Bergamot Oil, FCF. Note that the object of the experiment is to produce a representation of a fragrance type, not a finished fragrance product. Other ingredients may be added in smaller amounts, down to one drop, depending on their individual odour strengths and, in the later stages of the experiment, on how finely adjustments to the formula need to be made to achieve the best fragrance effect. It is always possible to add further drops of an

---

1. See *Plant Aromatics: Safety Reference Manuals*, researched and published by Martin Watt, Medical Aromatherapy Training Services, 7 Elm Court Park, Chelmsford Road, Blackmore, Essex CM4 0SE, from whom full details are available on request.

Table 8.1 — Recommended dilutions of some essential oils for perfume experiments

Note	Essential oil	Dilution %		
T	Aniseed Oil	10		
T	Basil Oil, Sweet	10		
B	Benzoin Resinoid	10		
T	Bergamot Oil	10		
T	Caraway Oil	10		
M	Chamomile Oil, German	10		
M	Chamomile Oil, Roman	10		1
M	Cinnamon Bark Oil	10		
M	Clove Bud Oil	10		
T	Coriander Oil	10		1
M	Cypress Oil	10		
T	Eucalyptus Oil (*globulus* type)	10		
M	Frankincense (Olibanum) Oil	10		
T	Galbanum Oil		5	1
M	Geranium Oil	10		
M	Jasmin Absolute	10		
M	Juniper Oil	10		
B	Labdanum Resinoid or Absolute	10		
T	Lavandin Oil	10		
T	Lavender Oil	10		
T	Lavender Oil, Spike	10		
T	Lemon Oil	10		
T	Lemongrass Oil	10		
T	Mandarin Oil	10		
M	Marjoram Oil	10		
T	Myrrh Oil	10		
T	Neroli Oil	10		
T	Orange Oil, Sweet	10		
B	Patchouli Oil		5	1
T	Pine Oil, *pumilionis*	10		
M	Rose Absolute	10		
T	Rose Otto, Turkish		5	1
T/M	Rosemary Oil	10		
M/B	Sage Oil, Clary		5	
T	Sage Oil, Dalmatian	10		
B	Sandalwood Oil, East Indian	10		
B	Tarragon (Estragon) Oil	10		1
M	Ti-Tree Oil	10		
T	Thyme Oil, White	10		
M	Tuberose Absolute	10		
B	Vetivert Oil	10		
T/M	Ylang-Ylang Oil, Extra	10	5	

ingredient, but of course once added, an ingredient cannot be retrieved. Ingredients should be mixed by gentle but thorough swirling of the sample bottle.

Eau de Cologne-type fragrance

Bergamot Oil, FCF	10%	30 drops
Neroli Oil	10%	
Orange Oil, Sweet	10%	
Lemon Oil	10%	
Lavender Oil	10%	
Rosemary Oil	10%	
Thyme Oil	10%	(single drops only)
Sage Oil, Clary	10%	(single drops only)
Geranium Oil	10%	(single drops only)

A commercial Eau de Cologne may be used in this experiment as a fragrance goal, by comparison, using labelled smelling strips in triangle tests, but close correspondence between the odours of an experimental blend and the commercial fragrance should not be anticipated, if only because of the marked difference between the solvents. Small smelling strip dips only of the experimental fragrance should be taken for evaluation tests, and dips of the fragrance being used as a standard should be of comparable size.

Table 8.2 — Experiment 1: Example of an Eau de Cologne-type fragrance experiment

No.	Essential oil	Strength	Sequence of adding drops		Odour effect
1	Bergamot Oil, FCF	10%	30 + 2 + 1	= 33	
2	Neroli Oil	10%	5 + 5 + 4 + 2 + 1 =	17	Fresher, more floral
3	Orange Oil, Sweet	10%	5 + 5 + 5 + 1 =	16	More mellow
4	Lemon Oil	10%	5 + 5 + 5 + 4 + 2 =	21	Fresher, sharper
5	Lavender Oil	10%	5 + 5 + 5 + 5 + 1 =	21	Fresher, more herbaceous
6	Rosemary Oil	10%	5 + 1 + 1 =	7	Slightly resinous
7	Thyme Oil	10%	1 =	1	Slightly more herbal
8	Sage Oil, Clary	10%	1 + 1 =	2	More fragrant
9	Geranium Oil	10%	1 + 1 =	2	More floral — rosy
			Total number of drops =	120	

Table 8.2 shows an example of an experiment based on the above formula illustrating how the results may be recorded and the odour effects of adding ingredients noted.

The odour effects of any of the ingredients 6 to 9 in the finished fragrance may be tested by replacement of their amounts with equal amounts of Jojoba Oil, in separate experiments. As shown in the above formula, additional drops of any ingredient may be added, as necessary, as an experiment proceeds. The total numbers of drops of ingredients used are recorded at the end of the experiment.

Experiment 2

To prepare a balanced blend of two essential oils

Jasmin Absolute	10%	20 drops
Rose Absolute	10%	

Single drops of the solution of Rose Absolute are mixed with the Jasmin Absolute solution, until, on smelling the resulting blend, neither odour can be detected individually. At the point of odour balance between two aromatic materials an unexpected odour effect is occasionally produced. This possibility is increased as the number of ingredients in balance is increased. Odour balance in perfumes is in this respect important but, to avoid an overall, featureless 'plateau' of fragrance, should not characterize the entire fragrance of a perfume, within which emphasis upon certain notes provides necessary contours of distinction.

Experiment 3

Effect of a third ingredient on a balanced blend of Rose and Jasmin

Blend from Experiment 2		20 drops
Sandalwood Oil	10%	

The effect of the Sandalwood will become apparent as drops of the 10% solution are mixed with the floral blend. In further experiments of the same kind, the Sandalwood may be replaced by Benzoin Resinoid 10%, Chamomile Oil, Roman 1%, Coriander Oil 1%, Labdanum Resinoid or Absolute 10%, in whatever proportions give the most interesting results.

Experiment 4

Herbal-type blend

Lavender Oil	10%	30 drops
Geranium Oil	10%	
Sage Oil, Clary	10%	
Chamomile Oil, German	10%	
Rosemary Oil	10%	
Patchouli Oil	10%	
Thyme Oil	10%	

For further experiments, several alternative ideas spring to mind as, for example, replacement of Lavender by Lavandin, Geranium by Rose Otto (1 per cent), Clary Sage by Sage and Patchouli by Pine — all, again, in appropriate amounts.

Experiment 5

Spice blend

Clove Oil	10%	30 drops
Coriander Oil	10%	
Cinnamon Bark Oil	10%	
Rose Otto	1%	
Ylang-Ylang Oil, Extra	10%	
Sage Oil, Clary	1%	

The proportions of Cinnamon Bark, Ylang-Ylang and Clary Sage should be kept small, otherwise they can easily overwhelm the odours of the other ingredients.

Just for added experience (though not for application to the skin) a feminine-type and a masculine-type fragrance may be attempted, as follows:

Feminine-type fragrance

Blend from Experiment 3	30 drops	(as main fragrance theme)
Blend from Experiment 1		(as top note)

Masculine-type fragrance

Spice Blend, Experiment 4	30 drops	(as main fragrance theme)
Blend from Experiment 1		(as top note)

A small proportion of Mandarin Oil 10 per cent is likely to improve the top note of this latter fragrance. The Spice Blend may be replaced by the Herbal-Type Blend of experiment 4 or both may be tried together in different proportions.

Finally, a reminder that anything more ambitious in the way of fragrance experiments should follow a definite plan, as illustrated in the following example (fig. 8.1):

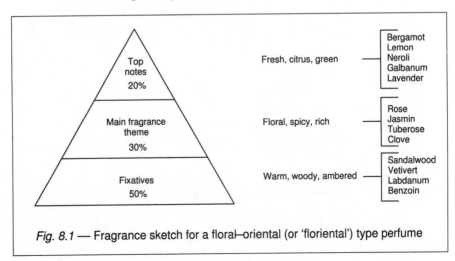

Fig. 8.1 — Fragrance sketch for a floral–oriental (or 'floriental') type perfume

Chapter 9

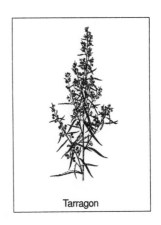

Tarragon

Personal Fragrances

9.1 Enfleurage and Floral Extraits

There was once a process, known as *enfleurage*, now obsolete as a commercial undertaking, which began with the individual placing of scented flowers, fresh from an early morning's harvest, on the surface of specially prepared animal fat spread over both sides of a rectangular glass plate. The fat, a mixture of purified suet and lard, was preserved by the addition of a small proportion (about 0·3 per cent) of benzoin. Benzoin contains from 19 to 29% of free organic acids, of which benzoic acid is the main preservative agent. The glass plate, surrounded by a wooden frame, was of dimensions 0·6 m × 0.3 m, an assembly known as a *chassis*. The only flowers suitable for enfleurage were those, such as jasmin and tuberose, which continue their production of essential oil for at least 24 hours after removal from the plant.

Many other chassis were similarly charged with flowers, all of the same kind, following which they were placed one above another to form tall stacks. The stacks were allowed to stand for 24, 48 or 72 hours, depending on how long the flowers continued to produce essential oil before they began to wilt and develop unpleasant odours. During the period of contact with the fat (called the enfleurage *graisse*), essential oil slowly flowed from the oil glands of the flowers, down the petals, to be absorbed by the graisse.

At the end of the correct period of time, the chassis were taken down and the flowers removed *(defleurage)*. The chassis were then turned over and charged with freshly picked flowers, and the entire process was repeated until no more were available. By this time, the graisse would have become saturated with essential oil, forming an enfleurage *pommade*.

To extract the essential oil absorbed by the fat, the pommade was transferred to a *batteuse*, a large cylindrical vessel fitted with paddles secured to a vertical revolving shaft, wherein it was vigorously stirred with alcohol warmed sufficiently to melt the pommade. This caused the molten pommade to break up into minute globules, suspended in the alcohol, thus greatly increasing the total surface area of the pommade. Under these conditions the alcohol extracted the essential oil from the pommade efficiently, but dissolved very little of the fat at the same time. One extraction was not, however, sufficient for the alcohol to dissolve most of the essential oil contained in the pommade, and so repeated extraction, using fresh alcohol, was necessary to obtain an economic yield. The alcoholic solutions were chilled to precipitate the small amounts of dissolved fatty matter, which was then removed by filtration. The filtrate, an alcoholic solution of the essential oil obtained from the flowers, was known as an *extrait*, meaning extract, although it was in fact an extract solution.

During defleurage, small amounts of essential oil-charged graisse would on each occasion cling to the flowers, accumulating an unacceptable total loss of the final product if simply thrown away. These flowers were therefore collected and extracted with a volatile hydrocarbon solvent, followed by extraction of the residue with alcohol after recovery of the solvent, to produce a *chassis absolute*. Chassis absolutes were less costly than the finer enfleurage absolutes, and possessed a somewhat fatty odour, which rendered them useful as ingredients for the preparation of otherwise largely synthetic reproductions of flower fragrances.

Extraits were for many years the main sources of the perfumer's natural flower fragrances for the composition of 'handkerchief' perfumes for personal use. They were blended with one another, and with preparations of musk, civet, ambergris and other materials, to create the popular perfumes of the Victorian era, which were mainly of floral or oriental character. Concentrated true floral extracts were manufactured by gently distilling the extraits in a vacuum to recover the alcohol. Once all the alcohol had been evaporated, the product remaining as a residue was known as an *enfleurage absolute*.

As we have noted, the great classic perfumes of the late nineteenth and the earlier years of the twentieth century were created by introducing carefully adjusted proportions of newly discovered aroma chemicals into existing formulae for perfumes composed entirely of natural ingredients. In this way, the completely novel, exciting notes of the chemicals were blended perfectly with the 'naturals' to produce highly attractive fragrance profiles of the finest quality.

9.2 Extrait Perfumes and Toilet Waters

As applied to perfumes, the word 'extrait' today refers not to the extraits of old, which have long vanished from perfumery, but to the products we call 'perfumes', i.e. the strongest, alcoholic, personal fragrances which are sold to the public. Alcoholic products of the same or similar fragrance to the corresponding extraits are the various types of toilet waters, which are are of weaker fragrance and alcoholic strength. Many of these perfumes are also of lighter fragrance character.

The modern era of perfumery may be said to date from the beginning of the twentieth century, when perfumers were at the threshold of realizing the fragrance potential of chemicals such as coumarin, vanillin, the ionones, heliotropine, the 'rose alcohols', linalöl, the fatty aldehydes, synthetic musk substitutes and a whole variety of esters, some providing fruity notes never before available at affordable prices.

The effect of the new synthetics on perfumery grew to be profound in terms of creative opportunity, particularly for those perfumers prepared to take the risk of breaking free from the shackles of convention to explore the new vistas for fragrance innovation concealed by the severity of odour of some of them. Careful dilution and aesthetically sensitive blending of the new materials brought bountiful rewards in terms of originality and commercial success to these intrepid pioneers, the fruits of whose labours inspire the most promising of trainee perfumers today, even as the great works of other arts inspire the artists of tomorrow.

Essential oils are generally easier to use as perfume ingredients than aromatic chemicals, even those which occur in nature as their major constituents. They are also frequently effective in smaller dosages. These facts have to be balanced against the advantages of the relative uniformity of quality of perfumery chemicals from a given manufacturer. In very general terms, the twentieth century has seen a decline in the proportions of natural materials and an increase in those of aroma chemicals in perfumes of all sectors of perfumery, including fine fragrance. A further important feature has been the 'reworking' or reformulating of perfumes created many years ago, but which remain popular today, in order to substitute materials which will be readily available for the foreseeable future as alternatives for ingredients that have disappeared from regular supply. This kind of substitution inevitably results in some alteration of the fragrance profile of a perfume, and, however much care is taken to reproduce the original with precision, the difference is almost always noticeable; by the time of the nth reworking it may be quite profound. Unfortunately, such was the quality of some of the original ingredients, such as the enfleurage absolutes, that their contributions simply cannot now be matched. The enforced reworking of a perfume is evidently in some instances regarded as an opportunity for cheapening the formula, with results that are better left to the imagination than experienced.

Regarding toilet waters, confusion still exists as to the meanings of such descriptions as 'Eau de Toilette', 'Parfum de Toilette', 'Cologne', 'Eau de Parfum', etc., especially as to the proportions of perfume compounds that they contain. Articles in the fashion magazines sometimes pontificate on the subject, but really to no avail, as individual manufacturers are strictly nonconformist, there being no inspired revelation to which to conform. Perhaps in these times of regulatory enthusiasm we should value such minor eccentricities while they have yet to be drawn to the attention of those whose mission in life it is even to regulate the size of the humble sausage.

Water is cheaper than alcohol and the two solvents are completely miscible. For these reasons, water finds use as a diluent for alcohol in toilet waters. Thus, the inscription '80°' on one of these products means that the alcohol it contains is 80 per cent pure ethanol of perfumery grade and 20 per cent purified water, by volume. The use of water for this purpose, while cutting manufacturing costs, reduces the solubility of perfume compounds, particularly those containing essential oils rich in terpenes, such as the citrus oils. If this problem is likely to arise in a product, it may be solved by replacing any terpene-rich essential oils included in the formula by the corresponding oils from which the terpenes have been removed.

Terpeneless essential oils can be prepared by vacuum fractionation of the complete oils, when the monoterpenes distil over, leaving the oxygenates, which constitute the required terpeneless product, together with the sesquiterpenes the oil contains. Alternatively, to obtain an almost completely terpeneless oil, the complete oil may be agitated with a solvent, such as triacetin (the glycerin, or glyceryl, ester of acetic acid, which is odourless). This will dissolve the oxygenates, but only minute amounts of terpenes, and the solution produced will hardly mix at all with the terpenes, which on separation form an upper layer. The lower layer is removed and vacuum-fractionated to recover the triacetin, leaving the terpeneless oil in the 'pot'. Terpeneless essential oils are stronger, and in the case of citrus oils much stronger, in characteristic odour than the corresponding complete oils, and are more resistant to attack by oxygen and much more miscible with alcohol diluted with water. They are, however, less 'natural' in odour character and more costly than the complete oils.

Toilet waters for men form an important and growing sector of the personal fragrance market. They developed originally from novel fragrance concepts, such as Eau de Cologne, Bay Rum and Fougère Royale, and by the 'masculinization' of perfumes originally created for women, particularly in the chypre and oriental categories (*see* pp. 233-5). Men's fragrance products include shaving lotions, antiperspirants, deodorants and splash colognes, in the better qualities of which are found essential oils from herbs, such as lavender, rosemary and artemisia, from woods, such as sandalwood, cedarwood, rosewood, etc., from citrus fruit peels, from roots, such vetivert, and from leaves, such as patchouli. These are frequently associated with animalic and mossy notes or examples of the latest 'oceanic' or 'marine' odour tones. These fragrances are traditionally less floral, more herbaceous, woody and citrus than perfumes for women, although there has in recent years been some movement towards acceptability of rather more emphasized floral character in comparison with men's fragrances of earlier years. The present author feels that this trend was initiated in the modern fougère fragrances (*see* p. 235) where rosy notes of geranium and nuances of hawthorn were accentuated to produce quite stunning effects, necessarily well removed from feminine associations.

Perfume solvents used as alternatives to alcohol include synthetic oils, such as the esters isopropyl palmitate and isopropyl myristate, both of which are odourless when pure and of low viscosity. These solvents are, however, virtually nonvolatile at skin temperature. Certain silicone oils are both odourless and volatile and are good solvents for terpenes, though not nearly so good in this respect for some of the oxygenated constituents of essential oils and resinoids, also some aroma chemicals. A further disadvantage is that the volatile silicones possess hardly any of the marked 'lifting' power of alcohol but they are less flammable than alcohol and reportedly nontoxic. The disadvantages of volatile silicones as perfume solvents can, however, be overcome, to produce elegant perfumes with seductive skin-feel and no cooling effect whatsoever. Silicone perfume solvents are appreciated where the use of alcohol is objectionable as, for example, in strictly Moslem communities. They are more costly than ethanol, though this need not necessarily be a disadvantage in the area of top-quality products. Certain vegetable oils, such as Jojoba Oil, can be used as perfume solvents, but these oils are totally nonvolatile, tending to suppress top notes and to some extent to act as fixatives.

Other media for the presentation of skin perfumes include heavily scented toilet soaps, talcum powder, foam bath detergents and liquid soaps intended for use as skin cleansers. These last-named products are popular in developing countries, where they are purpose-formulated to act also as personal fragrances. Water, with which perfume compounds are practically immiscible, can be made to dissolve most perfume oils with the aid of special dispersing agents called *solubilizers*. The solutions formed are, however, not true solutions, as the dissolved particles are larger than molecular size. They are colloidal solutions, which can be shown to be capable of scattering light, which true solutions do not. These solutions are nevertheless transparent and are, of course, nonflammable. A disadvantage of water-based perfumes is that, as water is less volatile than alcohol, they dry out rather slowly on the skin.

9.3 Fragrance Quality

The more flamboyant examples of feminine headwear are sometimes referred to as 'creations', in appreciation of the originality of their design or their resplendency of appearance. The word *creation*, as used in the context of art, denotes the bringing together by the artist of forms, colours, musical notes, words, mathematical symbols —

even atoms — into some novel arrangement, structure or proportions never before given existence or probably never even contemplated. Before a work of artistic expression, such as a sculpture, painting, musical composition, complex mathematical equation or molecular structure is produced, the elements of the art already exist. It is the originality of their assembly into a form capable of being appreciated aesthetically which determines whether or not the result may be regarded as an act of creation: this is always a matter of individual or collective human opinion and judgement.

A mixture of aromatic materials may with justification amount to a work of art if these elements have been blended in harmonious combination, as the instruments of an orchestra are harmonized in the playing of a symphony from a musical score. If formulated according to a preconceived plan, the blend is then a perfume. To be also a work of art, the perfume would have necessarily been inspired by some form of sensory experience and executed with that unique association of perception, feeling and discipline of approach that sets apart the artist in fragrance from the mere compounder of pleasant smells. If, in addition, the perfume were to display novelty of fragrance profile, then it would rank as a creation of the perfumer's art: a candidate for eventual recognition as a classic.

Perfumes for use as personal fragrances are classified commercially as either fine or mass market fragrances, according to retail price levels, which are generally accepted as reflecting fragrance quality. In practical terms, therefore, a fine fragrance would be expected to be composed of a higher proportion of natural ingredients than a mass-market fragrance, and this is a reasonable assumption: the top-quality essential oils, absolutes and resinoids used in fine fragrance creation are costly and cannot be replaced by synthetic equivalents without at least some sacrifice of fragrance quality. It is in the end very much a matter of *how* a perfumer uses the materials at his disposal that determines the quality of the final result, in the same way that it is *how* a chef uses everyday foodstuffs that results in either '*Cabillaud au Gratin et Pommes Frites*' or plain 'cod and chips'. Masterpieces are, however, to be found among mass-market fragrances as well as in the fine fragrance sector of perfumery.

There is an obvious quality difference between a natural Jasmin Absolute and a jasmin base which can be bought at a fifth of the price, and the question arises whether, given complete freedom of choice of materials whatever the cost, a perfumer would choose nothing but 'naturals' to create the world's finest perfume. For an answer, we turn to the more recent history of perfumery, to the time when perfumes of this very kind were giving way to new fragrance ideas in which a growing variety of aroma chemicals was playing an increasingly important role, stimulating users of personal perfume to adopt revolutionary fragrance preferences which led naturally to those of today. In the creation of modern perfumes, current consumer preferences are closely studied in order to maximize the likelihood of their success in the marketplace. For the realization of this goal, both natural materials and synthetics are essential. The perfection of symphonic orchestration demands brassy stridency and percussive punctuation to be interwoven with the mellow richness of strings and woodwind: the perfection of fragrance expression similarly demands the orchestration of relatively featureless but exciting chemical notes with the blended contours of nature's own perfumes.

The traditional fragrance preferences of the East are quite different from those of the Western world, and in certain Asian countries there is strong preference among influential connoisseurs for personal fragrances to be of very largely natural composition, aroma chemicals entering into a formulation only where ingredients of natural origin cannot supply highly favoured fragrance representations. Cost, within these highly cultured societies, is of far lesser importance than the assurance of personal fragrance of supreme quality. Under social conditions where the best can be afforded as a matter of routine, demands for high quality are preserved and are met by the ready availability and advertising of high-quality products, so tending to influence public taste more generally: for the better in helping to perpetuate the best of cultural traditions; for the worse in encouraging the manufacture, purchase and use of cheap copies of far-famed originals. The blatant copying of perfumes reduces the income from sales, and hence profit, of the long-established creators of the originals, who are as capable as ever they were of fragrance innovation at the classical level of perfumery, by reason of their concentrated creative effort maintained over many years. There are still perfumistic Rembrandts and Constables in this world, their creations commercially motivated maybe, but having yet further contributions to make to the inspiration of future practioners of the art of fragrance composition.

9.4 Perfumes of a Gentler Age

Queen Victoria came to the throne of England in 1837, some years before the advent of the first aromatic chemicals. Prior to and well into Victoria's reign, perfumes were composed entirely of materials of natural origin, mostly in the form of extraits, tinctures and essential oils bearing fragrances from far and wide.

Among perfumes of this era, those representing the scents of single flowers and of bouquets of flowers were all the rage, the most fashionable representing Rose, Jasmin, Orange Blossom and Violet, and combinations of these notes, modified and augmented by the essential oils of vetivert, cinnamon bark, patchouli leaves, bergamot fruits and other nonfloral sources of fragrance. Carefully purified, aromatic plant exudates, such as benzoin, frankincense, myrrh and labdanum, together with tinctures of ambergris, civet and musk, were used for their fixative properties to make the perfumes more long-lasting. Long experience revealed that the finest blenders — that is, ingredients for fusing together different notes to produce a single, complex fragrance impression — were the animal products, tinctures of which needed to be introduced selectively into a perfume and then in only very small proportions for the realization of their optimum effects. With musk, the amounts were found to be so small that the unequalled fixative property of this material could not be explained in terms of scientific principles and, in fact, the fixative action of musk remains a mystery to this day. Similarly unaccountable is the fact that mere traces of musk also increase the diffusion into the air of a perfume applied to the skin. This is also a property of the aroma chemical muscone, a compound identical to the natural muscone which is mainly responsible for the pleasant aspect of the odour of natural musk, the less attractive aspect of which is given by nitrogen-containing constituents such as muscopyridine.

Civet, like musk, presents to the nose notes both pleasant and unpleasant, the former donated by civettone, a constituent of delightful, musky odour when really pure and similar in chemical constitution to muscone. The repulsively lavatorial notes of raw civet, as freshly obtained from the animal, leave nothing at all to the imagination, the name of the principal culprit, skatole, being only too well deserved. Yet natural civet, prepared for use in perfumery, cannot be equalled for its ability to impart 'life' to the fragrances of delicate floral (e.g. lily-of-the-valley) and certain other perfume compositions, such as Chypre. Civet finds use also as an excellent fixative for perfumes of these types.

Ambergris is (or, rather, was) totally different in its properties from both musk and civet, possessing a cool, barely animalic odour recalling the smell of the sea and the musty atmospheres associated with old churches and solicitors' offices. It is a material of great complexity which was used, before its decline as a contribution to saving the sperm whale from extinction, for its superior properties as a fixative and blender. Further circumstances discouraging the use of natural ambergris in perfumery were the irregularities of its supply and quality. It seems almost unbelievable today that there were once experts who specialized in evaluating the quality of just one of the animal products of perfumery, which were truly jewels of the perfumer's palette. A further surprising fact is that the best of synthetic substitutes for natural ambergris, identical in chemical composition and molecular structure to its chief odorous constituent, are obtained by chemical treatment of the practically odourless sclareol remaining in clary sage herb following steam distillation to obtain Clary Sage Oil, and subsequent drying of the exhausted material. Even more surprising is the assurance of French producers of the essential oil, who labour high up in the foothills of the Alpes Maritimes, north of Grasse, that profit from the entire business of planting, growing, distilling and then selling the residual vegetation of clary sage for aroma chemical production comes not from any of these operations, but from the final sale of the completely exhausted residue to manufacturers of compost.

The perfumes of today are created with knowledge of preceding perfumes, passed down from master perfumer to trainee and gathered thereafter through experience in the practical business of perfume creation. They are reflections of public taste in fragrance to which, for commercial reasons, perfumers have constantly to respond. The great classic perfumes of the first fifty years of the twentieth century are descended from fragrance ideas of the nineteenth, wherein the transition from 'all-natural' to 'natural + synthetic' perfumes took place, and to some extent from one another, a perfume of one kind inspiring the development of another of a different kind. This transition, and its development in the modern era, may be illustrated by comparing a formula for a perfume of the mid-nineteenth century with one for a perfume of the same type from the early years of the twentieth century, and these with a formula for a modern composition, again of the same kind. For the purposes of this book these formulae will be given in terms of the names of well-known fragrance products of natural origin and the odour notes of aroma chemicals included in the later formulae.

From a comparison of formulae 1 and 2 (table 9.1), it would be wrong to conclude that the synthetic lilac, heliotrope and musk notes are entirely responsible for the large differences in the proportions of the extraits and most of the other ingredients, as it is always possible to formulate a perfume representing a given natural fragrance in a number of different ways. The increase in the proportions of the rose and jasmin extraits, decrease of tuberose and orange blossom and absence of acacia (known today as cassie) extraits in formula 2, for instance, are probably, at least in part, compensating adjustments for the use in this formula of synthetic lilac, as a mixture of aroma chemicals of around 100 per cent strength, as against the much weaker strength of the extraits. In formula 3, the one natural product, Ylang-Ylang Oil, imparts to an otherwise totally synthetic perfume a desirable touch of naturalness. In this formula, the synthetic lilac is not, of course, out of place, though since it is possible to produce a convincing lilac-type perfume without lilac-smelling chemicals, its inclusion in the formula is more a genuflection to tradition than an absolutely necessity.

It is interesting that lilac fragrances, labelled as such, have never been popular. Perhaps the myth of misfortune attached to the presence of lilac blossoms in a room has something to do with this. In spite of this quite unreasonable belief, one quite exceptional lilac perfume, masquerading as 'apple blossom', enjoyed well-deserved commercial success some years ago.

Table 9.1 — Lilac

Ingredient	1: Mid-19th century	2: Early 20th century	3: Modern formula
Extrait of Jasmin	7·97	38·58	–
Extrait of Rose	13·00	38·58	–
Extrait of Tuberose	46·40	14·75	–
Extrait of Orange Blossom	22·10	2·30	–
Extrait of Acacia Blossom	2·00	–	–
Tincture of Orris	4·00	0·25	–
Tincture of Vanilla	2·50	–	–
Tincture of Styrax	0·40	–	–
Tincture of Civet	1·50	0·23	–
Tincture of Musk	–	1·05	–
Oil of Ylang-Ylang	0·03	0·36	3·00
Oil of Coriander	0·03	–	–
Oil of Bergamot	0·02	0·20	–
Oil of Lemon	0·02	–	–
Oil of Bitter Almond, 10%	0·03	–	–
Fragrance notes of synthetic origin			
Lilac	–	3·40	4·17
Heliotrope	–	0·20	10·35
Musk	–	0·10	10·75
Coriander	–	–	2·00
Jasmin	–	–	7·00
Hyacinth	–	–	6·50
Lily-of-the-Valley	–	–	21·80
Carnation	–	–	8·90
Rose	–	–	22·40
Violet	–	–	3·13
	100·00	100·00	100·00

The perfume represented by formula 3 would be considerably improved by the partial replacement of the jasmin and rose synthetics by the natural absolutes, and the violet by a proportion of Orris Oil, distilled from the dried rhizomes of the Florentine iris plant. The lily-of-the-valley aspect of the fragrance could be refined by partial or total replacement by a superior lily-of-the-valley base, the genuine absolute, if available, being of unremarkable odour value. All of these adjustments would, of course, increase the cost of the perfume.

Since aroma chemicals are concentrated in comparison with the dilute condition of extracts and tinctures, formula 3 represents a much stronger product than either of the others.

9.5 The Classification of Perfumes

Systems of classification are devised to bring order where there would otherwise be chaos; to pave the way for relationships and differences to be seen among items, materials or objects of a given kind which in the absence of classification would have to be considered in isolation from one another. Classification makes life easier, by allowing us to deal with whatever is classified at first in a simple way, and that understood to progress our understanding by consideration of more detailed subdivisions of classification. For example, when studying perfumery we classify perfume ingredients as being of natural origin or synthetic — a very simple but neccessary beginning. Next, we classify the 'naturals' into essential oils, aromatic extracts and resinoids, and then the essential oils into those distilled and those expressed. Why? Because this opens the door to differentiation between these families of products in terms of their composition and properties and to appreciation of similarities between them as, for instance, the fact that they all contain aromatic and hence volatile constituents, quite apart from anything else. We classify the constituents of essential oils as terpenes and oxygenates, and the terpenes as monoterpenes and sesquiterpenes, so opening a further door beyond which lie the wonderful vistas of the chemistry of aromatic materials — and this of course relates to the study of aroma chemicals and their properties, and it is not now difficult to envisage where all this will lead, provided we have the vision, dedication and stamina to continue. Classification leads to understanding, and understanding to the construction in the mind of those systems of mental reference points which when correctly related to one another comprise our comprehension of an entire subject.

Essential to comprehension is memory, and the interrelationship of memories which is necessary to understanding. Memory serves special purposes in studies of aromatic materials and perfumes, first as a storage system for those odour percepts or experiences we know as odour notes — the elements of odour appreciation and evaluation — second, to enable us to recognize relationships between odour notes, such as similarities and differences and odour effects produced by combinations of notes; and third, for our appreciation and understanding of the complex odour impression of accords and perfumes. How do we pave the way for all these ideas to lodge in our memory? By classification, which facilitates study; by practical experience stimulated by study; and by practice, which reinforces memory and aids recall. This brings us to the subject of learning, which we shall discuss in the next and final chapter of this book.

We shall now consider the most universally recognized perfume types, to each of which has been assigned a two-letter code for easy reference, on the subject of classic perfumes. The letters **M** and **F** refer to the intended gender of usage of the different perfume types, although of course these days such a segregation is not observed to the extent that it once was — an example of cultural progress, it may be supposed.

Citrus Perfume Type **[CT] [M] [F]**

Citrus-type perfumes originated with the invention of a masculine toilet water in Milan, early in the eighteenth century. The inventor was probably one Jean-Paul Feminis, who is thought to have passed on his secret formula to his nephew, Jean-Antoine Farina. Farina moved to Cologne, where he manufactured and sold the product under the appropriate name of 'Eau de Cologne'. In 1906, Farina moved his business to Paris, where it was eventually sold to the perfumery house of Roger & Gallet, who to this day make the same Eau de Cologne under the name of Farina.

Traditional Eau de Cologne is not a perfume in the true sense of the word, for its characteristic fragrance has little lasting power. It is intended for liberal application to the skin as a means of refreshment, physically by the cooling effect of evaporation of the alcohol it contains, and psychologically by virtue of its light and refreshing fragrance. The ingredients of the classic Eaux de Cologne are obtained entirely from natural sources. They comprise citrus oils, with Neroli, Lavender and Rosemary Oils, and perhaps a touch of one of the spice oils. Cheaper brands of Eau de Cologne are formulated with complete or partial synthetic replacements for the essential oils, such as citral (plus limonene to prevent sensitization of the skin) for the lemon note, methyl anthranilate for the Neroli and linalöl and its acetate for both Neroli and Lavender.

Various aspects of the Eau de Cologne fragrance profile, bergamot and lavender in particular, appear in the top notes of countless feminine and masculine fragrances, while Lavender Oil of high quality is valued not for its characteristic odour profile alone, but equally for its freshening effect on the top note of almost any perfume.

Floral Perfume Type **[FL] [F]**

The floral fragrance theme in perfumery today encompasses notes of most fragrant flowers, lending itself to almost infinite variation in respect of the combinations of the flowers represented. Among these, the notes of rose, jasmin, neroli, violet and lily-of-the-valley make the most frequent contributions, notes of such flowers as tuberose, hyacinth and narcissus being reserved to produce other fragrance effects, such as heavy narcotic sweetness (tuberose) and various suggestions of greenness (as with hyacinth and narcissus). Floral notes in perfumes are often accompanied by notes of nonfloral character (e.g. suggestions of leafy and earthy nuances) to transform them into closer representations of the living plants in their natural surroundings or to create imaginative, abstract fragrance concepts.

The first perfume of the floral type to be accorded classic status was François Coty's 'L'Origan', launched in 1905, although at the time and for many years afterwards it was regarded as being of the

Oriental type (*see* pp. 234–5), being heavily floral with a distinctly balsamic base. Today, 'L'Origan' is usually placed in the 'floriental' subdivision of the floral category, together with the more modern classics 'Oscar de la Renta' (Stern, 1976) and 'Poison' (Dior, 1985).

The 'floral bouquet' fragrance concept was defined by the perfume 'Quelques Fleurs', introduced by Houbigant in 1912, a perfume from the concepts of which are descended many others in great variety.

Few perfumes of the 'single flower' subclass have attained great popularity. The prototype, here, is usually named as Coty's 'Muguet des Bois', launched in 1936, but it was Dior's 'Diorissimo' which gained recognized classical status. There are some very beautiful muguet, or lily-of-the-valley, perfumes, promotions of which adorn the perfume shops of France during the annual Flower Festival in the spring, and some of the relatively few perfume shops in England, too. It is instructive to compare the fragrance of a good quality muguet perfume with that exhaled by the living flowers. The difference is striking, having arisen from the stylistic nature of the muguet perfumes of old. These were perfumers' interpretations of the lily-of-the-valley fragrance rather than attempts to reproduce the true scent of the flowers, which is rose-like with delicate suggestions of lemon and fresh greenery.

Outstanding among 'green' variants of the floral bouquet class is Balmain's 'Vent Vert', launched in 1945 and clearly displaying the evocatively beautiful, agrestic notes of galbanum. The latest (1996) floral-type perfume to be accorded classical status is 'Amarige', introduced by Givenchy in 1991.

Aldehydic Perfume Type [AL] [F]

Perfumes of the aldehydic type are descended ultimately from the great 'No. 5' of Chanel, launched in 1921 (*see* p. 192). They well exemplify how certain notes, unpleasant in the concentrated state, can become first of all more tolerable if sufficiently diluted and, second, very attractive, even in excess of the 'normal' safe limit of usage as perfume ingredients, when suitably blended with other notes with skill and creative flair. 'Chanel No. 5' was the first personal fragrance to be characterized by notes of synthetic chemicals, tamed and beautified by superb orchestration with precious essential oils and absolutes exclusive to the realms of fine perfumery.

Perfumes of the aldehydic type display a smooth and unique fragrance note of 'nutty' character which shines forth from the composition, lending a warm and very beautiful tonality to the entire profile; a diffusive, elegant and forever fashionable effect.

Chypre Perfume Type [CH] [M] [F]

The Chypre (pronounced 'sheepra') perfume type has an interesting history. In the twelfth century, a crusader returning from the conquest of Cyprus is reputed to have brought to Europe a perfume named

'Eau de Chypre', *Chypre* being the French name for Cyprus. The perfume became popular, to the extent of inspiring the creation of many different variants of the fragrance. Eventually, declining popularity caused the disappearance of 'Eau de Chypre', interest in it faded and the formula became lost and forgotten.

In the early years of the twentieth century, François Coty became interested in the possible composition of 'Eau de Chypre', but, with no trace of any record of its composition or fragrance, was unable to attempt a reproduction. He was, however, inspired to attempt a recreation of the perfume, relying on knowledge of the aromatic plants in use in Cyprus at the time of the Crusades. In 1917, the House of Coty launched the result of its owner's creative genius in the form of a perfume named 'Le Chypre', which became a great success, to the extent that other perfumers undertook the extremely difficult task of discovering its secrets, relying on their noses and analytical methods which would today be regarded as hopelessly crude and time-consuming, as no doubt the techniques of today will be so considered a century from now.

A perfume of the classic Chypre-type is based on Coty's original perfume, in which oakmoss in the base was contrasted with bergamot in the top note, the two being linked by notes of rose, jasmin and other flowers. Touches of civet are considered essential in a Chypre-type perfume, lending radiance and additional fixation to perfection of the fragrance. Once the elements of the composition of 'Le Chypre' became generally known among perfumers, it was found that the fundamental accord characteristic of this perfume was capable of wide variation, to yield perfumes of the same type in which notes of particular kinds, such as floral, green, fruity, animalic, etc., were accentuated to lend distinction and originality to the basic composition.

For many years following the introduction of 'Le Chypre', perfumes of this type were created almost exclusively for women. This situation began to change, at first rather tentatively, in the 1960s, gaining momentum thereafter until, in the late 1970s, there occurred a great surge in the development of men's toiletries. The commercial potential of Chypre-type fragrances in the men's toiletry market began to be realized and before long there emerged from the perfumeries of the western world a whole succession of masculine toilet waters of this type, in great variety. The popularity of the Chypre-type fragrance motif is at the time of writing in decline. no doubt to be renewed at some time in the future by the daring launch of a sparkling re-creation.

Oriental Perfume Type [OR] [M] [F]

The first notable perfume of the Oriental type was the well-loved 'Jicky' of Guerlain, launched in 1889. Characteristic of a perfume of this type is the light, fresh character of the top note, which is almost always donated by the essential oils of Bergamot and other citrus fruits as the main contributors. The heart of an Oriental perfume is characteristically heavy, and made exceptionally long-lasting by the presence of essential oils such as Vetivert, Patchouli and Sandalwood, together with ambra notes and synthetic representatives of the other animal extracts formerly used as perfume ingredients. The floral elements of Oriental-type perfumes include the sweet, heavy notes of Jasmin and Tuberose, modified by traditional spices and balsams.

Masculine fragrances of the Oriental type are less sweet and floral than those for women, with greater emphasis on notes of citrus oils, herbs such as clary sage and lavender, and woody and ambra notes in the base.

Lavender Perfume Type [LV] [M]

Here again we have a perfume type of early origin. Toilet waters of distinction named 'Lavender' were first introduced by the perfumeries of Atkinson in 1910 and Yardley in 1913. These fragrances afforded softer and sweeter alternatives to Eau de Cologne, and were much favoured by our grandmothers of a generation or so ago.

We have already noted the importance of lavender as an agent for imparting freshness in the top notes of perfumes of other types. The lavender theme was developed in a much more long-lasting, fresh, woody Fougère direction in the classic masculine toilet water for men 'Silvestre', launched by Victor in 1946. This product inspired the creation of several further fragrances of related profile, displaying notes of citrus oils, rosemary, rosewood and other exotic woods, oakmoss and tonka, the last-named as an absolute rich in coumarin.

Fougère Perfume Type [FG] [M]

The ability of Lavender Oil of the finest quality to project freshness and distinction is fully expressed in fragrances of the Fougère ('fern') type, which originated with the toilet soap 'Fougère Royale', introduced by Houbigant in 1882 (*see* p. 186). Subsequently, the Fougère theme was taken in a feminine direction with Elizabeth Arden's 'Blue Grass' of 1935. In the same year came also 'Canoe', by the Spanish perfumery of Dana, which developed another similar feminine fragrance, 'Ambush', launched in 1959.

Then, in 1964, there suddenly burst into the men's market an arresting new product, the commercial reverberations of which continue to this day. Fabergé's 'Brut for Men' is a fragrance in which the theme of 'Canoe' and 'Ambush' is fully expressed in the masculine gender, taking for the first time the masculine fragrance market in a decidedly floral direction, this without any suggestion of the dreaded effeminacy which had for so many years excluded any form of floral intrusion into the masculine domain.

9.6 Classics of Perfume Creation

The author would stress that mention by name of commercial fragrances in this part of Chapter 9, and elsewhere in the book, is made entirely for the purposes of illustration and is in no way intended to overlook the excellence of other products of equal merit. It is also important to note that superiority of quality and fragrance innovation is to be found also among mass-market perfumes, price being in many instances a misleading indicator of inspired creative artistry.

In the following tables, which are supplemented by cross-references for ease of use in the shop or salon, the main features of examples of perfumes regarded as classics are briefly described. Since the status of a perfume as regards artistic merit is, in common with the works of all other arts, a matter of opinion, the author regrets any omissions dear to the hearts of individual readers, perhaps calling to mind persons and places of long ago. Great perfumes are rare and immortal treasures: creations of the great masters of fragrance perfection, their fragrances the stuff of dreams. We must cherish them all our days.

Table 9.2 — Classic feminine fragrances

Year	Fragrance	Type	House of origin	Top notes	Middle notes	Basic notes
1889	Jicky	OR	Guerlain	Lemon, Lavender, Rosemary	Jasmin, Heliotrope, Vetivert	Balsamic, Ambra
1905	L'Origan	FL	Coty	Bergamot, Pepper, Coriander	Clove, Carnation, Jasmin, Rose	Sandalwood, Balsamic, Musk
1912	Quelques Fleurs	FL	Houbigant	Bergamot, Neroli, aldehydic	Floral, green	Floral, Sandalwood, powdery
1917	Le Chypre	CH	Coty	Bergamot, Neroli, fruity	Rose, Jasmin, Carnation	Woody, Oakmoss, Ambra
1921	No. 5	AL	Chanel	Aldehydic, Bergamot, Neroli	Rose, Gardenia, Jasmin, aldehydic	Vetivert, balsamic, musky
1925	Shalimar	OR	Guerlain	Bergamot, Lemon, floral	Floral, Patchouli, woody	Balsamic, Ambra, powdery
1925	Crêpe de Chine	CH	Millot	Citrus, Neroli, aldehydic	Carnation, Gardenia, Rose, Jasmin	Vetivert, Oakmoss, Musk
1927	Arpège	AL	Lanvin	Aldehydic, citrus, fruity	Jasmin, Lily-of-the-Valley, Rose	Woody, powdery, animalic
1928	Soir de Paris	FL	Bourjois	Violet, green, aldehydic	Linden blossom, Rose, Carnation	Vetivert, balsamic, powdery
1932	Je Reviens	AL	Worth	Aldehydic, Neroli, Bergamot	Carnation, spicy, fruity	Woody, chypre-like
1935	Joy	FL	Patou	Floral, green, Peach	Rose, Jasmin, Lily-of-the-Valley	Sandalwood, musky, powdery
1937	Shocking	OR	Schiaparelli	Aldehydic, floral, fruity	Rose, spicy, green	Ambra, mossy, balsamic
1942	Muguet des Bois	FL	Coty	Green, Bergamot, aldehydic	Lily-of-the-Valley	Floral, woody

Table 9.2 (contd.) — Classic feminine fragrances

Year	Fragrance	Type	House of origin	Top notes	Middle notes	Basic notes
1944	Femme	CH	Rochas	Floral, Peach, Bergamot	Jasmin, Rose, Carnation	Mossy, balsamic, powdery
1945	Vent Vert	FL	Balmain	Galbanum, citrus, floral	Green, Narcissus, Lily-of-the-Valley	Oakmoss, woody, musky
1946	Ma Griffe	CH	Carven	Green, citrus, Gardenia	Gardenia, citronella, Rose	Powdery, mossy, balsamic
1947	Miss Dior	CH	Dior	Aldehydic, green, fruity	Jasmin, Carnation, Lily-of-the-Valley	Ambra, mossy, leather
1947	L'Air du Temps	FL	Ricci	Citrus, Neroli, Carnation	Clove, Rose, Gardenia	Sandalwood, Musk, Ambra
1952	Youth Dew	OR	Lauder	Citrus, spicy, aldehydic	Carnation, spicy, fruity	Balsamic, Ambra, woody
1955	Intimate	CH	Revlon	Aldehydic, floral, green	Jasmin, fruity, woody	Mossy, balsamic, animalic
1956	Diorissimo	FL	Dior	Green, Bergamot, floral	Lily-of-the-Valley, Jasmin, Rose	Sandalwood, floral, balsamic
1959	Cabochard	CH	Grès	Hyacinth, Jasmin, spicy	Rose, Gardenia, Tuberose	Oakmoss, Ambra, leather
1960	Madame Rochas	AL	Rochas	Aldehydic, floral, citrus	Rose, Lily-of-the-Valley, aldehydic	Woody, mossy, Ambra
1961	Calèche	AL	Hermès	Aldehydic, citrus, resinous	Floral, Lily-of-the-Valley, Violet	Woody, musky, leather
1964	Y	CH	St Laurent	Aldehydic, fruity, floral	Rose, Jasmin, Tuberose, green	Patchouli, Ambra, balsamic
1966	Fidji	FL	Laroche	Galbanum, Hyacinth, Bergamot	Carnation, Rose, Jasmin	Woody, Ambra, musky
1967	Climat	AL	Lancôme	Aldehydic, floral, Peach, citrus	Lily-of-the-Valley, Rose, Jasmin	Vetivert, Ambra, powdery
1969	Calandre	AL	Rabanne	Aldehydic, green, Bergamot	Rose, Jasmin, Lily-of-the-Valley	Woody, leather, Oakmoss
1969	Estée Super	FL	Lauder	Aldehydic, fruity	Lily-of-the-Valley, Rose, Jasmin, Carnation	Cedarwood, animalic
1970	Chamade	AL	Guerlain	Galbanum, citrus, Hyacinth	Aldehydic, floral, spicy	Benzoin, woody, Ambra
1970	No. 19	FL	Chanel	Galbanum; floral, Bergamot	Floral, woody, aldehydic	Vetivert, Oakmoss, leather, powdery
1972	Alliage	CH	Lauder	Green, Pineapple, citrus	Jasmin, conifer, spicy	Oakmoss, woody, animalic
1972	Diorella	FL	Dior	Lemon, Bergamot, green	Floral, spicy, green	Oakmoss, woody, spicy
1973	Coriandre	CH	Couturier	Aldehydic, Coriander, Neroli	Rose, Jasmin, spicy	Patchouli, Oakmoss, woody
1973	Charlie	FL	Revlon	Citrus, green, floral	Jasmin, floral	Woody, Oakmoss, balsamic
1975	Chloé	FL	Lagerfeld	Green, Peach, Aldehydic	White flowers, green	Sandalwood, animalic, balsamic
1976	Oscar de la Renta	FL	Stern	Aldehydic, green, Peach	Tuberose, Lily-of-the-Valley, Orange Flower	Woody, Oakmoss, musky, powdery

Table 9.2 (contd.) — Classic feminine fragrances

Year	Fragrance	Type	House of origin	Top notes	Middle notes	Basic notes
1976	First	FL	Van Cleef & Arpels	Aldehydic, fruity, green	Jasmin, floral, spicy	Woody, animalic, Ambra
1977	Opium	OR	St Laurent	Aldehydic, citrus, spicy	Floral, spicy, fruity	Balsamic, Ambra, Musky
1978	Lauren	FL	Cosmair	Green, fruity, floral	Cyclamen, Lily-of-the-Valley, Tuberose	Musky, woody, balsamic, powdery
1979	Anaïs Anaïs	FL	Cacharel	Green, Jasmin, citrus	Jasmin, Lily-of-the-Valley, spicy	Woody, Oakmoss, powdery
1981	Nocturnes	AL	Caron	Aldehydic, citrus, green, floral	Lily-of-the-Valley, aldehydic	Balsamic, Vetivert, powdery
1981	Must de Cartier	OR	Cartier	Citrus, aldehydic, fruity, floral	Jasmin, spicy, leather	Balsamic, woody, powdery
1981	Giorgio	FL	Beverly Hills	Neroli, green, aldehydic, floral	Tuberose, Jasmin, Gardenia	Woody, musky, powdery
1985	Poison	FL	Dior	Spicy, fruity, floral	Tuberose, Rose, spicy, fruity	Heliotrope, woody, powdery
1989	Joop!	OR	Joop	Citrus, aldehydic	Lily-of-the-Valley, floral	Woody, animalic, balsamic
1989	Samsara	OR	Guerlain	Floral, citrus	Floral, Sandalwood	Sandalwood, Ambra, balsamic
1991	Amarige	FL	Givenchy	Neroli, citrus, green	Mimosa, Gardenia, fruity	Woody, Ambra, balsamic

Table 9.3 — Classic masculine fragrances

Year	Fragrance	Type	House of origin	Top notes	Middle notes	Basic notes
1714	Kölnisch Wasser	CT	Farina Gegenüber	Citrus, Petitgrain, Neroli	Carnation, Rose, Rosemary	Musk
1882	Fougère Royale	FG	Houbigant	Lavender, Spike, citrus, Clary Sage	Spicy, Geranium, Heliotrope	Oakmoss, balsamic powdery
1910	English Lavender	LV	Atkinson	Lavender, Spike, Rosemary, citrus	Sage, Clary Sage	Oakmoss, Tonka
1924	Knize Ten	CH	Knize	Citrus, Rosemary, Petitgrain	Geranium, woody, floral	Leather, animalic, powdery
1937	Old Spice	OR	Shulton	Orange Peel, spicy, aldehydic	Floral, Carnation, spicy	Woody, powdery, balsamic
1946	Silvestre	LV	Victor	Lavender, citrus, green	Conifer, Carnation, spicy, floral	Woody, Oakmoss, powdery
1957	Vétiver	CH	Carven	Citrus, Petitgrain, spicy	Woody, herbaceous, Carnation	Mossy, woody, powdery
1957	Sandalwood	FG	Arden	Lavender, citrus, Petitgrain	Sandalwood, Geranium, woody	Mossy, Ambra, balsamic
1959	Tabac Original	CT	Mäurer & Wirtz	Citrus, Lavender, aldehydic	Floral, woody	Tobacco, Ambra, powdery
1960	Prestige Dry Herb	CT	Wolff & Sohn	Galbanum, citrus	Floral, spicy	Mossy, Ambra, Tonka
1964	Brut for Men	FG	Fabergé	Lavender, Bergamot, Basil	Hawthorn, Geranium, woody	Musky, Heliotrope, powdery

Table 9.3 (contd.) — Classic masculine fragrances

Year	Fragrance	Type	House of origin	Top notes	Middle notes	Basic notes
1966	Aramis	CH	Aramis	Artemisia, spicy, aldehydic, green	Woody, spicy, floral	Leather, animalic, mossy
1966	Eau Sauvage	CT	Dior	Bergamot, Basil, floral	Jasmin, woody, spicy	Woody, Oakmoss, powdery
1970	Royal Copenhagen	OR	Swank	Citrus, aldehydic, green	Floral, Patchouli, woody	Mossy, Tonka, Heliotrope, powdery
1973	Paco Rabanne pour Homme	FG	Rabanne	Lavender, citrus, spicy, green	Floral, spicy, Clary Sage	Mossy, Cedarwood, Ambra
1974	Gentleman	CH	Givenchy	Bergamot, fruity, floral	Woody, spicy, floral, balsamic	Woody, mossy, Ambra, leather
1976	Halston Z14	CH	Halston	Bergamot, green, spicy	Jasmin, woody, Patchouli	Ambra, leather, woody, mossy
1978	Lagerfeld	OR	Lagerfeld	Bergamot, green, spicy, aldehydic	Floral, tobacco, Cedarwood, Patchouli	Ambra, balsamic, powdery
1978	Azzaro pour Homme	FG	Azzaro	Lavender, citrus, Basil	Woody, Patchouli	Oakmoss, Ambra, leather
1978	Van Cleef & Arpels	CH	Van Cleef & Arpels	Bergamot, herbaceous, spicy, green	Artemisia, spicy, floral, woody	Leather, mossy, animalic
1978	Devin	CH	Aramis	Galbanum, citrus, spicy, aldehydic	Floral, spicy, Pine, green	Woody, leather, mossy, Ambra
1978	Polo	CH	Cosmair	Artemisia, green, citrus	Pine, spicy, floral	Leather, mossy, woody
1980	Macassar	CH	Rochas	Citrus, Artemisia, green	Carnation, Vetivert, Jasmin, spicy	Woody, mossy, leather
1982	Drakkar Noir	CH	Laroche	Artemisia, green, Bergamot	Spicy, Pine, floral	Mossy, Patchouli, woody
1984	Armani pour Homme	CT	Armani	Citrus, herbaceous, Basil	Spicy, floral, Lavender	Woody, mossy, musky
1986	Zino Davidoff	FG	Davidoff	Citrus, Clary Sage, Lavender	Floral, herbaceous	Woody, balsamic, powdery
1988	Fahrenheit	CH	Dior	Violet, citrus, green, herbaceous	Floral, woody	Ambra, leather, Tonka
1988	Cool Water	FG	Davidoff	Citrus, Neroli, green, spicy	Clary Sage, floral	Cedarwood, Oakmoss, Ambra
1988	Jazz	FG	St Laurent	Lavender, citrus, Basil	Spicy, herbaceous, floral	Leather, woody, Ambra

Table 9.4 — Classic perfumes: cross-referenced by name of perfume

Perfume	House of origin	Feminine or Masculine	Type*	Date introduced
Alliage	Lauder	F	CH	1972
Amarige	Givenchy	F	FL	1991
Anaïs Anaïs	Cacharel	F	FL	1979
Aramis	Aramis	M	CH	1966
Armani pour Homme	Armani	M	CT	1984
Arpège	Lanvin	F	AL	1927
Azzaro pour Homme	Azzaro	M	FG	1978
Brut for Men	Fabergé	M	FG	1964
Cabochard	Grès	F	CH	1959
Calandre	Rabanne	F	AL	1969
Calèche	Hermès	F	AL	1961
Chamade	Guerlain	F	AL	1970
Charlie	Revlon	F	FL	1973
Chloé	Lagerfield	F	FL	1975
Climat	Lancôme	F	AL	1967
Cool Water	Davidoff	M	FG	1988
Coriandre	Couturier	F	CH	1973
Crêpe de Chine	Millot	F	CH	1925
Devin	Aramis	M	Ch	1978
Diorella	Dior	F	FL	1972
Diorissimo	Dior	F	FL	1956
Drakkar Noir	Laroche	M	CH	1982
Eau Sauvage	Dior	M	CT	1966
English Lavender	Atkinson	M	LV	1910
Estée Super	Lauder	F	FL	1969
Fahrenheit	Dior	M	CH	1988
Femme	Rochas	F	CH	1944
Fidji	Laroche	F	FL	1966
First	Van Cleef & Arpels	F	FL	1976
Fougère Royale	Houbigant	M	FG	1882
Gentleman	Givenchy	M	CH	1974
Giorgio	Beverly Hills	F	FL	1981

* AL Aldehydic type; CT Citrus type; FL Floral type; CH Chypre type; OR Oriental type; LV Lavender type; FG Fougère type

Table 9.4 (contd.) — Classic perfumes: cross-referenced by name of perfume

Perfume	House of origin	Feminine or Masculine	Type	Date introduced
Halston Z14	Halston	M	CH	1976
Intimate	Revlon	F	CH	1955
Jazz	St. Laurent	M	FG	1988
Je Reviens	Worth	F	AL	1932
Jicky	Guerlain	F	OR	1889
Joop!	Joop	F	OR	1989
Joy	Patou	F	FL	1935
Knize Ten	Knize	M	CH	1924
Kölnisch Wasser	Farina Gegenüber	M	CT	1714
Lagerfeld	Lagerfield	M	OR	1978
L'Air du Temps	Ricci	F	FL	1947
L auren	Cosmair	F	FL	1978
Le Chypre	Coty	F	CH	1917
L'Origan	Coty	F	FL	1905
Macassar	Rochas	M	CH	1980
Madame Rochas	Rochas	F	AL	1960
Ma Griffe	Carven	F	CH	1946
Miss Dior	Dior	F	CH	1947
Muguet des Bois	Coty	F	FL	1942
Must de Cartier	Cartier	F	OR	1981
Nocturnes	Caron	F	AL	1981
No. 5	Chanel	F	AL	1921
No. 19	Chanel	F	FL	1970
Old Spice	Shulton	M	OR	1937
Opium	St. Laurent	F	OR	1977
Oscar de la Renta	Stern	F	FL	1976
Paco Rabanne pour Homme	Rabanne	M	FG	1973
Poison	Dior	F	FL	1985
Polo	Cosmair	M	CH	1978
Prestige Dry Herb	Wolff & Sohn	M	CT	1960
Quelques Fleurs	Houbigant	F	FL	1912
Royal Copenhagen	Swank	M	OR	1970

Table 9.4 (contd.) — Classic perfumes: cross-referenced by name of perfume

Perfume	House of origin	Feminine or Masculine	Type	Date introduced
Samsara	Guerlain	F	OR	1989
Sandalwood	Arden	M	FG	1957
Shalimar	Guerlain	F	OR	1925
Shocking	Schiaperelli	F	OR	1937
Silvestre	Victor	M	LV	1946
Soir de Paris	Bourjois	F	FL	1928
Tabac Original	Mäurer & Wirtz	M	CT	1959
Van Cleef & Arpels	Van Cleef & Arpels	M	CH	1978
Vent Vert	Balmain	F	FL	1945
Vétiver	Carven	M	CH	1957
Y	St. Laurent	F	CH	1964
Youth Dew	Lauder	F	OR	1952
Zino Davidoff	Davidoff	M	FG	1986

Table 9.5 — Classic perfumes: cross-referenced by perfume type

Perfume	Feminine or Masculine	House of origin	Date introduced
Citrus perfume type			
Armani pour Homme	M	Armani	1984
Eau Sauvage	M	Dior	1966
Kölnisch Wasser	M	Farina Gegenüber	1714
Prestige Dry Herb	M	Wolff & Sohn	1960
Tabac Original	M	Mäurer & Wirtz	1959
Floral perfume type			
Amarige	F	Givenchy	1991
Anaïs Anaïs	F	Cacharel	1979
Charlie	F	Revlon	1973
Chloé	F	Lagerfeld	1975
Diorella	F	Dior	1972
Diorissimo	F	Dior	1956
Estée Super	F	Lauder	1969
Fidji	F	Laroche	1966
First	F	Van Cleef & Arpels	1976
Giorgio	F	Beverley Hills	1981

Table 9.5 (contd.) — Classic perfumes: cross-referenced by perfume type

Perfume	Feminine or Masculine	House of origin	Date introduced
Joy	F	Patou	1935
L'Air du Temps	F	Ricci	1947
Lauren	F	Cosmair	1978
L'Origan	F	Coty	1905
Muguet des Bois	F	Coty	1942
No. 19	F	Chanel	1970
Oscar de la Renta	F	Stern	1976
Poison	F	Dior	1985
Quelques Fleurs	F	Houbigant	1912
Soir de Paris	F	Bourjois	1928
Vent Vert	F	Balmain	1945
Aldehydic perfume type			
Arpège	F	Lanvin	1927
Calandre	F	Rabanne	1969
Calèche	F	Hermès	1961
Chamade	F	Guerlain	1970
Climat	F	Lancôme	1967
Je Reviens	F	Worth	1932
Madame Rochas	F	Rochas	1960
Nocturnes	F	Caron	1981
No. 5	F	Chanel	1921
Chypre perfume type			
Alliage	F	Lauder	1972
Aramis	M	Aramis	1966
Cabochard	F	Grès	1959
Coriandre	F	Couturier	1973
Crêpe de Chine	F	Millot	1925
Devin	M	Aramis	1978
Drakkar Noir	M	Laroche	1982
Fahrenheit	M	Dior	1988
Femme	F	Rochas	1944
Gentleman	M	Givenchy	1974
Halston Z14	M	Halston	1976
Intimate	F	Revlon	1955
Knize Ten	M	Knize	1924
Le Chypre	F	Coty	1917
Macassar	M	Rochas	1980
Ma Griffe	F	Carven	1946

Table 9.5 (contd.) — Classic perfumes: cross-referenced by perfume type

Perfume	Feminine or Masculine	House of origin	Date introduced
Miss Dior	F	Dior	1947
Polo	M	Cosmair	1978
Van Cleef & Arpels	M	Van Cleef & Arpels	1978
Vétiver	M	Carven	1957
Y	F	St Laurent	1964
Oriental perfume type			
Jicky	F	Guerlain	1889
Joop!	F	Joop	1989
Lagerfeld	M	Lagerfeld	1978
Must de Cartier	F	Cartier	1981
Old Spice	M	Shulton	1937
Opium	F	St Laurent	1977
Royal Copenhagen	M	Swank	1970
Samsara	F	Guerlain	1989
Shalimar	F	Guerlain	1925
Shocking	F	Schiaparelli	1937
Youth Dew	F	Lauder	1952
Lavender perfume type			
English Lavender	M	Atkinson	1910
Silvestre	M	Victor	1946
Fougère perfume type			
Azzaro pour Homme	M	Azzaro	1978
Brut for Men	M	Fabergé	1964
Cool Water	M	Davidoff	1988
Fougère Royale	M	Houbigant	1882
Jazz	M	St Laurent	1988
Paco Rabanne pour Homme	M	Rabanne	1973
Sandalwood	M	Arden	1957
Zino Davidoff	M	Davidoff	1986

The powerful and insistently diffusive fragrance creations of the 1980s are today giving way to softer, more delicate and more 'natural' trends. The preceding eras of perfumery, we should recognize, bore witness to a rise in public esteem of perfumes of certain, identifiable kinds, some of which were sooner or later accorded classical status. These perfumes rose to outstanding levels of appreciation, not only of their fragrance qualities alone, but of the totality of aesthetic experience they afforded through the agencies of the senses of sight and touch. They were, are and will remain, outstanding products of the commercial art of perfumery of our time.

The quality determining role of natural products in the earlier classic fragrances, and in many others, has been recognized by perfumers ever since the coming of aroma chemicals to perfumery. Now, we have the distinct possibility that research into the composition of natural odours through headspace analysis will come to full fruition in the foreseeable future. This prospect will certainly be augmented by further development of the 'electronic nose' for the investigation and permanent recording of odour impressions. Quite suddenly it seems, in terms of technological evolution, the essential oils and perfume industries now approach the threshold of practical realization of what were, even a year or so ago, impossible dreams: the almost total synthetic reproduction of the fragrances of nature and the elimination of subjectivity from odour evaluation, both demanding the availability of synthetic chemicals of ultra-high purity.

There are, however, possible alternatives to a totally synthetic world of perfumery which are of the greatest interest to users of essential oils in alternative or supplementary medicine. One of these, already in use or under intensive investigation, is the well-established microculture of individual, identical plants; another is the closely controlled tissue culture of essential oil-bearing cells, with subsequent processing to yield natural products of constant quality.

A field of aroma chemical production of growing interest is the microbial conversion of natural isolates, such as terpenes, into useful aroma materials, just as yeasts ferment bland sugar solutions, transforming them into products of spiritually exciting quality.

It is today true that never before in the history of science and technology have opportunities been so ripe for the successful investigation of natural sources of fragrance, and for application of the discoveries certain to be made to the benefit of mankind.

9.7 Essential Oils, Perfumes and the Retailer

The following notes apply to members of staff working in shops and stores where *personal service to the customer*, an important application of total quality management, is regarded as the basis for successful business. They summarize means whereby the mutual benefits of good personal chemistry between the salesperson and the customer may be maximized.

9.7.1 Principles of Service to the Customer

1. Premises must be clean and tidy.
2. Display of products should be distinctive, informative, attractive and uncluttered.
3. There should always be a sufficiency of stock for immediate needs ready to hand. All stock should be kept in a clean and tidy condition.

4. Essential oils and perfumes must be stored
   a) in a cool place, preferably at an even temperature
   b) protected from light
   c) under dry conditions
5. The sales environment should be welcoming and lead from the front door to the point of sale.
6. Sales persons should be
   a) alert
   b) attentive
   c) interested in people and in selling
   d) unprejudiced towards customers or particular products
   e) well informed on products offered for sale
   f) well informed on prices
   g) courteous and tactful without being gushing (the days of the effusive "Would modom like ----?" are long past)
   h) presentable in appearance and manner

9.7.2 A Systematic Approach to the Selling of Perfume

The selling of *personal fragrances* to customers seeking advice requires a certain technique of approach and testing if the customer is to derive a maximum of satisfaction from a purchase. This involves the following procedures:

a) Items of stock should always be in perfect condition; they should never be used for window display
b) Perfume testers should be kept clean, and dipstick-type testers kept free from evaporation residues
c) Customers for personal fragrance should be encouraged to select three perfumes from which a final choice will be made
d) The chosen perfumes should be applied, in succession, to the customer's pulse spots and within the bend of one arm
e) The customer should be asked to evaluate the top notes, but it should be mentioned that they will not last and that the final decision should rest upon the evaluation of the main fragrance theme of the perfume, which will quickly follow
f) The customer should be asked to select one of the perfumes by smelling all of them from the skin, occasionally, over a period of 24 hours
g) The customer's ability to afford a perfume should never be doubted, but if price seems to be a problem the customer should be tactfully offered a *corresponding* toilet water
h) If there is a choice of sizes, the customer should first be offered one size larger than the smallest
i) In completing the sale, the customer should be advised on the conditions under which the perfume should be stored

The above notes notwithstanding, it is a fact that in this country perfumes are most frequently purchased as gifts for other people. If in this case advice is sought by the purchaser, the sales person should enquire as to the a fragrance preferences of the prospective recipient, and then suggest a perfume of the same a fragrance family.

The reasons for personal testing of perfumes are that residues of sebum and those from the evaporation of sweat present on the skin surface are never of the same composition from one person to another, and that certain reactive perfume ingredients, such as aldehydes and ketones, can interact with constituents of these residues, such as amino acids. Amino acids enter the blood stream as a result of the breakdown of proteins by digestion in the small intestine. They are required for tissue growth and repair. Excess amounts of amino acids in the blood are eliminated partly via the sweat glands in the blood filtrate that we know as sweat. With reference to the 'lone pair' amine structure in sect. 3.10 (p. 75), a typical amino acid has the organic acid functional group -COOH bonded to the hydrocarbon chain, R. The hydrogen atoms *bonded to nitrogen* are reactive with, for example, the oxygen atom of an aldehyde, such as aldehyde C_8 or C_{10} (fig. 3.7, p. 60) to form a molecule of water. A double bond forms between the nitrogen atom of the amino group and the carbon atom of the aldehyde to which the oxygen atom was bonded. In the following equation, the general structural formula for an aldehyde has been reversed for convenience:

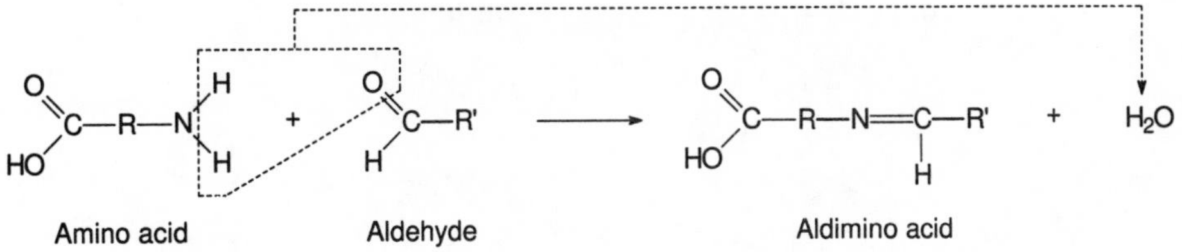

Amino acid   Aldehyde   Aldimino acid

Fig. 9.1 — Formation of an aldimino acid, as may occur when a fragrance interacts with aldehydes in sweat

The odour of the aldimino acid, if odorous, would be quite different from that of the aldehyde from which it was formed. Amino acids are odourless.

Since the proportions of amino acids in the sweat residues of different persons are never exactly the same and since the nature of those present depends on diet, it can be understood how the removal of traces of very powerfully odorous aldehydes, as occur in essential oils, from a perfume on the skin by the above reaction can have a noticeable effect on the a fragrance, which will vary from person to person. Usually such changes of a fragrance are slight, and if noticeable are acceptable, but this is not always so, and it is better for the customer to discover any adverse change of a fragrance before rather than after making a purchase.

A very small proportion of would-be users of a fragrance by application to the skin are unable to do so in consequence of the development of unacceptable, adverse odour changes with all perfumes. This problem can be overcome by using skin perfumes as they were originally intended to be used — on the handkerchief or, these days, on a paper tissue.

Chapter 10

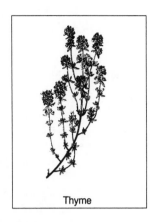

Thyme

Burning the Midnight Oil

Introduction

There were times, not so long ago, when the gift of a chemistry set to a youngster would often lead to an ever-widening interest in home experiments conducted in the garage, garden shed or, best of all, in a fully-fitted home laboratory. Chemicals and simple apparatus were readily available from most local pharmacists, whose own interest in chemistry had, more likely than not, been kindled in the same way. The lives of those of us fortunate enough to have lived through at least the closing years of the 'home chemistry' era were enriched and, for the totally immersed, given direction, by the wonders of personal discovery.

All that is now gone, and with it incalculable opportunity for the useful and adventurous stimulation of young minds. Yet, with the ever-widening application of the results of chemical and biochemical research to human need, the practical value of chemistry continues to increase.

The human body is basically a genetically and environmentally determined system of interrelated, organized chemical systems. Any form of chemical treatment aiming to remedy or correct an irregular condition of the body, or of the personal entity residing within it, who depends upon the body for all the activities of day-to-day living, has therefore to be undertaken with at least a basic knowledge of the chemistry involved.

The chemistry of essential oils is complex, as anyone who has survived the preceding chapters will have noticed. The book is, of course, merely a guide, intended to accompany and perhaps supplement lectures on the subject. This final chapter is written particularly with those readers who may not, for one reason or another, have formed the *habit* of study while at school, who are now concerned to learn some chemistry relevant to the development of their professional careers, and who for that purpose are prepared to light the lamp and burn the midnight oil.

10.1 How to Begin

For whatever purpose you are studying the chemistry of essential oils, you will find regular smelling exercises a valuable aid to memorizing their properties and chemistry. Odours are, as we have noted before, evocative of past experience; an odour can bring forth recollections of the circumstances under which it was experienced at some time in the past, provided those circumstances were at the time sufficiently impressed upon the mind. It is therefore reasonable to expect that if an essential oil is thoughfully smelled, just occasionally, while studying its chemistry, mental associations will form between the name of the oil, its odour and the facts of its nature and properties which are the subject of the learning exercise. Thus when the name 'Clary Sage' crops up, the main aspects of the odour of Clary Sage Oil will spring to mind: fresh, light, herbaceous, ambra, together with names of constituents — linalöl, linalyl acetate, sclareol, etc., and aspects of its uses, safety, botanical and geographical sources. Similarly, if one is confronted with an apparently unfamiliar essential oil in common use, a quick sniff should trigger recognition, then identification and, following identification, at least the main facts about the oil that you have memorized. Facility of recall requires repeated practice, a subject to which we shall return later in this chapter. So, you will need a set of essential oils. This may be made available to you as part of your course; if not, then you may be able to purchase small bottles of individual oils from your local pharmacy. The address of a supplier of small quantities of essential oils, as well as smelling strips, is given in the Appendix.

Once on the threshold of a course of your choice, the first decision to be made about private study will be that of how much time to devote to each subject area included in the course per week. The author's experience of science-based courses is that a student's working week should consist of six days, and that the seventh, whichever day that may be, should be reserved for leisure-time activities. One whole day 'away from it all' is much more refreshing than two half-days.

In a full-time course at higher education diploma level, lectures and practical periods are usually timetabled to take place on weekdays during daytime, leaving evenings and weekends free for private study and leisure. In this case an acceptable total amount of study time per week would probably amount to no more than 30 hours; that is, five hours per night for six nights, inclusive of two short breaks of 15 minutes each night for refreshment. Some students may well need less study time, while some may actually prefer more, the best plan being to build up on the nightly hours to a tolerable level, say to three hours, then to extend the time as the need for regular revision grows.

An important truth to bear in mind is that you can achieve anything in this world which is sensibly within your reach, *provided* your desire for achievement is strong to the point of dedication. Under these circumstances, your life will become suffused with your ambition, not obsessively, but sufficiently for you to be prepared to go for every opportunity for fulfilment. You have to be prepared to work, and work hard, but you will find that your capacity to do so will be sustained by your determination to succeed.

The conditions under which you pursue your private studies should be simple and plain. An ordinary chair and desk, your lecture notes, books and writing equipment are all that you need. It is difficult to believe students who say they can study in a nice, warm room, enfolded in the depths of a comfortable armchair, or even better in the convivial atmosphere of the local hostelry. A normal sitting posture without discomfort, coupled with active study, are conditions which tend gently to tense the muscles involved in sitting on a chair, and this mild muscular tension tends to concentrate the mind on the task in hand.

10.2 Planning Your Studies

To plan your private studies, begin by looking through your course syllabus to gain a general perspective of what lies ahead. Note the different subjects and the amount of lecture and practical time to be devoted to each. Regard your course as an adventure, offering opportunities for personal discovery, remembering that you, in common with all other students, can learn anything with sufficient determination to do so. There will be mountains to climb, but the view from one of the peaks always beckons to the next. There is no pleasure like mastering a subject that you thought you could never understand.

Next, prepare your personal study timetable. Allocate a definite amount of study time per week to each main topic area, relative to its importance and quantity of content, as expressed by the total amount of time allowed for lectures and practical work shown by your course timetable.

Let us suppose that you enrol for a one-year, full-time, advanced course in aromatherapy, beauty therapy, perfumery or any other subject involving the chemistry of essential oils. Lectures and practical sessions occupy, say, 20 hours per week and the total number of weeks occupied by your course is 48. A total of four hours per week is devoted to organic chemistry and the chemistry of essential oils — not much, but there are other things to be done. You decide initially to study for three hours per evening for six evenings per week during term-time.

Total weekly study time =18 hours
Weekly study time for organic chemistry and chemistry of essential oils

$$= \frac{4}{20} \times 18 = 3 \cdot 6 \text{ (about } 3\frac{1}{2} \text{ hours)}$$

On the above basis, you could try three separate hours' study of chemistry, using the additional half-hour for revision, reducing your study time roughly in proportion to your existing knowledge of chemistry as, for example:

Recent good pass in Chemistry at GCSE level: 3 hours + $\frac{1}{2}$ hour revision
Recent good pass in Chemistry at 'A' level: 2 hours + $\frac{1}{2}$ hour revision
Recent degree or equivalent in Chemistry, or in a discipline where chemistry is of major importance: 2 hours + $\frac{1}{2}$ hour revision

Notice the need for revision at all levels of past success.

Take account also of any natural interest in chemistry that you may have — you can, of course, if you wish, devote more study time to chemistry than that recommended above, though *not at the expense of your studies of other subjects*. If exceptionally keen, you could even organize a 'sponsored swot' for charity, though whether such a marathon would do you any good would be questionable, even if at the end of it you were able to convince your sponsors that you had not fallen asleep!

It is surprising how quickly one's knowledge of a subject can deteriorate if it is not used. It is also surprising how much of it 'comes back' on dredging the depths of your memory through renewed study, perhaps after a lapse of time, on realizing that an abstruse subject such as chemistry can actually be useful and interesting to learn.

The effective study of a science-based subject involves the following basic processes:

1. *Learning the facts*, and how they relate to one another and to the subject as a whole
2. *Understanding the facts*, so that they can be used in practical situations
3. *Listing and remembering relevant examples*, to illustrate the facts
4. *Bringing the facts together* to form systems of facts and examples, i.e. *concepts*
5. *Revising facts and concepts* to revive your knowledge, then extending your knowledge by further study
6. *Using your knowledge* in practical situations and, for examination purposes, for answering questions from past examination papers

These processes will be the foundation stones of your learning, and so we will discuss them one by one.

1. <u>Learning the facts</u> of a subject usually involves attending relevant classes, then following these up by private study. Undoubtedly, the most beneficial kind of lecture for students undergoing a course of study is not a lecture at all, but a lesson in which, while much of the lecturer's available time is occupied with the giving, interpreting and explaining of the facts of the subject, the victims know that they can interrupt to ask questions occasionally without fear of admonishment. However, the sheer amount of subject-matter comprising many courses frequently means that a lecturer just has to lecture uninterrupted, allowing a brief period of time at the end for questions before rushing off to inflict a further discourse elsewhere. The very act of writing notes during a lecture helps to imprint the subject-matter on the mind, and at the same time provides sets of reference points indicating directions for further studies.

2. <u>Understanding the facts</u> of a subject is essential if the subject as a whole is to be learned and known. Learning involves, as we have noted, memorizing and interrelating the facts of a subject to form concepts. The bringing together and interrelating of concepts results in the formation of a body of understood knowledge, which amounts to the sum total of one's learning of a subject. Every lecture must be regarded as an opportunity for understanding, at the time of the lecture. At the end of the lecture, you should have the feeling that the whole occasion has been, for you, a hard-working and worthwhile experience. Making the best of a lecture in an academic situation means following the drift of what is being said, while at the same time taking adequate notes for later study.

3. <u>Listing and remembering relevant examples</u> is something to be done during later private study. A highlighter is very useful to make examples stand out from a mass of notes, so that the examples can be easily dissected out on a later occasion.

4. <u>Bringing the facts together</u> involves finding points of relationship between related, apparently unrelated or poorly related facts. Thus, for example, in forming the concept of the composition of an essential oil we might usefully make a start by listing the names of its chief constituents, or by studying a GLC trace of the oil on which peaks corresponding to important constituents have been identified.

Sensory evaluation is extremely useful in relating the composition of an essential oil to its odour profile, especially if samples of constituents of the oil also are available for smelling. It seems very likely that olfactroscopy, the study of odours using print-outs from an 'electronic nose', will soon be commonplace, and these should assist our objective conceptualization of odour profiles in general, being independent of the human olfactory system and the vagaries of human judgment.

Next, we come to the composition and molecular structure of individual constituents, as deduced from the results of mass spectroscopy and other instrumental aids to molecular structural determination and represented by structural formulae.

It is, by this time, hardly possible not to have formed, through careful study and through the making of additional notes and odour evaluation, at least an outline of the concept sought, which may be brought to completion as far as it is necessary to go with information on applications, safety in use, botanical and geographical sources, production methods, and so on.

The concept of an essential oil may usefully be represented in the form of a monograph of the kind that we shall presently recommend for a card index system. Then having produced a whole collection of concept monographs, you will find it easy to identify relationships between different essential oils with regard to applications, including those depending on odour (which itself depends on the nature and proportions of constituents); nature of constituents (depending on molecular structure); and molecular structure (depending on the valencies and arrangement of the constituent atoms of the molecules), until eventually the body of knowledge firmly in place in your mind may demand an answer to the question, 'How do essential oils work as aromatherapeutic or aromachologic agents or as perfume ingredients?', at which point it will be time to seek some explanations.

5. <u>Revising facts and concepts</u> will now present no difficulty if you have good sets of lecture notes and monographs. For revision purposes you will find it helpful to condense your lecture and textbook notes, and to keep the condensed version in a separate folder. This, you will find, will be enormously helpful when the examinations begin to loom, as by that time you will be thoroughly accustomed to serious study and will be able to revise from the condensed notes quickly and efficiently. Some students recondense their condensed notes until they have the essence of an entire course within the covers of a folder of modest thickness.

6. <u>Using your knowledge</u>. The knowledge you gain during a course involving essential oils can be applied to specific situations through practical work tailored to the particular purposes of the course: massage and odour diffusion in the case of aromatherapy; preparation and application of cosmetics in beauty therapy; creation of experimental blends in perfumery, etc. Practical work gives point to the theory and, of course, makes the subject-matter much more interesting and purposeful to learn. The careful and systematic recording of experimental and other practical work in a notebook or folder reserved for that purpose provides the notes you will require for revising before practical examinations, if set, and in either case the notes will provide a valuable aid towards effective revision.

10.3 Making Lecture Notes

Whatever the subject of a lecture, and however the lecture may be delivered, it is for the individual student to make the best of it. Lecture rooms today are mostly clean, bright and, if not exactly cheerful, are not usually in the state of impending collapse that some of them were years ago. But the physical state of the learning environment is not that important, as long as it will physically withstand occupation by students, is dry, and neither arctic in the winter nor tropical in the summer as regards temperature. The almost universal adoption of dustless boards in place of the blackboard has banished the blanketing clouds of chalk dust once raised by the most vigorous of lecturers at the end of a dissertation, and the overhead projector also is a great improvement, even if the images on the screen are usually distorted, and too small or obscure at distances of more than a few metres. Colleges already old half a century ago possessed a certain kind of atmosphere that the newer ones cannot hope to emulate. Memories of such places are treasured by those of us fortunate enough to have experienced them, the fact that many of them occupied grim, gloomy-looking buildings enhancing, rather than detracting from, their almost Dickensian character.

One such ancient establishment, alma mater to the present author, boasted a Great Hall of some size, along one side of which stood a row of pointed-arch, perpendicular Gothic windows facing a quadrangle. On the opposite side of the enclosure were lecture rooms having windows of similar architectural style. The experience of attending a lecture in one of these rooms on a darkening afternoon in depth of winter, the glowing windows of the Hall lending a backdrop of warmth to the cold without, and to whirling snowflakes falling silently to a thickening carpet below, was one to be reflected upon with rather more than a touch of nostalgia in the years to come.

The amount of detail to be taken down in the form of lecture notes is ultimately for the individual student to decide. Always bear in mind that the best notes (i.e. the notes from which you will gain maximum benefit during later study) will be those that are *legible* and that include all the essential features of the subject-matter exposed, together with any explanatory diagrams and examples. To make good notes does not require the recording of the lecturer's every utterance, including anecdotes, though the present writer would not be without his collection of lecturers' tales and quasi-eccentric expressions, hastily scribbled down during lectures before they were lost forever.

It is extremely difficult if not impossible to record a lecture verbatim. It is also unnecessary. On the other hand, students who make no lecture notes at all tend to do worse in examinations than those who make some notes. There is also the not unimportant point that lecturers give of their knowledge during lectures, and that for a student to be seen writing down even occasional notes during a lecture is an acknowledgement of that fact which the lecturer will notice and appreciate.

To compare the amount of labour involved and the resulting clarity of taking almost verbatim notes with those produced after some thought, and hence at least on the basis of some learning, during a lecture, here are two examples of notes taken from the same introductory lesson on essential oils.

[In the remainder of this chapter, comments on students' notes and on answers to examination questions will appear in italics and in square parentheses].

Essential Oils

Essent. oils are mixtures of volatile org. compounds produced by certain plants. Not known whether essent. oils are of any value to the plant or whether they are waste products of the plant's mbm. *[metabolism]*

Preparation of essent. oils

Obtained from plant sources mainly by steam dist., but essential oils of citrus fruits obtained by cold expression from the peel. (Exception: lime oil mostly distilled.)

Properties of essent. oils

Most essential oils used in pharm. *[pharmacy]* have med. *[medicinal]* props. but a few are used to cover the odours or flavours of unpleasant tasting preps. *[preparations]* or unpleasant smelling ointments or lotions. Lavender Oil B.P. is an ex. *[example]*. Because of their pleasant odours Lavender and other pleasant smelling essent. oils, e.g. Rose Otto, Geranium, Pine, Neroli and Bergamot, are used in perfumery. Essent. oils are readily oxidized and must be stored in securely closed containers, protected from light and in a cool place.

Composition of essent. oils

The consts. *[constituents]* of essent. oils are unsat. *[unsaturated]* hydrocarbons called terpenes and their oxygenated derivs. — terpenoids. Some oils contain aliphatic and benzenoid cpds. *[compounds]*. Occasionally cpds. of N or S are present. Terpenes are h'carbons *[hydrocarbons]* having the general formula $(C_5H_8)_n$, where n is 2,3 or 4; i.e. $C_{10}H_{16}$ monoterpenes, $C_{15}H_{24}$ sesquiterpenes. Diterpenes $C_{20}H_{32}$ are of very low volatility and so may be found in extracts but not in dist. essent. oils. Terpenes and terpenoids are widely distributed in nature.

The above notes were taken down at some considerable speed and probably incompletely understood at the time. It would have been far less of an onerous task, as well as clearer for learning purposes and revision, if they had been recorded in much shorter form, as follows:

Essential Oils

<u>Essent. Oils</u>:	Volatile org. cpds. prod. by certain plants May or may not be useful to plant.
<u>Prep.</u>:	Mainly steam dist., but citrus oils cold expression from peel (Lime Oil mainly dist.).
<u>Props.</u>:	Most pharmacy e.o. *[further abbreviation of 'essential oil(s)' as the expression is certain to crop up many times]* have med. props.
	Some used to cover unpleas. odours/flavours e.g. Lavender & Peppermint. Rose, Lavender, Neroli, etc. used in perfumery.
	E.o. readily oxidized so store in well-closed cont. *[containers]* prot. *[protected from]* light, cool pl. *[place]*
<u>Comp.</u>:	Unsat. h'carbons (terpenes) + oxygenated derivs – terpenoids. Some contain aliphatics and benzenoids, some N & S cpds.
	Terpenes $(C_5H_8)n$. n = 2,3 or 4. $C_{10}H_{16}$ monoterpenes, $C_{15}H_{24}$ sesquiterpenes. Diterpenes $C_{20}H_{32}$ v. low vol. so found in exts. *[extracts]* not e.o. Terpenes & terpenoids widely distributed in nature.

The sets of notes, above, were taken from about five minutes of the lecture time, whereafter the lecturer droned on to expand the subject in considerable detail. The amount of sheer drudgery involved in taking very full notes is plain to see. Also clear is the ease with which the writer of the second set of notes could use them for study in association with a textbook, popping in bits and pieces of further information here and there.

Notice that both students used abbreviations, having done so many times before. It is, of course, necessary to use abbreviations that will be understood on subsequent perusal of the notes. Nothing is more frustrating than coming across an abbreviation, invented on the spur of the moment during a lecture, the meaning of which has been completely forgotten. A quick marginal note at the time of use can prevent this from happening. Finally on this subject, a policy of *always double-spacing lecture notes* is very helpful, in leaving room for the insertion of additional information gathered from other sources, such as books, works of reference and articles and papers found in technical periodicals.

The making of personal recordings of lectures, if allowed, enables full attention to be given to understanding what is being said. It is, however, advisable also to make some notes at the time for later study in association with the recordings, and as a safeguard against loss of a recording through failure of the tape recorder or other cause. It is not unknown for a student, supposedly making a tape recording, to be blissfully unaware that the machine is not running. Permission to record lectures should, as a matter of courtesy, always be requested beforehand. If for any reason permission is refused, this should be accepted without question, and any further approach to the lecturer on the matter should be deferred until after completion of the lecture. In some institutions there is a strict rule forbidding the recording of lectures. If such a rule is in force, it should always be respected.

10.4 Study Method

Personal notes, if carefully and legibly written, are probably the best source of learning material for general use throughout a course. They are familiar, and should have been taken down with at least a basic understanding of the subject-matter at the time. They should represent the essence of a subject in terms of facts, reasons for and explanations of the facts, together with relevant examples. Recommended textbooks, particularly if there are alternatives, should be carefully perused before purchase to make sure that the contents are clear and well presented.

Lecture notes should be *used*, not simply read over and over again in the vain hope, never fulfilled, that the good stuff will go in and be absorbed, as happens to refreshment of the same description under more convivial circumstances. Your studies must be *active*, not passive. The simple procedure of reading through your notes carefully and with reflection, and highlighting important definitions, explanations, examples, etc. is one example of an active approach to study. Doing this can ease you into a few hours of profitable study in a quite painless way, even when you would rather be doing something else. When you subsequently go through notes so improved, your attention will quickly be drawn to what you *must* and *should* know of the subject, the rest of your notes representing what you *could*, with advantage, know if you have the time to learn it. Highlighting, if used sparingly, and employing different colours for different purposes, will increase the efficiency of your studies. Too much colour, and the result will take on a certain avant-garde appearance conducive more to appreciation as a work of art than to the purpose of learning.

During studies, passing thoughts and ideas relevant to the subject, as well as questions to be asked, should be noted down *as they come to mind*, in separate pages reserved for this purpose and kept at the back of the notes in your folder. Alternatively, and possibly better, you could write your lecture notes on only one side of your notepaper, leaving the left-hand or right-hand pages of your notes, as they appear on opening them, unused except for this purpose. Double-space your notes, and leave about 5 cm at the bottom blank for making additional notes. Closely written, cramped notes with no space for more are difficult to use.

For students making fairly full notes (old habits die hard!), it is useful, a week or so after starting a course, to begin to condense them, to 'distil the essence', so to speak, ready for pre-examination revision. Time passes so quickly when one is absorbed in lectures and studies week after week that it is necessary to adopt a sense of urgency towards learning and revision. Always try to study just that little bit harder than you feel is reasonable, so that on entering the examination room, chill thought, you *know* that your preparation has been as thorough as you could possibly have made it. You can do no more.

A further helpful mode of study, to make a change from the usual grind, is to choose a topic and then set yourself simple questions of the kind likely to crop up in the examinations and which require only short answers, bearing in mind that such questions could occur as parts of longer questions in examination papers on aromatherapy, beauty therapy or perfumery. Here are some examples taken from different questions on the subject of the citrus oils:

1. *Briefly describe the process used for the production of Berga-mot Oil.*
2. *State and explain the conditions to be used for the storage of citrus oils.*
3. *For what purpose(s) is Lemon Oil used in perfumery?*
4. *Name the aromatic products obtained from the bitter orange tree. Briefly describe their odours.*
5. *Account for the changes of odour which occur when Lemon Oil is exposed to the air on a smelling strip.*

This kind of exercise is most useful where a small group of students get together in a vacant lecture room for revision. One member of the group, appointed leader for the session, prepares the questions and writes them on the board — that is, unless all the markers have, wisely, been hidden or removed, in which case the questions are read out. Twenty minutes are then allowed for all members of the group to answer the questions, following which each member in turn reads out his or her answer to one of the questions. This is followed by discussion and verification of the correct answer in each case from notes and textbooks.

When working alone, there are many ways of usefully varying the monotony of studying from notes or textbooks. Here are a few suggestions:

1. Choose a topic, then prepare a simple scheme of essential information on the topic. An example is shown in figure 10.1.
2. Try to develop a train of thought from a chosen subject as, for example, in figure 10.2.

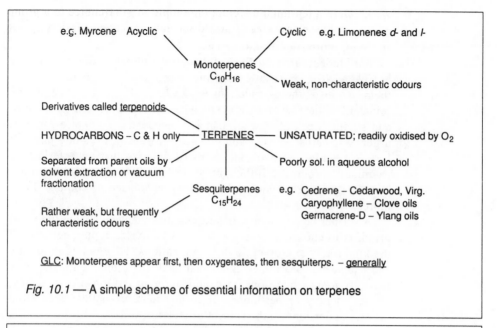

e.g. Myrcene   Acyclic

Cyclic   e.g. Limonenes *d-* and *l-*

Monoterpenes
$C_{10}H_{16}$

Weak, non-characteristic odours

Derivatives called <u>terpenoids</u>

HYDROCARBONS – C & H only —— TERPENES —— UNSATURATED; readily oxidised by O_2

Separated from parent oils by
solvent extraction or vacuum
fractionation

Poorly sol. in aqueous alcohol

Sesquiterpenes
$C_{15}H_{24}$

e.g. Cedrene – Cedarwood, Virg.
      Caryophyllene – Clove oils
      Germacrene-D – Ylang oils

Rather weak, but frequently
characteristic odours

<u>GLC</u>: Monoterpenes appear first, then oxygenates, then sesquiterps. – <u>generally</u>

Fig. 10.1 — A simple scheme of essential information on terpenes

ESTERS   R.COOR'

In essential oils:

e.g. Lavender Oil   — linalyl acetate
     Jasmin Abs.   — benzyl acetate
     Ylang-Ylang Oil   — benzyl acetate, methyl salicylate
     Roman Chamomile Oil — tiglates, angelates
                            :
                            :
                            :
                           etc.

Many easily <u>hydrolyzed:</u>

$$R.COOR' + H_2O \rightleftharpoons R.COOH + R'OH$$
ester   +   water   organic acid   +   alcohol

also:

$$R.COOH + H_2O \rightleftharpoons R.COO^- + H_3O^+$$
acid molecule water molecule   acid anion   oxonium ion

Can happen in <u>moist. essent. oils</u> over a period of time, also during <u>distillation</u> → increase <u>acid value</u> by
increased conc. H_3O^+.

Acid value — measure of free acid in an essent. oil. Should be <u>low</u>, increases with age of oil. Can
quickly increase if oil is poorly stored ∴ essential oils should be <u>dry</u>.

Many esters have fruity odours, used in perfumery, e.g. acetates of lower aliphatic alcohols, e.g. amyl
acetate (pear), ethyl butyrate (pineapple), amyl butyrate (banana), also tiglates in Roman Chamomile Oil.

Fig. 10.2 — A train of thought about esters

3. Give a ten-minute lecture on a topic of your choice to a group of your classmates. Suitable subjects might be as follows:

Distillation and properties of a chosen essential oil
Aldehydes in essential oils
Essential oils containing phenols
The question of 'vital force'
Rose Otto in perfumery

Preparing the notes for your lecture will be useful revision, but don't write them out in full, then bore everyone to death by reading them out verbatim. There is no better persuader to learning something thoroughly than knowing you have to teach it — you have to know your stuff, or watch out! Above all, enjoy the exercise and be ready for questions!

4. Devise a crossword puzzle on the theme of essential oils, providing suitable clues.
5. Write summaries of information, as illustrated in figures 10.1 and 10.2. This can be an ongoing exercise, affording ready means of quick revision and reference.

Use of a card-index system

Purchase a simple card-index system to hold about 100 cards, dimensions *no smaller* than 15 cm x 10 cm, and lined feint (faint parallel lines across).

Twice a week make out one card, giving details of an essential oil used in aromatherapy and/or perfumery, depending on the information you need. Arrange to have essential information on the front of the card and other information on the back. Leave room for notes to be added as and when opportunities arise. Shown in figure 10.3 are examples of possible arrangements for the information to appear on the cards for a student of aromatherapy.

Because of the increasing associations between aromatherapy and perfumery, it is becoming more and more important for students of either subject area to have a basic knowledge of the other.

10.5 Sensory Studies

Anyone using essential oils professionally needs to be familiar with their odours for purposes of identification and quality evaluation before deliveries are taken into stock. Such familiarity is a safeguard to the user, who may be faced with a wrongly labelled product or one of questionable quality, or who may inadvertently take the wrong container from the shelf, with potentially unfortunate results. A quick sniff at the contents before any are used should become as habitual to a user as it was to the pharmacist of old, who daily prepared medicines from the botanicals and chemicals lining the dispensary

Front side of card

YLANG-YLANG OIL, EXTRA

Pale yellow, mobile liquid having a powerful, "medicated" and floral odour

Aromatherapy applications
Antidepressant, hypotensive, hypnotic

Aromatherapy safe use restrictions
Not for babies or young children of age 12 years or less

Storage
Cool place, small headspace, protect from light

Notes

Back of card

YLANG-YLANG OIL, EXTRA

Collected as first fraction of fractional steam distillation of freshly picked flowers of *Cananga odorata*

Geographical source
Madagascar, Nossi-Bé, Comoro Is.
Chief constituents
Linalöl, linalyl acetate, eugenol, benzyl acetate, methyl salicylate, methyl benzoate, methyl *para*-cresol, geraniol, geranyl acetate, caryophyl-lene, germacrene-D
Perfumery applications
Jasmin, Carnation and other florals, as a lifting agent
Cost (give current cost and date; update as necessary)

IFRA restrictions
None (update if necessary)
Flash point
Above 62°C

Top notes
Powerful, medicated, floral
Body notes
Medicated, floral, fruity, spicy
Dryout
Balsamic, floral

Fig. 10.3— An example of an index card with details of an essential oil

shelves. In aromatherapeutic practice this precaution safeguards the patient, while in perfumery it can prevent considerable financial loss. For effective quality control the odours of all aromatic products in use must be *known*, to the extent that any of them can be identified by odour alone. Most aromatherapists are involved with aromachology, the study and applications of the psychological effects of odours, where knowledge of the odours of essential oils is fundamental to their use for the purpose of treatment. There is but one way to gain this knowledge, and that is through practical experience and regular testing.

Since in the everyday working situation there is no time (or need) to use smelling strips simply for identity checks, familiarization exercises should be conducted under the same conditions, that is, by 'smelling from the bottle'. Carefully note that for purposes of *quality evaluation* smelling strips *must* be used over periods of time sufficient to permit comparative evaluation of the entire odour profile of an essential oil.

To set up an identity test for practice, take five bottles of essential oils at random from your collection and, resisting the temptation to look at the labels, line them up in a row with the labels facing away from you. Now take each bottle in turn, carefully smell the contents, write down the name of the oil you think the odour represents, then check your result by reference to the label. If you are wrong on any occasion, wait until you have completed the test, then compare carefully the odour of the essential oil that you named with that of the oil you incorrectly identified.

A variation of this test for occasional use is to take a set of essential oils of related odour, e.g. Lavender, Lavandin, Spike Lavender, Clary Sage and Rosemary, for which purpose you will, of course, need to read the labels on the bottles. Now turn the bottles so that you cannot see the labels and line them up, randomizing their positions in the row. Try to identify the contents of each one by smelling and writing down your results. At the end of the test, carefully smell the oils from smelling strips to final dryout.

On at least two occasions per week of a one-year course you should study in detail the entire odour profile of an essential oil. The subject of odour profiling is discussed in Chapter 5.

Recommendations for the sensory quality control of essential oils in the salon appear in the booklet *Lecture Notes on Essential Oils*, noted in the Appendix.

10.6 The Crunch — Taking Written Examinations

An examination may be regarded as a process of quality control by filtration, in that the filtrate consists of those who, by virtue of their knowledge, the condition of the examiner's liver and perhaps rather more than a modicum of good luck, will not again be required to suffer the pangs of that particular stage of ritual purification deemed necessary to the achievement of their ultimate educational goal. It has, on the other hand, been suggested, though perhaps with tongue in cheek, that the whole unfortunate business is perpetuated simply for the purpose of keeping examiners' knowledge up to date by perusal of the answers of their victims.

One cannot know everything about a subject area that lecturers, examiners and everybody else thinks is necessary or at least highly desirable. Examinations, like race meetings, are very much occasions in which chance plays a major role: it is anyone's guess as to the topics on which questions will be asked, as it is as to whether or not "Examiners' Tipple" will win the 3.30. Hence those who do not pass may well do so at a further attempt. Fortunately, the modern systems for the assessment of candidates for the awards of diplomas and degrees take into consideration candidates' course work, dissertations, etc. and not simply what they know or appear to know at a certain time on a certain day — a much fairer and more reasonable state of affairs.

Though some students seem to take examinations in their stride, for most of us they are occasions of some dread — even of foreboding and approaching doom. Mild apprehension at the thought of sitting an examination is quite normal. It is an indication that the adrenaline is flowing in preparation for the efforts to be made, and soon fades once the invigilator has intoned the time-honoured dispensation, 'You may begin'. It is at this moment beneficial consciously to relax every voluntary muscle, from fingers to toes except, of course, those that are necessary to maintain a sitting position, and to take several slow deep breaths before turning to the examination paper. Some students report after an examination, 'My mind just went blank and I couldn't think of anything'. Such can be the effects of 'examination nerves'. The positive approach is to *use* the examination paper, regarding each question as the key, or trigger, which will unlock your knowledge of the subject-matter of the question. From the flow of concepts thereby released from your memory, you then choose those which are relevant to the question, allowing them to interact to form the expressions of your answer. Do not think for a moment that relaxing before commencing work will impair your capacity for recall — quite the opposite; it will provide the few moments of calm contemplation you need to make a start on the paper, and once you have started writing you are on the way to completing the examination successfully.

Regarding a strategy for obtaining the maximum total marks for your efforts, you will need to know *in advance of an examination* what the instructions will be in reference to the total time allowed for answering the questions and the number of questions to be attempted in that time. If you answer more than the stated number of questions, your answers to those beyond that number will be ignored by the examiner. In most examinations you will be required to *begin each answer on a separate sheet of paper*. This instruction is given not because examiners hold shares in paper manufacturing companies, though such investments might well be profitable, but because very frequently the questions are set by more than one examiner (even an examiner cannot be expected to know all there is to know about a subject!) and so the answers have to be distributed accordingly after the examination for marking.

Past examination papers are a most useful source of confidence to students taking an examination course and are available from most examining boards. It is an excellent idea to obtain copies of the papers set for the past three or four examinations in a subject and, using whatever sources of information you need, to prepare 'model answers' which could gain high marks, or so you would hope.

'Mock' examinations can provide opportunities for practice under examination conditions and for assessment of the state of your knowledge, or lack of it, in time for any deficiencies to be corrected.

Let us take an imaginary situation in which you discover, on perusal of past papers that a written examination that you are to take comprises a paper of two-and-a-half hours' duration in which five questions are to be attempted out of a choice of, say, eight. Then the time you should allow for answering each question should be

$$\frac{150}{5} - 3 = 27 \text{ and } not \text{ 30 minutes}$$

The three minutes' 'spare time' allowed in respect of each question are for the following purposes:

a) The brief period of relaxation, noted above
b) Reading through *the whole* of the examination paper and choosing the questions you will attempt
c) The writing of an 'answer plan' for each answer
d) A quick read-through of your answers near the end of the examination to correct any small errors
e) Recovery from any disruptive incidents

Regarding (c) above, once you have decided on the first question you will answer, draw a line across the answer paper, about 10 cm from the top and, preferably using pencil, *quickly* make a list of the main points of your answer, in any order, as they come to mind. Then write your answer, in a suitable order of main points, marking off the points on your answer plan as you go along.

Do not over-run your time.
Similarly, plan your answers for the other questions you have chosen.

If you have not completed your answer to a question at the end of the allotted time, stop writing, make sure there is space for completion of your answer and immediately begin your answer plan for the next question that you will answer, on a fresh sheet of paper.

Draw a neat line through each of your answer plans as you complete your answers

Proceed in this way until you have used up the total time that you have allowed for answering all the questions (135 minutes in the case of our example). Use the remaining time for (d) above.

Regarding (e) above, it is easy despite all precautions to forget some vital item of writing equipment needed for an examination, and even if you remember everything, your brand new pen, carefully tested beforehand, may refuse to work. Invigilators are very much on the candidate's side when potential disasters arise and will usually have spare pens, etc. available on loan. It is, however, surprising just how long it can take to attract an invigilator's attention, explain what has happened, have the problem solved and then settle down again, *so always carry spares*.

The most disturbing in the way of disruptive incidents that happen during an examination is usually no worse than a sudden, noisy invasion of the sanctum by students who have not seen the signs 'SILENCE — EXAMINATION IN PROGRESS' displayed without, or who have chosen to ignore them.

10.7 Model Answers to Examination Questions

In this final section of Chapter 10, we shall aim to illustrate how examination questions in the general area of the chemistry of essential oils can be answered with reasonable economy of words. Examiners hope that candidates will show a good standard of English when answering examination papers, will write legibly and will answer the questions that they have set rather than easier ones that candidates would rather the examiners had set.

1. Question on the storage of essential oils

a) What are the conditions under which citrus oils must be stored to preserve their quality?
b) State and explain the consequences of poor storage

Notes
A simple enough question, but one demanding full reasoning for good marks. Explanations of storage conditions can be left to Part (*b*), which specifically asks for them to be discussed.

Start with a definition of the expression 'citrus oils', to show you know what they are, and give a few examples.

Model answer
a) Citrus oils are the essential oils produced from the outer rinds of citrus fruits, mostly by mechanical expression. Examples are the oils of Bergamot, Lemon and Sweet Orange.

Citrus oils must be stored under a minimum headspace of air, or preferably under nitrogen, to minimize their deterioration by oxidation, in a refrigerator to slow down the rate of the oxidation that slowly takes place even under cool conditions, protected from light, which catalyses their spoilage, and in tightly sealed containers to prevent evaporation and admission of air, containing oxygen.

b) All of the citrus oils contain very high proportions of monoterpenes, $C_{10}H_{16}$, which are readily oxidized by oxygen from the air. An example is *d*-limonene, which oxygen can oxidize to limonene oxide and carvone:

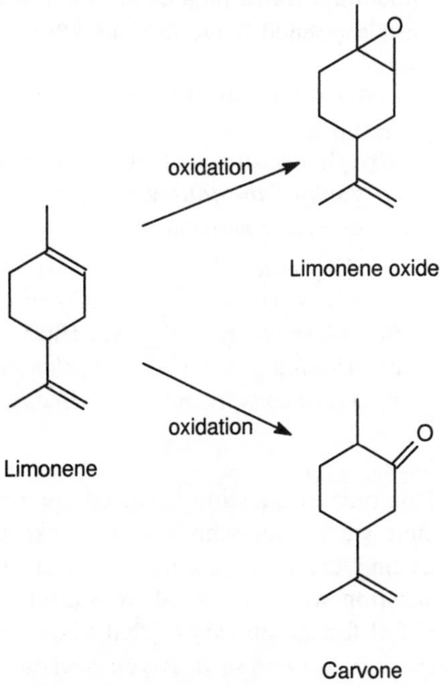

Fig. 10.4 — Oxidation of limonene

Limonene has a weak, paraffin-like odour which contributes little to the characteristic odours of the essential oils in which it occurs. The odours of limonene oxide and carvone are, respectively, pine-like and caraway-like, and quite strong. When limonene is oxidized, therefore, unwanted changes of composition and odour occur in an essential oil containing this terpene. These changes render the oil unfit for use.

Monoterpenes can also polymerize, particular under oxidizing conditions, to form odourless, resinous polymers.

The above reactions do not affect the oxygenated constituents of a citrus oil, which are responsible for its characteristic odour. Monoterpenes such as limonene can, however, form unstable terpene peroxides, which quickly break down to form hydrogen peroxide, H_2O_2. This is a powerful oxidizing agent, which can attack readily oxidizable constituents of citrus oils, such as the fatty aldehydes C_8 to C_{10}, oxidizing them to the corresponding carboxylic acids. These can slowly react with alcohols, such as linalöl in Bergamot Oil, to form esters. Such changes, too, alter the composition and odour of any essential oil, causing rapid deterioration.

The rate of deterioration of an essential oil is approximately halved by each 10°C fall in temperature, hence cool storage for all citrus oils, and is greatly reduced by protection from light, particularly sunlight, containing UVL, which has a photocatalytic effect on the deterioration of citrus and other essential oils.

2. A ten-part question on a variety of topics

Briefly explain, and exemplify where possible, what is meant by each of the following terms, as they are used in reference to aromatic materials:

i. *Body note*	vi. *Fixation*
ii. *Monoterpene*	vii. *Rectification*
iii. *Odour purity*	viii. *Hydrolysis*
iv. *Absolute*	ix. *Phototoxicity*
v. *Trace constituent*	x. *Headspace analysis*

Notes

This type of question is siezed upon with joy by students who 'know their stuff', but who may not take too kindly to the necessity for writing the more usual, longer answers. It is, indeed, the kind of question which is 'good for starters', though there lurks within it a pitfall for the unwary — that of *overrunning the allocated time to be spent in answering it*. If you overrun your answer time you will have that much less time for answering the other questions you have chosen, in respect of which you may well give better answers, having by the time you answer them gained some confidence by answering the first one. Remember that you can answer the parts of a multiple-part question in any order, *provided* you number your answers correctly, unless there is an instruction to the contrary.

Model answer

i. '<u>Body note</u>' refers to the characteristic odour of an essential oil, given mainly by the combined odours of oxygenated constituents of intermediate volatility, when the oil is allowed to evaporate from a smelling strip, e.g. cineole in *Eucalyptus globulus* Oil.

ii. <u>Monoterpene</u> - an unsaturated hydrocarbon, formula $C_{10}H_{16}$. Monoterpenes have cyclic (e.g.limonenes) or acyclic (e.g. myrcene) molecular structures and occur widely in essential oils. They have weak, noncharacteristic odours, poor solubility in aqueous alcohol and are readily oxidized by oxygen.

iii. <u>Odour purity</u> in reference to an essential oil or aroma chemical is the extent to which the odour of the material matches that of a standard sample of the same material of the same grade, at all stages of evaporation.

iv. <u>An absolute</u> is an extract of a natural source produced by extraction of the source with a volatile, hydrocarbon solvent, evaporation of the solvent to produce a concrete and extraction of the concrete with pure ethanol. Recovery of the alcohol by vacuum distillation leaves a residue of absolute, e.g. Jasmin Absolute.

v. With reference to an essential oil, a <u>trace constituent</u> is a constituent present at a level of 0·01 per cent or less, e.g. *cis*-3-hexenol:

$$CH_3{-}CH_2{-}\underset{\underset{\textstyle H}{|}}{C}{=}\underset{\underset{\textstyle H}{|}}{C}{-}CH_2{-}CH_2OH$$

powerful green odour

Powerfully odorous trace constituents often determine the quality of an essential oil, such as Nutmeg Oil, or even determine the overall character of its odour, as in Galbanum Oil, containing pyrazines.

vi. <u>Fixation</u> is the property of certain materials, such as Sandalwood Oil, to prolong the evaporation of a perfume, such as a personal fragrance. This may be a result of hydrogen bonding e.g. in a perfume, between molecules of santalol in Sandalwood Oil and 'rose alcohols', or larger molecules impeding the escape of smaller ones during evaporation.

[There are other possible explanations of fixation, but in answering a question of this kind it would take too long to discuss them all, even briefly. The two most likely causes of fixation have therefore been given as good value for marks.]

vii. <u>Rectification</u> is the redistillation in steam or in a vacuum of an essential oil to remove nonvolatile matter; e.g. of spice oils imported as the crude products.

viii. <u>Hydrolysis</u> - decomposition of a compound, such as an ester, e.g. geranyl formate in Geranium oil, by water. General equation:

$$R.COOR' + H_2O \rightleftharpoons R.COOH + R'OH$$

ester + water   carboxylic acid   alcohol

Essential oils must be water-free to prevent their deterioration through hydrolysis of any esters they contain.

ix. <u>Phototoxicity</u> - the property of a material, such as bergaptene in Bergamot Oil, to cause skin damage (Berloque dermatitis with bergaptene) when exposed to the UVL of sunlight.

x. <u>Headspace analysis</u> is the analysis by GLC of odorous vapour from a source such as a flower, which has been desorbed from an adsorbent used to capture the vapour from the source.

3. A five-part question on basic and applied chemistry

The following are the names of different chemical families of organic compounds:

i.   *Alcohols*   iv. *Phenols*
ii. *Esters*   v. *Ketones*
iii. *Aldehydes*

In respect of __each__ of the above families:
a) *write down the name of the family, as given above;*
b) *write a general formula representing all members of the family;*
c) *give the prefixes and/or suffixes used in writing the systematic names of all members of the family;*
d) *give one example of a constituent of an essential oil which is a member of that family;*
e) *name one essential oil containing the constituent you have named.*

Notes

This is a complex question, designed to test candidates' knowledge of some simple, basic chemical nomenclature and of constituents of essential oils, The most clear and tidy way of presenting your answer to a question of this type would be by means of a table. The question does not instruct you to 'Write your answer in tabular form', or to 'Tabulate your answer to this question', but there is no reason why you should not do so.

Notice that the first column will consist of (*a*) above — the family names — and that parts (*b*) and (*c*) are concerned with the different functional groups of atoms in the molecules of different chemical families. Parts (*d*) and (*e*) ask for examples; hence the column headings in the following answer:

Model answer

Chemical family				Examples	
(a)	(b)	(c)		(d)	(e)
Family name	*General formula*	*Chemical name*		*Constituent*	*Essential oil*
		prefix	*suffix*		
Alcohols	R-OH*	Hydroxy- *or*	-ol	Linalöl	Rosewood Oil
Esters	R-COOR'	None	-yl *and* -ate	Geranyl acetate	Palmarosa Oil
Aldehydes	R-CHO	None	-al	Citral	Lemongrass Oil
Phenols	R-OH†	None	-ol	Thymol	Thyme Oil
Ketones	R-CO-R'	None	-one	Zingerone	Ginger Oil

* Where -OH is not bonded directly to a benzene ring
† Where -OH is bonded directly to a benzene ring

4. A five-part question referring to a specific essential oil and the corresponding absolute

Carefully explain the following:
a) The composition of the essential oil obtained from the flowering tops of Lavandula officinalis *is different from that of the absolute obtained from the same botanical source.*
b) Steam distillation, and not water distillation, is used for the production of Lavender Oil.
c) Samples of the Lavender Oil from different suppliers do not have the same odour profile.
d) Lavender Oil is almost colourless, while the absolute is dark green in colour.
e) Lavender Oil, but not Lavender absolute, is used to impart freshness to the top notes of perfumes.

Notes
The question refers to Lavender Oil and Lavender Absolute, and this information can be used to begin the answer. The question is straightforward but, as in Question 2, there will be a tendency to run out of time by giving too much detail. A concise answer, containing all the essential information and that is strictly relevant to the question, should therefore be given.

Model answer

a) <u>*Lavandula officinalis*</u> is the plant from which the Lavender Oil and Lavender Absolute of commerce are obtained.

The essential oil is produced by steam distillation, a process in which steam under pressure from a boiler enters a distillation vessel packed with lavender herb, at a temperature of about 110°C. Under these conditions water molecules condense on the flowers and leaves, releasing latent heat enough to vaporize the essential oil exuding from the oil cells. During steam distillation, esters, such as linalyl acetate, hydrolyse only minimally to the parent alcohols and carboxylic acids, which are volatile, while certain glycosides hydrolyse to nonvolatile sugars and volatiles such as terpenes. These volatiles are present in the essential oil obtained by condensation of the vapours from the still.

Lavender Absolute, produced by solvent extraction, contains the essential oil from the plant as well as nonvolatile wax and pigments. The composition of the essential oil in the absolute is very little changed from its composition in the plant because it does not come into contact with hot steam.

b) Water distillation is a much slower process than steam distillation, and so a Lavender Oil produced by the former method would suffer the consequence of a much longer residence time in the still and therefore much more hydrolysis of esters. Since the quality of Lavender Oil is judged by its content of esters and its odour, which depends largely though not entirely on its ester content, an oil produced by water distillation under ordinary atmospheric pressure would be unlikely to be acceptable.

c) There are many different qualities of Lavender Oil available. These quality differences arise from differences in soil quality and climatic conditions under which the plants are grown in different parts of the world, from differences in the altitude at which growing and processing take place, and from differences in processing techniques. The higher the altitude, the lower is the distillation temeprature and the higher is the ester content, resulting in less hydrolysis of the esters present. Some suppliers of Lavender Oil blend oils of different quality to produce a standard quality, acceptable to most of their customers. It is therefore very unlikely that two samples of even the same grade of Lavender Oil from different suppliers will be found to have exactly the same odour profile.

d) Lavender herb contains the green pigment chlorophyll, essential to photosynthesis in the living plant. Chlorophyll is nonvolatile, and so does not distil over with the essential oil. Chlorophyll is, however, soluble in the solvents used for manufacturing Lavender Absolute, and so imparts to the absolute a green colour.

e) Lavender Oil contains a substantial proportion of monoterpenes, which Lavender Absolute does not. These terpenes tend to have a 'lifting' action on the body notes of the oil. Also, Lavender Oil contains no coumarin, present at a substantial level in the absolute, a constituent having fixative action on the body notes of the absolute. Hence Lavender Oil is more volatile than the absolute and has an altogether much fresher and lighter odour profile.

5. A general question on quality by reference to an essential oil of candidates' choice

What are the most important criteria by which the quality of an essential oil may be judged?
How is the required information obtained?
Illustrate your answer by reference to one essential oil of your choice.

Notes
There is a free choice of an essential oil to illustrate an answer to this question, and so choose an oil with which you are thoroughly familiar. The most obvious thing to do when you are given an essential oil for quality evaluation is to have a good look at it, so begin your answer with visual inspection. Then will come odour, quickly followed by composition, at which point you will be lucky to have any time left for more.

Model answer

I will choose Lemongrass Oil to illustrate my answer to this question.

1. Appearance

A representative sample of the oil is taken and inspected visually in comparison with a standard sample of the same oil. The oil should be of a pale to dark yellow or amber colour, but the colour of the test sample should be close to that of the standard to be acceptable. It is slightly viscous, but should not show turbidity, which may indicate the presence of water. Water should be absent from essential oils containing aldehydes, such as the citral of Lemongrass Oil, which are unstable in the presence of water.

2. Odour profile

The odour profile of a sample of Lemongrass Oil is evaluated by comparison with a standard sample over 24 hours. Two 1 cm dips of the test sample are taken on smelling strips and one 1 cm dip of the standard sample. The strips are identified by marking with the name of the oil and the words 'test', or 'standard', whichever is correct. They are also labelled A,B and C in succession. The strips are held in the hand in the form of a fan and are then turned over so that identification marks cannot be seen by the evaluator. They are then shuffled so that the evaluator does not know which is which. The impregnated ends of the strips are then smelled briefly in turn, and the strip which is different in odour from the other two is identified. If the strip selected is the standard strip, it is then decided whether or not the difference in odour is sufficient for the test sample of Lemongrass Oil to be rejected. If none of the strips is found different in odour from the other two, the test sample is further evaluated after eight hours by setting it aside with the standard strips, and then again after 48 hours in the same way. If in any of the tests one of the test strips is found different in odour from the other two the test is judged invalid and is repeated.

The first of the three smelling tests is for evaluation of the top note of the essential oil, which in the case of Lemongrass should be strong, fresh, sharp and lemony.

The second test is for evaluation of the body notes, which in a good sample are strong, lemony, slightly fruity, slightly oily-green and herbaceous.

The final test, of the dryout, should show fainter, fresh, lemony-fruity notes without oiliness.

If the test sample shows no significant odour differences from the standard at all stages of evaporation, it is acceptable on odour quality.

As the odour evaluation test is subjective, it should preferably be carried out by more than one person. The 'electronic nose' is used in industry to reduce the subjectivity of odour evaluation tests.

3. Composition

A sample of the essential oil is subjected to analysis by gas– liquid chromatography and the chromatogram is compared with that of a standard sample of the same oil chromatographed under identical conditions. All major and minor peaks should correspond in their positions, and the percentage of citral, as given by the integrator readout should, after applying the corresponding correction factor, be within the limits of the specification for the oil. The percentages of other major and of minor constituents should not differ greatly from the standard, no constituents usually found in the oil should be missing and there should be no additional peaks indicating the possibility of adulteration.

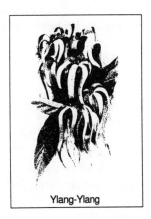
Ylang-Ylang

GLOSSARY

Words set in SMALL CAPS *are defined elsewhere in the Glossary.*

ABSOLUTE
In perfumery, an aromatic extract prepared by repeated washing of a melted CON-
CRETE with warm ALCOHOL (ethanol) in a BATTEUSE. The alcoholic solution so
formed is then dewaxed by chilling to reduce its solubility in the alcohol sufficiently
to precipitate the wax, which is then removed by filtration. The alcohol is recovered
from the filtrate by DISTILLATION under reduced pressure. The absolute remains as a
residue representing the highest CONCENTRATION of, and closest approach to the quality of, the corresponding natural fragrance in general use in perfumery.

ABSORPTION
A process of soaking, as water is absorbed by a sponge. (Cf. ADSORPTION.)

ACCORD
A harmonious blend of a small number of aromatic materials.

ACETAL
The organic product of a CHEMICAL REACTION between an ALCOHOL and an ALDE-
HYDE.

ACID
A COMPOUND which can donate hydrogen IONS, as hydrogen chloride in contact with
water donates hydrogen IONS to water MOLECULES to form OXONIUM IONS.

ACID VALUE
A measure of the proportion (or CONCENTRATION) of free ACID present in a product,
such as an ESSENTIAL OIL, measured as the number of milligrams of potassium hydroxide required to neutralize the free acid in one gram of the sample.

ACIDIC
Having the properties of an ACID, as in the case of an aqueous solution containing a higher CONCENTRATION of OXONIUM IONS than HYDROXIDE IONS. A solution of *p*H less than 7·0.

ACYCLIC
Not in the form of a ring as, for example, a STRAIGHT-CHAIN or BRANCHED-CHAIN MOLECULAR STRUCTURE.

ADSORBENT
A substance to which certain MOLECULES will stick, as molecules of certain ink dyes stick to cotton fibres, making the stain difficult to remove.

ADSORPTION
The adherence of MOLECULES to a surface of some kind by the formation of relatively weak intermolecular bonds. (Cf. ABSORPTION).

ADULTERANT
An impurity accidentally or deliberately introduced into a product, rendering it of inferior quality.

AGARBATHIE
An Indian incense stick.

AGEING
The process of allowing a product to mature. In perfumery, refers to the mellowing of a perfume COMPOUND over a period of about a month, by allowing it to stand in a closed vessel in a cool place of even temperature. This allows REACTIVE ingredients of the perfume to interact to the point of equilibrium, at which the fragrance of the perfume is at the peak of its perfection.

AGLYCON
Any product of the HYDROLYSIS of a GLYCOSIDE other than a sugar. The hydrolysis of glycosides during the DISTILLATION of an ESSENTIAL OIL may introduce into the oil constituents which, as such, may not occur in the oil naturally. These are VOLATILE aglycons, which are mainly of TERPENOID constitution.

AGRESTIC
Pertaining to the countryside, especially as regards odour.

ALBEDO
The pith, or inner rind, of a citrus fruit.

ALCOHOL
An organic COMPOUND characterized by the presence in its MOLECULES of one or more hydroxy- FUNCTIONAL GROUPs bonded directly to a HYDROCARBON structure other than a BENZENE RING.

ALCOHOLYSIS

A reversible REACTION between an ALCOHOL and an ESTER of which the result is the interchange of the HYDROCARBON part of the alcohol MOLECULES with the alcohol part of the ester molecules. Thus, in the maturing of finished, alcoholic perfumes, the ethanol used as a diluent can react, slowly and incompletely, with, for example, esters of TERPENOID alcohols, such as geraniol, citronellol and nerol.

ALDEHYDE

An organic COMPOUND characterized by the presence in its MOLECULES of a CARBONYL GROUP of atoms and a hydrogen ATOM bonded to the carbon atom of the carbonyl group. A compound of general formula R.CHO, where R represents a hydrogen atom, HYDROCARBON, or substituted hydrocarbon RADICAL.

ALDEHYDIC

In perfumery, a fragrance NOTE typical of *fatty* ALDEHYDES: powerful, fatty or waxy, and becoming pleasant only in very low CONCENTRATION. Also descriptive of a perfume characterized by emphasis on aldehydic notes set within a rich, floral BASE. The prototype of aldehydic perfumes is the famous "No. 5", launched by Chanel in 1921.

ALKALI

A COMPOUND which when dissolved in water gives rise to a higher CONCENTRATION of HYDROXIDE IONS than OXONIUM IONS. Examples are sodium, potassium and calcium hydroxides and the gas ammonia.

ALKALINE

Any substance which when dissolved in water gives a solution of pH greater than 7·0.

ALKANE

A saturated HYDROCARBON, of the kind found in natural gas and petroleum and having the general formula C_nH_{2n+2}. The highly volatile alkane hexane, C_6H_{14}, is one of the solvents used for the extraction of aromatic botanical materials in the preparation of CONCRETES and RESINOIDS.

ALKENE

An unsaturated HYDROCARBON the MOLECULES of which each contain one or more double COVALENT BONDS. The simplest alkenes have the general formula C_nH_{2n}. TERPENES are alkenes of the general formula $(C_5H_8)_n$ which are important constituents of ESSENTIAL OILS.

ALKYNE

An unsaturated HYDROCARBON the MOLECULES of which each contain one or more triple COVALENT BONDS. The simplest alkynes have the general formula C_nH_{2n-2}. Alkynes and their DERIVATIVES are uncommon as constituents of ESSENTIAL OILS.

ALLERGEN

A substance which causes an allergic reaction as, for example, reddening and irritation of the skin following sensitization by contact with the same allergen. A substance to which some persons are allergic may not give rise to sensitization in others.

ALTERNATIVE MEDICINE

Any form of medical diagnosis and treatment which is not generally regarded as orthodox, i.e. conforming to long-established principles.

AMBER

A fossil resin, unrelated to amber*gris*. The description 'amber' is, however, commonly used in perfumery to refer to a powdery, vanilla-like NOTE having some relationship to the odour of natural ambergris.

AMBERGRIS

A soft black, unpleasant-smelling abdominal secretion of the sperm whale, released into the sea by the normal process of elimination or when the animal dies. The material is thought to be produced as an excretion in response to irritation by the sharp, indigestible beaks of cuttlefish, which lodge in the internal intestinal folds. On release from the animal, ambergris rises to the surface of the sea, where it may drift about for many years, becoming harder, lighter in colour and losing its unpleasant odour. Now rarely used, ambergris is said to have been the finest blending agent known to perfumery.

AMBRA

A term used in perfumery to refer to an odour of AMBERGRIS as, for example, the odours of preparations of ambergris-smelling fragrance bases, labdanum and of certain AROMA CHEMICALS.

AMINE

An organic COMPOUND the MOLECULES of which are characterized by the presence of one or more amino-, NH_2, FUNCTIONAL GROUPS.

AMINO ACID

A CARBOXYLIC ACID the MOLECULES of which are characterized by the presence of one or more amino- groups, in addition to a CARBOXYL GROUP. Amino acid molecules are the 'building blocks' for PROTEIN SYNTHESIS in living plant or animal cells.

ANALYSIS

In chemistry, any process for determining the composition of a substance. Examples are the analysis of an ESSENTIAL OIL by GLC and the subsequent DETERMINATION of the composition of one of its constituents by MASS SPECTROMETRY.

ANIMALIC

A term used in perfumery to refer to an odour associated with an animal source, such as CIVET, or to a NOTE of animal excreta as may be given by certain plants, such as the heavy note of indole in Jasmin ABSOLUTE or Orange Flower ABSOLUTE.

ANTIOXIDANT

An agent capable of preventing, or reducing the rate of, OXIDATION. The ORGANIC COMPOUNDS butylated hydroxyanisole (BHA) and butylated hydroxytoluene (BHT) are antioxidants commonly used, in traces, to protect CITRUS OILS from deterioration.

ARCHIMEDEAN SCREW
A device having the form of the shaft of a wood screw, used for transporting material through a tube in the manner of a mincing machine.

AROMA CHEMICAL
Any chemical having a useful odour and which is harmless and legal when properly used as a fragrance or flavour ingredient.

AROMACHOLOGY
The study of pyschological effects of odours, particularly those of ESSENTIAL OILS used in AROMATHERAPY.

AROMATHERAPY
The use of ESSENTIAL OILS for the treatment of human disorders. Essential oils should not be taken internally except under the supervision of a duly qualified medical practitioner.

ARTEFACT
In reference to GAS–LIQUID CHROMATOGRAPHY, this term refers to any product of chemical change to a constituent of a sample under ANALYSIS, brought about by the conditions of the analysis. Artefacts are revealed as peaks on a CHROMATOGRAM which do not correspond to true constituents of the sample. They are frequently the result of partial decomposition of true constituents in the HEATING BLOCK.

ASYMMETRIC CARBON ATOM
A carbon ATOM bonded to four different atoms or groups of atoms.

ATOM
The smallest particle of an element which can take part in a chemical change.

ATOMIC NUMBER
The number of PROTONS in the NUCLEUS of an ATOM, which is equal to the number of ELECTRONS that the atom contains.

ATOMIC WEIGHT
As a close approximation, the ratio of the weight of one ATOM of an element to the weight of a hydrogen atom taken as one atomic weight unit. For accurate scientific work, atomic *masses* are used, where the atomic mass of an element is the ratio of the mass of one atom of the element to $\frac{1}{12}$ of the mass of one atom of the ISOTOPE CARBON-12.

AVOGADRO'S LAW
A principle of chemical science first put forward by the professor of physics at Turin University, Amedeo Avogadro, in 1811, and which has subsequently been upheld by experiment to the present day. Avogadro's law states that under the same conditions of temperature and pressure, equal volumes of all gases contain the same number of MOLECULES (6×10^{23}, approx. per mole). It implies that the amount of space occu-

pied by the actual molecules of a gas is negligible as compared with the volume occupied by the gas.

AZULENES
Members of a family of dark blue, practically odourless, VOLATILE, unsaturated CYCLIC HYDROCARBONS occurring in ESSENTIAL OILS obtained by DISTILLATION from certain plants, such as chamomiles, some species of artemisia and pepper.

BALANCE
See ODOUR BALANCE.

BASE
In perfumery, a perfume ingredient specially formulated to represent a natural source or a blend of natural sources of fragrance, or an abstract fragrance concept.

In chemistry, a simple definition of a base is that it is a substance which will react with an ACID to form a salt and water only. More scientifically, a base may be defined as an ATOM, ION or molecule capable of accepting a PROTON (HYDROGEN ION).

BASE LINE
A horizontal line drawn on a graph (such as a CHROMATOGRAM or SPECTROGRAM) by a pen recorder when receiving no signal from the instrument to which it is connected.

BASIC NOTE
A fragrance NOTE of extended persistence; an aromatic material of very low VOLATILITY.

BATTIE
An AGARBATHIE.

BATTEUSE
A large, cylindrical vessel, standing upright and fitted with a vertical stirrer, used for breaking up a mass of a molten CONCRETE immersed in warm ethanol. Once the concrete has been dispersed in the ALCOHOL in the form of small globules, the alcohol can extract the ESSENTIAL OIL it contains efficiently, forming an alcoholic EXTRACT solution ready for the next stage in the preparation of an ABSOLUTE.

BENZENE RING
Term used in reference to the MOLECULAR STRUCTURE of the unsaturated, CYCLIC HYDROCARBON, benzene, C_6H_6.

BENZENOID COMPOUND
A COMPOUND the MOLECULES of which each contain one or more BENZENE RINGS.

BODY NOTE
See MIDDLE NOTE.

BOILING POINT
The temperature at which a liquid boils. Scientifically, the maximum, constant temperature at which a liquid can evaporate at a given pressure, provided it is not in the superheated condition.

BOND
See CHEMICAL BOND

BRANCHED CHAIN
In chemistry, any branching arrangement of the ATOMS in a MOLECULE as, for example, in the molecules of thymol and limonene.

BRIDGED MOLECULAR STRUCTURE
A molecular ring structure, having a skeleton usually of carbon ATOMS, in which one or more additional carbon atoms are bonded across the ring. Alpha- and beta-pinenes are examples of MONOTERPENES having bridged MOLECULAR STRUCTURES.

BURETTE
A graduated tube, commonly of 1 cm internal diameter and 50 cm^3 capacity, used in the analytical technique of TITRATION

CAMBIUM
The ring of green, living tissue situated beneath the bark of a woody stem or tree-trunk, and containing vessels for transporting aqueous solutions of mineral salts from the roots to the leaves, and of elaborated nutrients from the leaves to the roots.

CAPILLARY GLC
A refinement of the analytical technique of GAS–LIQUID CHROMATOGRAPHY, in which the column consists of a long (e.g. 50 m), coiled tube of very fine internal diameter, internally coated with a thin layer of nonVOLATILE STATIONARY PHASE material, such as a SILICONE oil.

CARAMELLIC
Term descriptive of the odour of caramel, as given by molten sugar when heated to a high temperature.

CARBON-12
The ISOTOPE of the element carbon having an atomic mass of 12 precisely.

CARBONYL GROUP
The divalent group of atoms consisting of a carbon ATOM joined to an oxygen atom by a DOUBLE BOND: >C=O

CARBOXYL GROUP
The monovalent group of atoms consisting of a carbon ATOM joined to an oxygen atom by a DOUBLE BOND and to a HYDROXY– GROUP:

CARBOXYLIC ACID
An organic ACID characterized by the presence in each of its MOLECULES of one or more carboxyl FUNCTIONAL GROUPS. *See also* CARBOXYL GROUP.

CARRIER GAS
A gas, chemically inert to all other substances involved, used to transport samples of VAPOUR through the column of a gas–liquid chromatograph (*see* GAS–LIQUID CHROMATOGRAPHY). Nitrogen or helium are commonly used for this purpose and form the MOVING PHASE of the system.

CARRIER OIL
A FIXED OIL of vegetable origin, such as Jojoba Oil, Avocado Pear Oil or Grapeseed Oil, used in AROMATHERAPY as a solvent and diluent for ESSENTIAL OILS.

CASTOREUM
The dried, glandular secretion of the beaver, *Castor fiber*, used in perfumery as an ingredient of 'leather'-type fragrances, and formerly to some extent as a MUSK substitute.

CATALYST
A substance which can alter the speed (rate) of a CHEMICAL REACTION and which remains unchanged in mass and composition at the end of the reaction.

CENSER
See THURIBLE.

CHAMAZULENE
A member of the chemical family of AZULENES found as constituents of Chamomile and other ESSENTIAL OILS.

CHASSIS
The arrangement of rectangular glass plate and surrounding wooden frame used in the ENFLEURAGE process.

CHEMICAL BOND
A force of attraction holding ATOMS together in the MOLECULES of a molecular COMPOUND, IONS together in an ionic compound and, to a lesser extent, the molecules of a polar compound, such as water, ALCOHOLS, etc. by hydrogen bonding (*see* HYDROGEN BOND).

CHEMICAL EQUILIBRIUM
A state of balance which exists in a reversible CHEMICAL REACTION, or system in DISSOCIATION when the speed (rate) of the forward reaction or dissociation is equal to that of the reverse reaction or association.

CHEMICAL PROPERTIES
Those properties of an ELEMENT or COMPOUND which are shown when the substance undergoes some change of composition as, for example, decomposition by heat, OXI-DATION, HYDROLYSIS or REACTION with another substance.

CHEMICAL PURITY
The extent to which a chemical, such as an AROMA CHEMICAL, consists of MOLECULES or ion-aggregates of that chemical only; usually expressed as a percentage, e.g. alpha-iso-methyl ionone, 98%, the other 2% consisting of acceptable impurities (which nevertheless contribute to the odour profile of the product).

CHEMICAL REACTION
Any rearrangement of ATOMS or IONS in which energy, usually but not exclusively heat, is either lost or gained.

CHEMICAL TEST
A test involving a change in the composition of the subject material, such as during DETERMINATIONS of the percentage of ALCOHOLS, ESTERS, etc. in an ESSENTIAL OIL, or in a test for *p*H using an INDICATOR

CHLOROPHYLL
The mixture of magnesium-containing organic pigments — chlorophyll a (green) and chlorophyll b (yellowish-green) found in green plants and which is necessary for PHOTOSYNTHESIS.

CHROMATOGRAM
The graph of DETECTOR response against time drawn by a pen recorder in response to electrical signals originating from the detector of a gas–liquid chromatograph (*see* GAS–LIQUID CHROMATOGRAPHY). It takes the form of a series of peaks corresponding to the constituents of a mixture of VOLATILES, such as an ESSENTIAL OIL or perfume COMPOUND.

CHROMOSOME
One of a number of microscopic, thread-like structures present in the cell nuclei of animals and plants. Chromosomes carry inherited information in the form of GENES. The nature and sequence of the genes carried by the chromosomes of an organism determine the characteristics of form and constitution inherited by the organism from its parents from generation to generation.

CHYPRE
The French word for 'Cyprus'. In perfumery, a type of perfume characterized by a HARMONY of the notes of Oakmoss, Sandalwood and MUSK in the BASE, floral middle notes, such as those of Rose and Jasmin, and a top NOTE of Bergamot and other CITRUS OILS. The first chypre-type perfume was 'Le Chypre', launched by Coty in 1917.

cis/trans ISOMERISM

The occurrence of two different geometrical forms of MOLECULES of the same unsaturated COMPOUND. In the *cis-*, or (Z-) form, identical ATOMS or groups of atoms are on the same side of a DOUBLE BOND. In the *trans-*, or (E-) form, the same groups of atoms are on opposite sides of the double bond, as in the following example, where a and b represent different atoms or groups of atoms:

$$\underset{b}{\overset{a}{>}}C=C\underset{b}{\overset{a}{<}} \qquad \underset{b}{\overset{a}{>}}C=C\underset{a}{\overset{b}{<}}$$

cis- or (Z-)　　　　　*trans-* or (E-)

cis/trans Isomerism is not possible in the following cases:

$$\underset{a}{\overset{a}{>}}C=C\underset{b}{\overset{b}{<}} \qquad \underset{b}{\overset{a}{>}}C=C\underset{b}{\overset{b}{<}}$$

The occurrence of *cis/trans* ISOMERS shows that free rotation of two carbon atoms joined by a double bond is not possible, as it is if they are joined by a single bond.

CITRUS OIL

An ESSENTIAL OIL obtained from the oil glands of the FLAVEDO of a citrus fruit.

CIVET

In perfumery, the glandular secretion obtained from the civet, *Viverra civetta*, and other species of *Viverra*, animals related to the weasel.

CLASSIC PERFUME

A perfume accorded the distinction of representing the highest level of fragrance creation. A supreme example of the perfumer's art.

COEUR

The French word for 'heart'. The heart or main fragrance theme of a perfume, particularly in reference to a perfume for personal use.

COHOBATION

A process of redistillation of DISTILLATION waters in order to recover dissolved ESSENTIAL OIL.

COLATION

The removal of contaminating, insoluble particles from a liquid by straining through muslin, cotton wool, tow, etc. A process of coarse filtration.

COLLOIDAL SOLUTION (or **COLLOIDAL SOL**)

A dispersion of ultra-fine particles in a continous medium as, for example, of solubilised MICELLES of an oil in water. Colloidal particles, though invisible, will scatter light, so that a beam of light, itself invisible in a dust-free room, can be seen if passed through a colloidal solution.

COLUMN

In GLC, the long tube, containing the STATIONARY PHASE, through which the CARRIER GAS transports the vaporized sample for separation of constituents.

In FRACTIONAL DISTILLATION, a FRACTIONATING COLUMN.

COMPOUND

In chemistry, a substance composed of ATOMS of two or more ELEMENTS bonded together in fixed and definite proportions by mass.

In perfumery, a finished perfume composition in concentrated form. *See also* 'JUICE'.

CONCENTRATION

A process of increasing the proportion of a required substance present in a mixture, or, the weight per unit volume of a substance present in a mixture as, for example, the concentration in grams per litre of an ALKALI or ACID in a STANDARD SOLUTION.

CONCRETE

In perfumery, an aromatic, waxy or fatty EXTRACT prepared by washing a natural, aromatic source material with a pure, VOLATILE HYDROCARBON solvent, such as hexane, followed by recovery of the solvent. Most concretes are amorphous, solid or semi-solid masses containing ESSENTIAL OIL, natural wax and pigments from the source.

CONDENSATION

The change of state of a substance from gas or VAPOUR to liquid or solid. As used in ORGANIC CHEMISTRY, condensation is a term of indefinite meaning, usually referring to a process of SYNTHESIS between two reactants, in which a COVALENT BOND is formed between a carbon ATOM of one REACTANT MOLECULE and a carbon atom of the other, with the elimination of a small MOLECULE of some kind, such as water.

CONDENSER

In distillation, a cooling device for removing sufficient heat from the distillation vapour to enable it to change to the liquid state (or to the solid state if, as in the case of Orris Oil, the product is solid at room temperature).

COPPICED

The regrowth of a tree in the form of thin stems after felling to leave a stump.

CORPS

A prepared fat, such as a mixture of purified suet or lard, as used in the ENFLEURAGE process.

CORRECTION FACTOR

A figure by which the recorded percentage of a constituent of a mixture of VOLATILES, as given by GLC ANALYSIS, has to be multiplied to find its true percentage in the mixture.

COSOLVENT

A solvent which increases the solubility of a solute in the principal solvent of a solution. Water, for example, dissolves about 9% of its weight of phenylethyl alcohol at ordinary room temperature. The addition of increasing amounts of ethanol to water progressively increases the solubility of the AROMA CHEMICAL.

COVALENT BOND

A BOND between two ATOMS consisting of a shared pair of ELECTRONS. *See also* DOUBLE BOND.

COVALENT COMPOUND

A COMPOUND consisting of ATOMS of two or more ELEMENTS joined by COVALENT BONDS.

CREATIVITY

In perfumery, the artistic composition of an *original* perfume from aromatic raw materials.

CROTON OIL

A FIXED OIL obtained from the seeds of *Crotum tiglium*, a tree cultivated in Southeast Asia, and once used in medicine in minute doses as a powerful cathartic and counter-irritant. Not suitable as a carrier oil for aromatherapeutic purposes.

CYCLIC

In chemistry, descriptive of a MOLECULE containing one or more rings of ATOMS, such as the molecules of benzene and cyclohexane.

d-

See DEXTROROTATORY.

DEFLEURAGE

The removal of spent flowers from the CHASSIS in the ENFLEURAGE process.

DÉPART

Abbreviation for the French expression 'note de départ', meaning 'TOP NOTE' (*see also* NOTE).

DERIVATIVE

In perfumery, a single constituent or a mixture of constituents, separated from an ESSENTIAL OIL or aromatic EXTRACT. Linalöl, isolated from Rosewood Oil, terpeneless Petitgrain Oil and petitgrain TERPENES are examples of derivatives.

DERMATOLOGY
The study of the HISTOLOGY, physiology and pathology of the skin and the treatment of skin diseases.

DESORPTION
The detachment of adsorbed ATOMS or MOLECULES (*see* ADSORPTION) from an AD-SORBENT as, for example, following the HEADSPACE capture of a flower fragrance for ANALYSIS of the desorbed VAPOUR by CAPILLARY GLC.

DETECTOR
A device which responds to a change of some kind in its environment as, for example, a change of temperature, pressure, electrical conductivity (as with the FLAME IONIZA-TION DETECTOR used in GLC) or radiation of some kind. Electrical signals from a detector of an analytical instrument, such as a gas–liquid chromatograph (*see* GAS–LIQUID CHROMATOGRAPHY), are transmitted, after amplification, to a computer and pen recorder for the purposes of visual display and permanent recording of the analytical results.

DETERMINATION
In chemistry, any process of ANALYSIS leading to a QUANTITATIVE result.

DEXTROROTATORY
The property of a material, such as *d*-limonene, to rotate the plane of polarized light in a clockwise direction.

DIFFUSION
The spontaneous spreading out of a gas or VAPOUR, or of a solute placed in a solvent in which it is soluble, to become evenly distributed throughout the whole of the available space.

DISSOCIATION
A chemical process in which MOLECULES split into smaller groups of ATOMS or molecules, or into IONS. An example is the dissociation of water molecules into HYDROGEN IONS and HYDROXIDE IONS; another is the dissociation of molecules of ACIDS into ions on contact with water.

DISTILLATE
Any product of DISTILLATION collected in the RECEIVER of a still.

DISTILLATION
The process of vaporizing a substance in a distillation vessel and collecting the product of cooling the VAPOUR in a separate vessel or, in the case of REFLUX DISTIL-LATION, in the same vessel.

DOUBLE BOND
A linkage between two ATOMS, consisting of two bonding pairs of ELECTRONS.

DRY DOWN

The final residue of odour remaining after the almost total EVAPORATION of an aromatic material or perfume.

DRYOUT

See DRY DOWN.

(E-)

Abbreviation, used in chemistry, for the German word *entgegen*, meaning 'opposed to', in reference to the *trans-* form of a pair of geometrical isomers [*see cis/trans* ISOMERISM and also *(Z-)*].

ELECTRON

A negatively charged particle, of mass approximately $\frac{1}{2000}$ of that of a PROTON.

'ELECTRONIC NOSE'

An electronic instrument for the characterization of odours independently of the human nose.

ELECTRON SHELL

A region of space around the NUCLEUS of an ATOM containing one or more ELECTRON orbitals. *See* ORBITAL.

ELECTROVALENCY

The combining power of an ATOM, numerically equal to the number of electrons that it can lose or gain to form an ION.

ELEMENT

A substance composed of atoms, the nuclei of all of which contain the same number of PROTONS. It follows that the ATOMS of an element will all contain the same number of ELECTRONS, external to the NUCLEUS, equal to the number of protons. This number is unaffected by the presence of NEUTRONS in the nuclei of the atoms. ISOTOPES of the same element therefore have identical CHEMICAL PROPERTIES.

EMOLLIENT

A material capable of restoring the flexibility and elasticity of the skin.

EMPATAGE

In ENFLEURAGE, the process of spreading the GRAISSE on the glass plate of a CHASSIS.

EMPIRICAL FORMULA

The simplest formula expressing the composition of a chemical COMPOUND. For example, the MOLECULAR FORMULA for ethanol is C_2H_5OH, corresponding to the empirical formula C_2H_6O.

ENANTIOMER (or ENANTIOMORPH)

An OPTICAL ISOMER.

ENANTIOMORPHISM
The existence of OPTICAL ISOMERS of the same chemical COMPOUND.

END ODOUR
See DRY DOWN.

END POINT
The point during a TITRATION at which neither of the REACTANTS is in excess, as at the point of neutrality when an ALKALI is titrated with an ACID.

ENFLEURAGE
The process of absorbing the fragrance (as ESSENTIAL OIL) from living flowers of the same kind into specially purified, preserved fat over a period of many hours. Enfleurage has been commercially obsolete since the 1960s.

ENZYME
A biochemical CATALYST, such as the zymase of yeast used in fermenting certain natural sugars to ethanol and carbon dioxide in the brewing industry.

EQUILIBRIUM
A state of balance. *See* CHEMICAL EQUILIBRIUM.

ESSENTIAL OIL
The term 'essential oil' is frequently used quite loosely, to refer to any fragrant product from a natural source, whether distilled, extracted or expressed. Most commercial essential oils do not, in fact, conform to a strict definition, which may be stated as follows:
   An essential oil is a totally VOLATILE product, obtained from a natural source of a single species, which corresponds to that species in chemical composition and odour.

ESTER
The organic product of a REACTION between an ALCOHOL or PHENOL and a CARBOXYLIC ACID.
   The MOLECULES of an ester contain the FUNCTIONAL GROUP

ESTERIFICATION
The type of REACTION by which an ESTER is synthesized from an ALCOHOL or PHENOL and a CARBOXYLIC ACID.

ESTER VALUE
A figure expressing the percentage of an ESTER, or of all esters calculated as the most important ester, in an ESSENTIAL OIL.

ETHER
An ORGANIC COMPOUND the MOLECULES of which are characterized by the presence of an oxygen ATOM bonded to two HYDROCARBON chains, ring systems or other hydrocarbon MOLECULAR STRUCTURES.

EVAPORATION

The physical change of a liquid or solid to the VAPOUR state.

EVOCATIVE PROPERTY

The property of a certain kind of sensation, such as a particular odour, to cause immediate and vivid recall of the circumstances with which the same sensation, or a very similar one, was emotionally associated at some time in the past.

'EXTENDING'

The practice of increasing the quantity of an aromatic material by the addition of a cheaper material without altering the properties, in particular the odour and appearance, of the material to a generally perceptible extent.

EXTRACT

The soluble matter obtained from a natural source, such as jasmin flowers, by washing with a pure, VOLATILE solvent and subsequent recovery of the solvent by DISTILLATION, usually under reduced pressure. The CONCRETES, ABSOLUTES and RESINOIDS of perfumery are examples of extracts.

EXPRESSION PROCESS

A mechanical process of SCARIFICATION or compression for obtaining the ESSENTIAL OILS from citrus fruits, or the juice from any fruit.

EXUDATE

A resinous product, such as benzoin, FRANKINCENSE or myrrh, produced by the CAMBIUM of a woody plant, either naturally or in response to wounding or removal of bark.

FATTY ALDEHYDE

A STRAIGHT CHAIN or BRANCHED CHAIN ALDEHYDE having the general formula $C_nH_{2n+1}.CHO$. MOLECULES of the fatty aldehydes commonly used in perfumery contain from 7 to 14 carbon ATOMS. *See also* ALDEHYDIC.

FERMENTATION

A process of the partial decomposition of organic matter, catalysed by ENZYMES as in the fermentation of grape sugar (dextrose) by the zymase of yeast in the making of wine. Useful perfume ingredients can be produced by the bacterial fermentation of certain TERPENES.

FID

see FLAME IONIZATION DETECTOR.

FINE FRAGRANCE

A fragrance of the highest quality. *See also* CLASSIC PERFUME.

FIXATION

The technique of prolonging the lasting power of the main fragrance theme of a perfume.

FIXATIVE
A material, such as Sandalwood Oil, capable of prolonging the effects of the main fragrance theme of a perfume. RESINOIDS are excellent fixatives by virtue of their content of odourless resin.

FIXED OIL
An oil, such as a VEGETABLE OIL, which is nonVOLATILE at ordinary temperatures and atmospheric pressure.

FLAME IONIZATION DETECTOR (FID)
A device for detecting the VAPOURS of constituents of mixtures of VOLATILES, such as ESSENTIAL OILS or perfumes, which have been separated by a GLC column. The separated vapours pass through a small flame of burning hydrogen, wherein they burn, causing changes of electrical conductivity between two electrodes at high POTENTIAL DIFFERENCE placed near to the flame. These changes are approximately proportional to the relative amounts of the constituents in the original sample. *See also* DETECTOR and CORRECTION FACTOR.

FLAVEDO
The coloured part of the rind of a citrus fruit.

FLORET
A small flower, usually one of a cluster, such as the florets of hyacinth or lilac blossom which together form complete flowers.

FLORIENTAL
An ORIENTAL type perfume displaying emphasis on floral NOTES, such as those of exotic flowers — jasmin, tuberose, gardenia, plumeria, etc.

FOND
The French word for 'BASE', or 'foundation', used in reference to the base of a perfume.

FORMULATION
The process of composing a formula for a product of some kind, such as a perfume.

FOUGÈRE
French word meaning 'fern'. A type of perfume based on a combination of oakmoss or treemoss and the AROMA CHEMICAL coumarin, and displaying emphasis on lavender in the TOP NOTE.

FRACTION
In chemical and perfume technology, a separately collected portion of the DISTILLATE from the DISTILLATION of an ESSENTIAL OIL or crude AROMA CHEMICAL.

FRACTIONAL DISTILLATION
A DISTILLATION process in which portions of the DISTILLATE having different boiling points, or ranges of BOILING POINT, are collected in separate RECEIVERS.

FRACTIONATING COLUMN

A hollow, vertical column, made of glass, stainless steel or other nonREACTIVE, non-absorbent material, used for separating FRACTIONS from the VAPOURS rising up the column from a DISTILLATION vessel beneath. Most fractionating columns are fitted internally with some form of solid, inert packing or device for increasing their efficiency.

FRACTIONATION

See FRACTIONAL DISTILLATION.

FRAGMENTATION PATTERN

The displayed results of the separation of fragments of the MOLECULES of a chemical COMPOUND bombarded by high-energy ELECTRONS in a mass spectrograph.

FRANKINCENSE

A resinous EXUDATE from the trunk of the tree *Boswellia carterii* and other species of *Boswellia*. Known also as OLIBANUM.

FREQUENCY

Number of complete vibrations (cycles) per second. Measured in HERTZ (Hz).

FUNCTIONAL GROUP

A group of bonded ATOMS or a single ATOM, which is the most chemically REACTIVE part of a MOLECULE.

FURANOCOUMARINS

DERIVATIVES of coumarin, certain of which are PHOTOTOXIC, found as constituents of CITRUS OILS and some other ESSENTIAL OILS. Known also as bergaptenes and methoxy-psoralens, although the latter is not an accurate description.

GAS–LIQUID CHROMATOGRAPHY

An analytical technique for separating the constituents of a minute sample of a mixture of VOLATILES, such as a natural aromatic material or a perfume, and recording the results of the ANALYSIS. The sample is vaporized and the constituents separated by virtue of differences in their solubilities in a nonvolatile absorbent coating the inner walls of a long capillary tube (the chromatography COLUMN) through which they pass. The vaporized sample is carried through the column in a slow stream of helium or nitrogen, and all constituents are kept in the vapour state by means of hot air circulating round the column. The results of the analysis are recorded as a series of peaks, drawn by a pen recorder, each one of which corresponds, with respect to its position, to a constituent of the sample. Chromatographs of ESSENTIAL OILS will be found on pages 152–171 of this book.

GEL

A COLLOIDAL SOLUTION in which the colloidal particles are combined with the solvent to form a semi-solid, such as a jelly.

GENE

A unit of the molecular GENETIC CODE, located on a CHROMOSOME. Sequences of genes provide the programme whereby specific anatomical and physiological features of an organism are passed on from one generation to the next.

GENETIC

Pertaining to the means whereby inherited characteristics of a living organism are transmitted from one generation to the next.

GENETIC CODE

The sequence of information, in the form of units of three organic, nitrogen-containing BASES called *codon*s, which, as present in GENES, determines the composition of all proteinaceous matter (*see* PROTEIN) in a plant or animal cell. Each codon codes for the biosynthesis of one specific AMINO ACID of the molecular chain of a protein.

GENOTYPE

The genetic constitution of an organism, as determined by its GENETIC CODE.

GEOMETRICAL ISOMERISM

See cis/trans ISOMERISM.

GLC

See GAS–LIQUID CHROMATOGRAPHY.

GLC MATCH

A mixture of aromatic materials prepared to conform to the results of ANALYSIS by GLC of a perfume COMPOUND or complex aromatic material such as a fragrance BASE.

GLC TRACE

A CHROMATOGRAM.

GLYCOSIDE

A member of a family of plant cell constituents which on HYDROLYSIS undergo partial decomposition to a sugar and another COMPOUND, called an AGLYCON. Some aglycons are VOLATILE and, if formed during the distillation of an ESSENTIAL OIL, appear as constituents of the oil.

GRAISSE

A French word, meaning 'grease', formerly used in perfumery in reference to the mixture of purified fats used in the ENFLEURAGE process.

'HALO EFFECT'

A perceived impression that the functional performance of a perfumed product is better than that of the same product which is either unperfumed or perfumed with a less suitable fragrance.

HARMONY

In perfumery, a pleasing blend of fragrance NOTES having a smooth, unified effect.

HEADSPACE
The space bounded by the walls of a container, the closure and the surface of its contents.

HEADSPACE ANALYSIS
ANALYSIS, by GAS–LIQUID CHROMATOGRAPHY, of the gas or VAPOUR present in a HEADSPACE.

HEARTWOOD
The internal, non-living part of a woody stem, branch or tree-trunk.

HEATING BLOCK
The part of a gas–liquid chromatograph (*see* GAS–LIQUID CHROMATOGRAPHY), situated at the entrance to the column, where injected samples for ANALYSIS are quickly vaporized by heat.

HEDONIC
Pertaining to pleasant and unpleasant sensations, or sensual pleasure.

HERBIVORE
A plant-eating animal.

HERTZ
Unit of FREQUENCY in cycles per second.

HISTOLOGY
The study of the fine structure of animal and plant tissues.

HOLISTIC MEDICINE
Any form of medicine in which treatment is decided after consideration of the condition of the entire organism to be treated, rather than by deduction from the symptoms of the disorder.

HOMOLOGOUS SERIES
A series of organic COMPOUNDS in which succesive MOLECULES differ only by a -CH_2-, or methylene, group of ATOMS.

HUMECTANT
A HYGROSCOPIC substance, such as glycerol (glycerine), which can moisturize the skin by absorbing water VAPOUR from the air and possibly also by promoting the upward movement of water to the skin from subcutaneous tissues.

HYDROCARBON
A COMPOUND composed of molecules consisting of atoms of carbon and hydrogen only.

HYDROGEN BOND

A weak, electrostatic BOND formed between oppositely charged parts of POLAR MOLE-
CULES, such as the oxygen ATOM of an ALCOHOL molecule and the hydroxy- hydrogen
atom of another MOLECULE of the same or a different alcohol.

HYDROGEN ION

A hydrogen ion is a PROTON as produced, for example, by the DISSOCIATION of a
molecule of an acid. In aqueous solution, a hydrogen ion combines immediately with
a water molecule to form an OXONIUM ION.

HYDROLYSIS

The decomposition of a COMPOUND by water. ESTERS, for example, may under suitable conditions be hydrolysed to the ALCOHOLS and carboxylic acids from which they
are derived.

HYDROXIDE ION

The negatively charged ION OH^-, produced by the IONIZATION of water MOLECULES
and characteristic of ALKALIS.

HYDROXY– GROUP

The FUNCTIONAL GROUP -OH, present in water MOLECULES and molecules of ALCO-
HOLS, and distinguished from the HYDROXIDE ION by its electronic configuration and
lack of negative charge.

HYGROSCOPIC

Water-attracting (cf. Hydroscopic, pertaining to underwater observations).

Hz

HERTZ

IFRA

International Fragrance Association. The voluntary body, based in Switzerland, which
advises the perfume industry on the safety of fragrance ingredients.

IMINE

An ORGANIC COMPOUND characterized by the presence in its MOLECULES of an imino,
>NH, FUNCTIONAL GROUP, as present in the indole molecule.

INDICATOR

A substance used, usually in very small amounts, to test for the presence or absence
of another substance, to estimate the extent to which a REACTION has taken place, to
determine the CONCENTRATION of a substance or to measure the *p*H of a solution.

INFLORESCENCE

A collection of FLORETS, together forming a complete flower, as found in the blossoms of hyacinths and members of the botanical family of *Compositae*, e.g. dandeli-
ons and daisies.

INFRARED SPECTROPHOTOMETRY (IRS)

An instrumental technique for measurement of the absorption of infrared radiation (heat rays) over a range of frequencies by the MOLECULES of a material, such as an AROMA CHEMICAL, ESSENTIAL OIL or perfume COMPOUND. The infrared SPECTRO-GRAM, which is the analytical result of the IRS of a material, is extremely useful for purposes of identification as, like a fingerprint, it is unique to that material under standardized conditions of ANALYSIS.

INJECTION PORT

The fine hole through which samples, of the order of less than one MICROLITRE, are injected into a gas–liquid chromatograph (see GAS–LIQUID CHROMATOGRAPHY).

INORGANIC CHEMISTRY

The study of the chemical behaviour of ELEMENTS, and of COMPOUNDS of elements, other than carbon, but including ionic compounds such as carbonates, and simple molecular compounds such as carbon dioxide.

INSTRUMENTAL ANALYSIS

ANALYSIS of any kind performed by an advanced analytical instrument, such as a chromatograph (*see* GAS–LIQUID CHROMATOGRAPHY) or spectrograph (*see* INFRARED SPECTROPHOTOMETRY).

INTEGRATOR

A dedicated computer of the kind used to calculate the results of ANALYSIS performed by GAS–LIQUID CHROMATOGRAPHY.

INTERFACE

The boundary between two immiscible (*see* MISCIBLE) liquids or solids, or between a liquid and a solid.

ION

An electrically charged ATOM or group of atoms, such as the sodium ION, Na^+, or the carbonate ion CO_3^{2-}.

ION-AGGREGATE

A collection of IONS of opposite charge, such as those occurring in common salt, Na^+Cl^-. In any ion-aggregate the sum total of the positive *charges* is equal to the sum-total of the negative charges, as in a crystal of sodium carbonate, $Na^+{}_2(CO_3)^{2-}.10H_2O$ in which example there is twice the number of sodium ions as carbonate ions.

IONIC ASSOCIATION

The *association* (NB *not* combination) of IONS to form an ionic COMPOUND, such as sodium chloride:

$$Na^+ \; + \; Cl^- \longrightarrow Na^+Cl^-$$

IONIC COMBINATION

The chemical interaction of a metallic ELEMENT with a non-metallic element to form an IONIC COMPOUND. The reaction involves ionization of atoms of the metal by electron loss to form positively charged metal IONS, and of atoms of the non-metal by gain of electrons lost by the metal atoms to form negatively charged non-metal ions. The oppositely charged ions then associate to form ION-AGGREGATES comprising the compound formed. *See* IONIZATION and IONIC ASSOCIATION.

IONIZATION

Any process of the formation of IONS, such as in the following examples:

$$Na \ - \ e^- \ \longrightarrow \ Na^+$$

$$Cl \ + \ e^- \ \longrightarrow \ Cl^-$$

$$H_2O \ \longrightarrow \ H^+ \ + \ OH^-$$

IRS

See INFRARED SPECTROPHOTOMETRY.

ISOLATE

A term usually employed to refer to a single constituent separated from a mixture of VOLATILES such as an ESSENTIAL OIL. Typical examples are citral from Lemongrass Oil and linalöl from Rosewood Oil.

ISOMER

One of two or more chemical COMPOUNDS, of which the MOLECULES contain the same number of ATOMS of the same ELEMENTS, but in which these atoms are combined or arranged in different ways. Examples of pairs of isomers are ethanol and dimethyl ether (C_2H_5OH and CH_3OCH_3, respectively), alpha- and beta-pinenes, in which the only difference is that of the position of the DOUBLE BOND in the molecules, the *cis-/trans-* isomers geraniol and nerol (see *cis-/trans* ISOMERISM) and the OPTICAL ISOMERS *d*- and *l*-limonene.

ISOMERISM

The existence of isomers. *See* ISOMER.

ISOTOPES

ATOMS of the same ELEMENT containing different numbers of NEUTRONS. The ISOTOPES of a given element have the same CHEMICAL PROPERTIES, but different PHYSICAL PROPERTIES, such as RELATIVE ATOMIC MASS and (hence) density.

'JUICE'

Anglicized version of the French word *jus*, meaning 'juice', used colloquially in reference to a perfume COMPOUND.

KETONE

An organic COMPOUND characterized by the presence in its MOLECULES of a carbonyl FUNCTIONAL GROUP bonded to two HYDROCARBON RADICALS: R.CO.R'.

KEY BASE

In perfumery, a mixture consisting of all the ingredients of a perfume COMPOUND which are essential to the specific character of the fragrance.

KEY INGREDIENT

In perfumery, an ingredient of a perfume essential to the specific character of its fragrance.

l-

See LAEVOROTATORY.

LACTONE

An ORGANIC COMPOUND characterized by the presence in its MOLECULES of an ESTER FUNCTIONAL GROUP as part of a ring system.

LAEVOROTATORY

The property of a material, such as an ESSENTIAL OIL, to rotate the plane of polarized light anticlockwise.

LATENT HEAT OF FUSION

The quantity of heat required to melt a given mass of a solid to liquid at the melting point. This same quantity of heat is given out by the same weight of the liquid when it solidifies at the MELTING POINT. The melting point of a solid may therefore be defined as that temperature at which the liquid and solid states of a substance can coexist: an EQUILIBRIUM temperature when the rate at which melting is taking place is equal to the rate of solidification.

LATENT HEAT OF VAPORIZATION

The heat required to vaporize a given mass of a liquid at the BOILING POINT. This same quantity of heat is given out by the same weight of the VAPOUR when it condenses, at the boiling point. The boiling point of a liquid may therefore be defined as the temperature at which the liquid and vapour states of a substance can coexist: an EQUILIBRIUM temperature when the rate at which vaporization is taking place is equal to the rate of CONDENSATION of the vapour.

An important contribution to our understanding of STEAM DISTILLATION was made some years ago by E.F.K. Denny, of the Bridestowe Estate, Tasmania, who from the results of his experiments concluded that the process works as efficiently as it does as the result of the release of latent heat as steam condenses around the margins of released ESSENTIAL OIL droplets on a charge of lavender or other essential oil-bearing material in the DISTILLATION vessel.

'LIFT'

The property of certain aromatic materials, such as YLANG-YLANG Oil, Extra, to render middle NOTES of a perfume perceptible in the TOP NOTE.

LONGITUDINAL WAVES

Alternate regions of compression and rarefaction propagated from a source through a medium of some kind, such as air or water in the case of sound waves.

MACERATION

The process of allowing a definite weight of extractable matter to soak, in a closed vessel for several days, in a definite weight of ALCOHOL of given strength to produce a crude TINCTURE. The tincture is filtered and adjusted to standard strength with respect to its odour or content of an active ingredient, allowed to mature and finally filtered bright ready for use. Tinctures are today almost obsolete in both perfumery and pharmacy.

'MARINE'

In perfumery, a NOTE of the sea or seashore. The term 'oceanic' is an alternative and more expressive term having a similar meaning.

MASS NUMBER

The sum of the numbers of PROTONS and NEUTRONS in the NUCLEUS of an ATOM.

MASS SPECTROMETRY

An instrumental analytical technique for determining the composition of a COMPOUND, usually an ORGANIC COMPOUND. *See also* FRAGMENTATION PATTERN.

MATCHING

The copying of a perfume or complex perfume ingredient for the purpose of duplicating its fragrance and other properties.

MATURATION

The AGEING of a finished alcoholic perfume until fully mellowed.

MELTING POINT

The temperature at which a solid changes to liquid.

MEMBRANE

In biology, a thin, flexible sheet of tissue, such as the epidermis of the skin or of a leaf.

META–

In chemistry, a prefix referring to positions in a BENZENE RING which are separated by one carbon ATOM of the ring as, for example, the 1,3- positions.

METASTABLE

A transient condition of a system or part of a system, such as exists in a supercooled liquid. A liquid in this condition remains liquid at temperatures below the melting point, and is an example of a substance in a metastable state. Certain AROMA CHEMICALS, having melting points a few degrees above normal room temperature, such as diphenyl oxide, $C_6H_5OC_6H_5$, melting point 26·5°C, frequently show this phenomenon. Solidification occurs on sufficiently disturbing the supercooled liquid or on adding to it a crystal of the solid.

MICELLES

Colloidal particles consisting of droplets of oil surrounded by MOLECULES or IONS of a SURFACTANT which prevent the droplets from coalescing. Soap and soapless detergents are surfactants which form micelles with oily dirt ready for washing away. *See also* SOLUBILIZER.

MICROLITRE

One millionth of a litre.

MIDDLE NOTE

A fragrant note of intermediate volatility and lasting power.

MISCIBLE

Capable of complete mutual dispersion in another substance. Liquid aromatic materials are in most cases mutually miscible in all proportions.

MOLAR

In chemistry, a molar solution is a solution containing one MOLE of a dissolved solute per litre of solution.

MOLARITY

The number of MOLES of a solute dissolved in one litre of a solution.

MOLE

In chemistry, the quantity of an ELEMENT or COMPOUND contained in its formula weight. Examples are as follows:

Substance	Molecular formula	Formula weight	= weight of 1 mole (g)
Oxygen	O_2	2×16	= 32
Water	H_2O	$2 \times 1 + 16$	= 18
Hexane	C_6H_{14}	$6 \times 12 + 14 \times 1$	= 86
Limonene	$C_{10}H_{16}$	$10 \times 12 + 16 \times 1$	= 136
Geraniol	$C_{10}H_{18}O$	$10 \times 12 + 18 \times 1 + 16$	= 154

MOLECULAR FORMULA

The formula expressing the true numbers of ATOMS of the different ELEMENTS present in a MOLECULE of a COMPOUND.

MOLECULAR GEOMETRY

The patterns of arrangement of the ATOMS in a MOLECULE.

MOLECULAR STRUCTURE
Term used in reference to the shape of a MOLECULE, as determined mainly by the nature and direction of the bonds holding its ATOMS together.

MOLECULAR WEIGHT
To a close approximation, the molecular weight of an ELEMENT or COMPOUND is the ratio of the weight of one MOLECULE of the substance to the weight of one ATOM of hydrogen taken as one ATOMIC WEIGHT unit.

MOLECULE
The smallest particle of an ELEMENT or COMPOUND which can exist on its own.

MONOMER
A chemical COMPOUND capable of undergoing polymerization.

MONOTERPENE
A TERPENE of MOLECULAR FORMULA $C_{10}H_{16}$.

MOSSY
An odour recalling Oakmoss or Treemoss ABSOLUTE: woody, green, earthy and 'MARINE' in character.

MOVING PHASE
In GAS–LIQUID CHROMATOGRAPHY, the CARRIER GAS.

MS
MASS SPECTROMETRY.

MUCUS
The glairy, colloidal solution produced by mucous cells (goblet cells) which covers a mucous MEMBRANE, keeping it moist.

MUSK
Natural musk is the dried, glandular secretion of the male musk deer, formerly used in perfumery as a FIXATIVE.

n-
Normal. In chemistry, a prefix denoting a straight-chain ORGANIC COMPOUND, as distinct from a BRANCHED-CHAIN structural ISOMER of the same compound.

NAPHTHENIC
An odour recalling that of naphthalene, the organic compound from which old-fashioned moth balls are made. Pure indole has a naphthenic odour.

'NATURE IDENTICAL'
Term designating a synthetic ORGANIC COMPOUND of the same composition and molecular structure as the same COMPOUND as it occurs in nature.

NERVOUS IMPULSE

A wave of electrical negativity which flows over a nerve fibre from the point of stimulation to a SYNAPSE.

NEUTRON

An electrically neutral particle of unit mass present in the nuclei of the ATOMS of all ELEMENTS other than hydrogen of unit atomic mass. The effect of the presence of neutrons in an atomic NUCLEUS containing more than one PROTON is to bind the protons together.

NITRILE

An ORGANIC COMPOUND characterized by the presence of a cyano, FUNCTIONAL GROUP: $-C\equiv N$

nm

Nanometre(s). A nanometre is one thousand millionth (10^{-9}) of a metre; a millionth of a millimetre.

NOODLES

In soap technology, noodles are small, rounded masses of unperfumed soap base.

NOTE

See ODOUR NOTE.

NUCLEUS

In chemistry, the positively charged, central body of an ATOM. In biology, a dense, organized, proteinaceous body (*see* PROTEIN) found in the PROTOPLASM of a plant or animal cell, containing hereditary material and controlling the metabolic activities of the cell.

'OCEANIC'

See 'MARINE'.

ODORANT

Any substance having an odour.

ODOUR BALANCE

The odour effect of a blend of aromatic materials in which none of the constituent fragrance NOTES is more prominent than any of the others.

ODOUR HARMONY

See HARMONY.

ODOUR MASKING

Rendering an unwanted odour imperceptible by means of a stronger odour, the effect of which is acceptable.

ODOUR NOTE
A distinctive odour impression, i.e. one which can be recognized and identified.

ODOUR PROFILE
A complete description of an odour in written, diagrammatic or graphical form, resulting from OLFACTORY evaluation or instrumental measurement.

ODOUR PURITY
The extent to which the odour of a test sample of an aromatic material or perfume conforms to the odour of a STANDARD SAMPLE of the same product.

ODOUR THRESHOLD
The least CONCENTRATION, or highest dilution, at which the odour of an ODORANT can be detected under standardized conditions.

OLEO-GUM RESIN
A plant EXUDATE consisting of a mixture of an ESSENTIAL OIL, water-soluble gum and resin. Several of these natural products are purified by SOLVENT EXTRACTION for use as RESINOIDS in perfumery.

OLÆOPTENE
The oily, odorous part of an essential oil, such as Rose Otto, which also contains VOLATILE, odourless matter in solution or as a crystalline deposit. *See also* STEAROPTENE.

OLEO-RESIN
A plant EXUDATE consisting of a mixture of ESSENTIAL OIL and resin. A small number of these products find use in perfumery as RESINOIDS after purification by SOLVENT EXTRACTION or other means.

OLFACTORY
Pertaining to the sense of smell.

OLFACTORY FATIGUE
Temporary loss of sensitivity to the odour of an ODORANT continuously smelled over a period of time. Fatigue to a certain odour leaves the nose fully sensitive to all other odours which it is able to detect. Recovery from olfactory fatigue is rapid and complete when the responsible odorant is no longer smelled.

OLFACTORY HAIRS
The submicroscopic, thread-like projections of primary OLFACTORY nerve fibres of the OLFACTORY ORGAN which support odour-sensitive sites for detecting the presence of odorous MOLECULES.

OLFACTORY ORGAN
The twin, odour-detecting MEMBRANES of the nose situated on either side of the nasal septum (the partition between the two nostrils) within the nasal cavity.

OLIBANUM
FRANKINCENSE.

OPTICAL ISOMERS
These are different optically active forms of the same chemical COMPOUND, in which the MOLECULE of one form is the mirror-image of that of the other form. One of a pair of optical isomers, the *d-* form, rotates the plane of polarized light in a clockwise direction, while the other ISOMER, the *l-* form, rotates it in an anticlockwise direction. Interesting examples are *d-* and *l-* carvones, occurring as the chief odorous constituents of Caraway Oil and Spearmint Oil, respectively, and possessing the odours characteristic of the parent oils. This example illustrates the fact that optical isomerism can give rise to odour differences between STEREOISOMERS.

OPTICAL ROTATION
Rotation of the plane of polarized light by transmission through an optically active substance. Almost all ESSENTIAL OILS show optical activity at least to some degree, arising from their content of optically active constituents.

ORBITAL
A region of space around the NUCLEUS of an ATOM where an unpaired ELECTRON or an electron pair is most likely to be found.

ORGAN
The traditional arrangement of shelving holding a perfumer's PALETTE of aromatic materials, so named for its resemblance to the console of a cinema organ. Now almost totally replaced by arrangements less conducive to creative thought.

ORGANIC ACID
See CARBOXYLIC ACID.

ORGANIC CHEMISTRY
The study of the chemical behaviour of COMPOUNDS of carbon, other than carbon-containing ionic compounds such as carbonates and simple molecular compounds such as carbon dioxide.

ORGANIC COMPOUND
A carbon COMPOUND other than a simple, ionic compound containing carbon, such as a carbonate or similar molecular compound such as carbon dioxide.

ORIENTAL
A type of perfume characterized by a heavy and very long-lasting fragrance. The perfume Shalimar, by Guerlain, launched in 1925, is a classic example of this fragrance type.

ORTHO–
In chemistry, the prefix *ortho–* refers to adjacent positions in a BENZENE RING as, for example, the 1,2- positions.

OXIDATION

A CHEMICAL REACTION in which oxygen combines with an ELEMENT or COMPOUND, or in which hydrogen is removed from a compound. A more fundamental concept is that oxidation is the loss of one or more ELECTRONS by an ATOM, ION or MOLECULE.

OXONIUM ION

The ION H_3O^+, formed by loss of a PROTON, H^+ (a hydrogen ion) from an ACID MOLECULE and its combination with a water molecule.

OXYGENATE

See OXYGENATED CONSTITUENT.

OXYGENATED CONSTITUENT

A constituent of an ESSENTIAL OIL or aromatic EXTRACT containing combined oxygen.

'OZONIC'

A fresh ODOUR NOTE, similar to the odour of ozone (O_3) often found in the fragrances of modern consumer products, such as domestic laundry detergents.

PALETTE

By analogy with the palette of colours of an artist, the range of aromatic materials available to a perfumer.

PARA—

In chemistry, the prefix *para—* refers to two positions in a BENZENE RING which are opposite to one another; i.e. separated by two carbon ATOMS as, for example, the 1,4-positions.

PARTITION

In physical chemistry, the distribution of a solute between two immiscible (*see* MISCI-BLE) solvents in contact with one another. Thus if an ESSENTIAL OIL is shaken with the solvents pentane and 50% aqueous methanol, both oxygenates and terpenes will become partitioned between both solvents, with most of the TERPENE content dissolved in the pentane and most of the OXYGENATE content in the weak methanol. The phenomenon of partition affords a means for the preparation of TERPENELESS ESSEN-TIAL OILS.

PATAGE

In the process of ENFLEURAGE patage is the inversion of the CHASSIS, following DEFLEURAGE so that the lower layer of GRAISSE is now the upper layer, ready for a fresh charge of flowers.

PATHOGENIC

Disease-producing.

PEAK AREA

The area of a peak on a CHROMATOGRAM, which is approximately proportional to the amount of the constituent that it represents in the product subjected to ANALYSIS.

PEAK HEIGHT

The vertical distance from the BASE LINE of a CHROMATOGRAM to the apex of a peak and which is proportional to the PEAK AREA .

PERIODIC TABLE

An arrangement of the chemical ELEMENTS in the order of their ATOMIC NUMBERS showing the regular recurrence of many of their properties, particularly CHEMICAL PROPERTIES. The most famous of periodic tables is that given by the great Russian chemist, Dmitri Ivanovitch Mendeleyev (1834-1907), who used it to postulate the existence of elements unknown at the time of its publication, but which were later discovered in nature.

***p*H**

A measure of the acidity or alkalinity of an aqueous solution, expressed as a numerical value on a scale from 0 (extremely acidic) to 14·0 (extremely alkaline). A *p*H value of 7·0 expresses neutrality. (Scientifically, the *p*H of a solution is measured as the logarithm to base 10 of the reciprocal of the hydrogen ion concentration in MOLES per litre.)

PERMANENT GAS

A gas, such as oxygen, nitrogen or hydrogen, which is difficult to liquefy.

PHENOL

The organic BENZENOID compound C_6H_5OH or any other COMPOUND of which the MOLECULES each have one or more HYDROXY GROUPS bonded directly to a BENZENE RING.

PHOTOCATALYSIS

A changing of the rate of a CHEMICAL REACTION by the incidence of light. ESSENTIAL OILS deteriorate very much faster when exposed to sunlight than they do in darkness.

PHOTOSYNTHESIS

The manufacture of the sugar glucose in the leaves of a green plant from carbon dioxide and water in the presence of CHLOROPHYLL, using sunlight as a source of energy and with the evolution of oxygen.

PHOTOTOXIC

This term describes the property of a substance to exert a toxic effect in the presence of light, particularly sunlight as, for example, bergaptene in Bergamot and some other ESSENTIAL OILS.

PHYSICAL PROPERTIES

Those properties of a substance which do not involve chemical change, such as melting point, BOILING POINT, SPECIFIC GRAVITY or REFRACTIVE INDEX.

PHYSICAL TEST

A test, such as the DETERMINATION of melting point or measurement of SPECIFIC GRAVITY, which does not involve a chemical change (change of composition).

PILOT-SCALE PROCESS
A process using apparatus of size intermediate between laboratory scale and industrial large scale, designed to facilitate determination of the conditions required for safe and efficient full-scale operation. Pilot-scale equipment is used, for example, for development of the full-scale manufacture of new AROMA CHEMICALS.

PLANE OF POLARIZATION
The set of parallel planes in which rays of light travel following POLARIZATION.

POLARIZATION
The filtration of rays of light orientated in all planes at right angles to their direction of travel, to allow only those rays orientated in a single set of parallel planes to pass through.

POLARISCOPE (or POLARIMETER)
An instrument for measuring the OPTICAL ROTATION of a transparent liquid or solid.

POLARIZER
An optical filter for polarizing light rays. *See also* POLARIZATION.

POLAR MOLECULE
A MOLECULE on which there is an uneven distribution of electrical charge, such as a water MOLECULE and molecules of ALCOHOLS, ALDEHYDES and CARBOXYLIC ACIDS.

POLYFUNCTIONAL
A term used in reference to a MOLECULE, such as that of vanillin, which contains FUNCTIONAL GROUPS of more than one kind.

POLYMER
A larger MOLECULE formed by the bonding together of small molecules, or parts of smaller molecules, of one or more MONOMERS; a COMPOUND of high MOLECULAR WEIGHT formed by the bonding of molecules of one or two compounds of low molecular weight.

POMMADE
The type of product resulting from ENFLEURAGE; it consists of GRAISSE which has become saturated with ESSENTIAL OIL exhaled by fragrant flowers.

POSITION ISOMERISM
ISOMERISM in which the ISOMERS differ in respect of the position of the FUNCTIONAL GROUP(s) in their MOLECULES.

POT
A DISTILLATION or REACTION vessel.

POTENTIAL DIFFERENCE
A difference of electrical charge between two points, such as the poles of an electrical cell or other source of current.

PROTEIN
A natural POLYMER of very high MOLECULAR WEIGHT, present in all living matter. A protein is formed by the linking together of AMINO ACID MOLECULES, with the elimination of water molecules.

PROTON
A positively charged particle of unit atomic mass, which occurs in the nuclei of all ATOMS.

PROTOPLASM
The complex, organized, colloidal contents of all living cells.

QUALITATIVE
A term descriptive of a test for identifying the ATOMS, IONS or MOLECULES present in a chemical COMPOUND or the components of a mixture.

QUANTITATIVE
A term descriptive of a test for determining the percentages of the ELEMENTS combined in a COMPOUND or of the components of a mixture.

RADICAL
An ATOM or group of atoms having one or more unpaired ELECTRONS; symbol R.

RASCHIG RINGS
Rings made of glass, ceramic or other nonREACTIVE material used in a FRACTIONATING COLUMN to increase the internal surface area available for condensing VAPOURS rising up the column.

REACTANT
See REAGENT.

REACTION
See CHEMICAL REACTION.

REACTION PATHWAY
A succession of CHEMICAL REACTION steps in which the product of one reaction is caused to undergo a further reaction to give an intermediate product until a required product is finally formed.

REACTIVE
In chemistry, a term applied to a substance which readily undergoes chemical change.

REAGENT
Any substance which can undergo a CHEMICAL REACTION. Applied mostly to chemicals used for testing purposes.

RECEIVER

In DISTILLATION, a vessel placed at the outlet of the condenser to collect the DISTIL-
LATE.

RECEPTOR

In biology, a cell or collection of cells capable of responding to a particular kind of
stimulus, such as odorous MOLECULES.

RECONSTITUTION

In perfumery, the synthetic or largely synthetic reproduction of an aromatic material
of natural origin. The term is also used to refer to the product of an exercise of this
kind.

REDUCTION

In chemistry, the opposite of OXIDATION: a CHEMICAL REACTION in which oxygen is
removed from a COMPOUND or in which hydrogen combines with an ELEMENT or
compound. More fundamentally, reduction is any reaction in which ELECTRONS combine with an ATOM, ION or MOLECULE.

REFLUX DISTILLATION

A process of DISTILLATION in which the distillation VAPOURS are condensed by a
vertical condenser and are continuously allowed to run back into the distillation vessel beneath. Used in chemical SYNTHESIS when a REACTION mixture has to be heated
for a time without loss of VOLATILE material by EVAPORATION, as in the manufacture
of AROMA CHEMICALS.

REFRACTIVE INDEX

In practical terms, a measure of the bending of parallel rays of light of a given
FREQUENCY when passed from a less dense medium into a denser medium. In more
precise, scientific terms, it is the ratio of the speed of light of given frequency in a
vacuum to the speed of light in a medium of some kind at a specified temperature. It
may be calculated using the following relationship:

$$\text{Refractive Index} = \frac{\text{sine of angle of incidence}}{\text{sine of angle of refraction}} \text{ at t}^\circ\text{C}$$

See SINE, *also* SNELL'S LAW.

REFRACTOMETER

An instrument for measuring REFRACTIVE INDEX.

RELATIVE ATOMIC MASS

The ratio of the mass of one ATOM of an ELEMENT to $\frac{1}{12}$ of the mass of an atom of the
ISOTOPE CARBON-12 taken as 12 atomic mass units precisely. *See also* ATOMIC
WEIGHT.

RELATIVE MOLECULAR MASS
The ratio of the mass of one MOLECULE of an ELEMENT or COMPOUND to $\frac{1}{12}$ of the mass of an ATOM of the ISOTOPE CARBON-12, taken as 12 atomic mass units precisely. *See also* MOLECULAR WEIGHT.

RESINOID
A purified, resinous plant EXUDATE, such as an OLEO-RESIN or oleo-gum resin.

RESOLVING POWER
In GAS–LIQUID CHROMATOGRAPHY, the least amount of a VOLATILE COMPOUND that a chromatograph can measure.

RESPIRATION
The production of energy in an animal or plant cell by the ENZYME-catalyzed combustion of foodstuffs, chiefly glucose.

RETENTION TIME
In GAS–LIQUID CHROMATOGRAPHY, the time which a vaporized COMPOUND takes to pass through the column.

REVERSIBLE REACTION
A CHEMICAL REACTION which can proceed in either direction according to prevailing conditions, such as the CONCENTRATIONS of the REACTANTS and products of the reaction.

REWORKING
In perfumery, the production of a close match of an original perfume, usually for the purpose of replacing ingredients which have become unavailable or too costly by equivalent materials likely to remain available for the foreseeable future.

R.I.
REFRACTIVE INDEX.

RIFM
Research Institute for Fragrance Materials. A voluntary organization, based in the United States, for testing the safety of perfume ingredients.

'ROSE ALCOHOLS'
The rose-smelling ALCOHOLS citronellol, geraniol, nerol and phenylethyl alcohol, which occur in Rose Otto.

SATURATED COMPOUND
An ORGANIC COMPOUND the MOLECULES of which contain no multiple BONDS. (Cf. UNSATURATED COMPOUND).

SATURATED SOLUTION
A solution containing as much of a solute as the solvent can hold at a stated temperature.

SCARIFICATION
A process of scraping as used, for example, in the mechanical expression of Bergamot Oil from the peel of the fruit.

SENSORY
In general, pertaining to the senses. In perfumery the term refers specifically to the sense of smell as, for example, in the expression 'sensory perception', meaning the process of smelling.

SEPTUM
In GAS–LIQUID CHROMATOGRAPHY, a small thin, flexible partition sealing off the IN-JECTION PORT, through which samples for ANALYSIS are injected into the HEATING BLOCK for vaporization.

SESQUITERPENE
A TERPENE of molecular formula $C_{15}H_{24}$ ($1\frac{1}{2} \times C_{10}H_{16}$).

S.G.
SPECIFIC GRAVITY.

SHELF LIFE
The period of time following manufacture during which a product remains fit for use.

SHOULDER
In GAS–LIQUID CHROMATOGRAPHY, the appearance of the apex of a smaller peak merged with the side of a larger peak due to imperfect separation of the corresponding VOLATILES.

SIDE CHAIN
A chain of ATOMS joined to a ring or straight-chain MOLECULAR STRUCTURE.

SIDE REACTION
An unwanted CHEMICAL REACTION, yielding an impurity, which takes place during a reaction for producing a required product.

SILICONE
An organic, silicon-containing, linear or CYCLIC POLYMER of general formula $(R_2SiO)_n$, where R is a HYDROCARBON RADICAL. Depending on the value of n and on MOLECULAR STRUCTURE, silicones take the form of oils, greases, rubbers, etc. which find use for many different purposes, e.g. as water repellents, foam suppressants, lubricants, SURFACTANTS, flexible tubing, electrical insulators, etc.

SINE

In the right-angled triangle ABC, the sine (abbreviated as *sin*) of the angle θ is the ratio $\frac{AC}{AB}$.

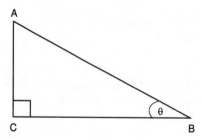

In the diagram below the REFRACTIVE INDEX of the ESSENTIAL OIL is

$$\frac{\sin i}{\sin r} = \frac{AC}{AB} \div \frac{A'C'}{A'B}$$

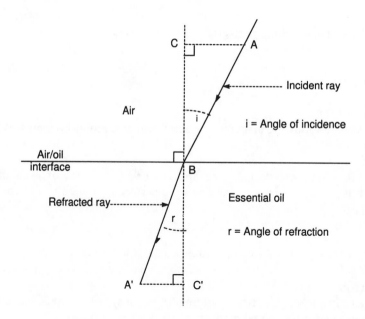

Rulers and protractors are unnecessary in the modern analytical laboratory, where computerized REFRACTOMETERS measure refractive indices automatically.

SITE-FITTING THEORY

A theory of odour detection developed by J.E. Amoore in the 1960s which suggested that stimulation of odour sensitive sites on the OLFACTORY HAIRS follows the fitting of odorous MOLECULES into cavities of opposite shape. The idea of site fitting is embodied in a modern theory of olfaction. (*See also* VIBRATIONAL THEORY.)

SKELETAL FORMULA

A formula for an ORGANIC COMPOUND in which BONDS between the carbon ATOMS are represented, but symbols for carbon atoms and for hydrogen atoms bonded to carbon atoms are generally omitted on the understanding that they are present. The conventional symbols are used to represent atoms of other elements present.

SNELL'S LAW

The natural law upon which measurements of REFRACTIVE INDEX are based. When a ray of light passes from a less dense medium to a denser medium the ratio of the SINE of the angle of incidence to the angle of refraction is constant for a given pair of media at constant temperature. This relationship was discovered by the Dutch physicist Willebrord Snell (1591-1626).

SOL

A COLLOIDAL SOLUTION.

SOLUBILIZER

A water soluble SURFACTANT capable of mediating the formation of a COLLOIDAL SOL in water of water-immiscible (*see* MISCIBLE) liquids such as perfume COMPOUNDS by the formation of MICELLES.

SOLUTE

The dissolved substance in a solution.

SOLVENT EXTRACTION

The separation of soluble matter from a natural source material by a pure, VOLATILE solvent, as in the preparation of EXTRACTS from aromatic sources, also of ABSOLUTES from CONCRETES.

SPECIFICATION

A statement of important properties of a product, to which all other samples or batches of the same product must conform to be acceptable.

SPECIFIC GRAVITY

The ratio of the weight of a substance to the weight of an equal volume of water measured at a stated temperature.

SPECTROGRAM

A graph or diagram of a spectrum, such as a spectrum resulting from the infrared spectrophotometric examination (*see* INFRARED SPECTROPHOTOMETRY) of an ESSENTIAL OIL, showing the degrees of absorption of infrared rays over a range of different WAVELENGTHS under standardized conditions. In infrared spectrophotometry, transmittance, the reciprocal of absorption, is recorded by the spectrometer.

STANDARD SAMPLE

A sample of a product which conforms to a SPECIFICATION for the product, and which is kept for comparison with batch samples for purposes of quality evaluation.

STANDARD SOLUTION

A solution containing a known weight of a given REAGENT in a known volume of solution. *See also* MOLAR and MOLARITY.

STATIONARY PHASE

In GAS–LIQUID CHROMATOGRAPHY, the general name give to the nonVOLATILE absorbent with which the interior of a capillary column (*see* CAPILLARY GLC) is coated. The stationary phase, in conjunction with the CARRIER GAS, effects separation of the vaporized constituents of a sample subjected to ANALYSIS.

STEAM DISTILLATION

A process of DISTILLATION in which steam under pressure is used to heat the charge and release and vaporize the VOLATILES that it contains. (*See also* LATENT HEAT OF VAPORIZATION).

STEAROPTENE

Any VOLATILE solid material which separates from an ESSENTIAL OIL following DISTILLATION, such as the mixture of colourless, waxy, odourless, crystalline HYDROCARBONS which separates from a genuine sample of Rose Otto on cooling in a refrigerator. *See also* OLÆOPTENE.

STEREOISOMERS

See OPTICAL ISOMERS.

STEREOSPECIFIC

Term used to designate a pure, synthetic stereoisomer, or to refer to a type of synthetic process which yields a pure stereoisomer.

STILL

Any form of DISTILLATION equipment, usually excepting that used for REFLUX DISTILLATION.

STILL HEAD

The removable top part of a DISTILLATION vessel leading to and in many cases continuous with, the VAPOUR pipe.

STILL NOTE

An unpleasant, vegetable-like or cabbagey NOTE commonly found in freshly distilled ESSENTIAL OILS, caused by the presence of traces of very highly odorous organic sulphides, such as dimethyl sulphide, $CH_3.S.CH_3$, formed by the partial HYDROLYSIS of proteinaceous matter (*see* PROTEIN). Still notes can be eliminated by brief aeration of an essential oil so affected. The presence of 'burnt' or 'smoky' NOTES in an essential oil which should not display them is indicative of scorching of the charge and hence of a poor quality product. 'Burnt' notes are not true still notes and cannot be eliminated. Birch Tar Oil and Cade Oil are produced by the destructive DISTILLATION of birch bark and juniper twigs, respectively. Both possess highly 'smoky' or 'burnt' odours but are not true essential oils. Guaiacwood Oil and Chinese Cedarwood Oil are examples of essential oils possessing characteristically slightly 'smoky' or 'burnt' notes when of completely acceptable quality.

STRAIGHT CHAIN
In organic chemistry, this term refers to a series of carbon ATOMS bonded together in succession.

'STRETCHING'
A form of adulteration of a costly aromatic material with cheaper material with the object of increasing the quantity without noticeably altering the odour character or strength. It should be noted that certain products so 'stretched' are perfectly usable as ingredients of consumer product perfumes, where the genuine counterparts would be too expensive to use or simply not available in sufficient quantities for bulk usage.

STRIAGE
The making of furrows in ENFLEURAGE GRAISSE following EMPATAGE to increase the surface area for ABSORPTION of flower fragrances (the natural ESSENTIAL OILS of fragrant flowers).

SUBJECTIVITY
Dependence on human judgment and opinion.

SUBLIMATION
In chemistry, the vaporization of a solid or the solidification of a gas or VAPOUR, without the appearance of the intermediate liquid phase.

SUBSTANTIVITY
In perfumery, the property of certain aromatic materials and perfumes to adhere to a surface, from which they are slowly released, yielding odour over very long periods of time. The term is used particularly in reference to lingering fragrance NOTES of a perfume in a product under in-use conditions. Examples are the 'fresh air', 'OZONIC' or 'MARINE'-type notes found in certain domestic laundry product fragrances, and in some fabric softeners, which survive the washing, rinsing, drying and airing sequence to render the linen clean-smelling.

SUBSTITUENT
An ATOM or group of atoms replacing a hydrogen atom in a MOLECULAR STRUCTURE, such as a hydroxy- FUNCTIONAL GROUP substituting for a hydrogen atom of a BEN-ZENE RING in a MOLECULE of a PHENOL.

SURFACTANT
A surface-active agent such as soap or a household detergent.

SURFACE ACTIVE AGENT
A substance which can reduce SURFACE TENSION; a SURFACTANT.

SURFACE TENSION

The stretching force acting at the surface of a liquid. The existence of surface tension at the surface of water is shown by the rapid bursting of bubbles formed by vigorous agitation of the water. The addition of a SURFACTANT reduces the stretching forces which break the bubbles, rendering them more permanent.

SYNAPSE

A narrow gap between the endings of two nerve fibres in close association, across which NERVOUS IMPULSES are transmitted chemically.

SYNTHESIS

The building up of a more complex chemical COMPOUND from ELEMENTS or from simpler compounds.

SYNTHETIC OIL

A term sometimes loosely applied to refer to an AROMA CHEMICAL, a perfume COMPOUND of synthetic composition or to an oily, odourless chemical, such as isopropyl palmitate or isopropyl stearate, which is nonVOLATILE under ordinary conditions of temperature and atmospheric pressure.

TEMPERATURE PROGRAMMING

In GLC, the computer-controlled increasing of temperature of the column at a predetermined rate to ensure that all components of a sample pass completely through it, and are not left behind to emerge during the next ANALYSIS.

TERPENE

An unsaturated HYDROCARBON of EMPIRICAL FORMULA $(C_5H_8)_n$, where n = 1 (hemiterpenes), 2 (MONOTERPENES), 3 (SESQUITERPENES), 4 (diterpenes), 5 (sesterterpenes) or 6 (triterpenes). Terpenes occurring in distilled ESSENTIAL OILS have n = 2 or 3, rarely 4. Higher, non-volatile, terpenes occur in plant EXTRACTS.

TERPENELESS ESSENTIAL OIL

An ESSENTIAL OIL from which all or part of the TERPENE content has been removed by VACUUM FRACTIONATION or SOLVENT EXTRACTION, or a combination of both processes.

TERPENOID

A DERIVATIVE of a TERPENE, such as citral, terpineol, linalyl acetate, etc. In industry, terpenoids are commonly referred to as terpenes.

TÊTE

A French word meaning 'head', used in perfumery to refer to the TOP NOTE of an ESSENTIAL OIL or perfume.

THERMAL DECOMPOSITION

A process of molecular fragmentation which occurs to a COMPOUND heated to a temperature high enough to break BONDS. The higher the temperature to which a compound is heated, the more violent are the vibrations of its MOLECULES until a temperature is reached when their structures begin to come apart.

THERMAL STRESS

A condition of molecular vibration, brought about by heating a COMPOUND, which tends to strain certain of the BONDS in their molecules to the point of structural breakdown.

THERMOSTATIC CONTROL

The automatic control of temperature within narrow limits by means of a thermostat. This form of control is applied to the column of a gas–liquid chromatograph (*see* GAS–LIQUID CHROMATOGRAPHY), which is contained in an oven fitted with a computer controlled thermostat and a fan to distribute heated air evenly throughout the length of the column. The oven temperature is usually set to increase progressively to a predetermined maximum during an ANALYSIS. *See also* TEMPERATURE PROGRAMMING.

THURIBLE (or CENSER)

A container for glowing charcoal and incense used for purposes of religious ceremony. The thurible is supported by chains, usually held by hand, although there are certain places of worship where very large thuribles are suspended from the ceiling. The charcoal heats the incense, causing vaporization and some THERMAL DECOMPOSITION of its constituents, so producing fragrant smoke. Swinging or looping of the thurible improves the air supply to the charcoal so that it does not burn out. A small door set in the body of the thurible provides for replenishment of the incense from time to time.

TINCTURE

In perfumery, an odour-standardized alcoholic solution of extractable matter from a source of aroma, prepared by MACERATION. Tinctures of MUSK, CIVET, Ambergris and CASTOREUM were once in regular use as perfume ingredients.

TITRATION

Measurement of the CONCENTRATION of the SOLUTE in a solution. The following are the essential steps:

   i. A BURETTE is filled to the zero mark with the required STANDARD SOLUTION.

   ii. An accurately measured volume of the solution whose concentration is to be found (the test solution) is transferred to a small flask.

   iii. The standard solution is slowly added from the burette to the test solution in the flask, with constant gentle mixing of the contents of the flask until, at the END POINT, a colour change or a sharp change of electrical resistance occurs, whereupon the volume of the standard solution added is measured. From this measurement, and knowing the concentration of the standard solution, the concentration (or titre) of the test solution may be calculated. Modern equipment for titration is automatic and computer-controlled; it performs all the required calculations and displays the results.

TOILET WATER

A fragrant product consisting of a weak solution (no more than about 8%) of a perfume COMPOUND dissolved in aqueous ALCOHOL, intended for liberal application to the skin after bathing as a means of physical and mental refreshment. As the product rapidly evaporates, it loses its most energetic MOLECULES (molecules of the alcohol-and-water BASE). The energy required for this EVAPORATION is heat, which is withdrawn from the skin. The skin thus quickly cools, and at the same time the refreshing fragrance of the perfume is perceived. The heat transferred to the evaporating product is known as LATENT HEAT OF VAPORIZATION.

TOP NOTE

The first SENSORY impression perceived on smelling an aromatic material, perfume or perfumed product. It consists of the VAPOURS of the most VOLATILE together with some proportion of the less volatile ingredients of the perfume.

TOTAL QUALITY MANAGEMENT (TQM)

A system of quality management aimed at the toal elimination of product rejects by making all employees of a manufacturing company personally responsible for the quality of their work. TQM, if correctly applied, extends to every single employee, from the chief executive to the trainee. It should be noted that systems of TQM can be applied with advantage to all areas of human activity.

TRANSPIRATION

The EVAPORATION of water from the leaves of a green plant. This process eliminates excess water from the plant, cools the leaves for maximum efficiency of PHOTOSYN-THESIS and assists the transport of water and dissolved nutrients from the root system to all other living parts of the plant.

TRANSVERSE WAVES

Waves, such as those of the sea, or of radiant energy, which travel in planes perpendicular to their direction of movement.

TRIANGLE TEST

A form of SENSORY test designed to reveal differences in the odours of standard and test samples of an aromatic material, perfume or flavour COMPOUND which may be very small yet important. Two smelling-strip dips of equal depth are taken from the test material, and one of the same depth from the standard, using strips inscribed with identification marks. The object of the test is to identify the strip smelling differently from the other two. The test is conducted by smelling the strips with their reference marks unseen, so that the tester is unaware of their identity. Since any given triangle test is highly subjective (*see* SUBJECTIVITY), it should be carried out by more than one person independently and the result discussed.

'TRICKLE DOWN' EFFECT

The diffusion of fragrance ideas originating in the FINE-FRAGRANCE sector of perfumery to the area of general perfumery and their appearance in mass-market products for domestic or personal care. Fragrance ideas may also 'trickle across' from one highly popular fragranced product to new products of the same or of a different kind. Very occasionally they even 'trickle up' as, for example, in the instance of a well-known fragrance initially appearing in a bath-time product being later refined and reintroduced as a fine fragrance for personal use.

TRIPLE BOND

A linkage between two ATOMS consisting of three bonding pairs of ELECTRONS.

UNSATURATED COMPOUND

A COMPOUND of which the MOLECULES each contain one or more double or triple bonds. (Cf. SATURATED COMPOUND).

VACUUM FRACTIONATION

FRACTIONAL DISTILLATION carried out in a vacuum to reduce the BOILING POINT of the charge to a temperature at which THERMAL STRESS will not occur.

VACUUM STRIPPING

Removal of the last traces of a VOLATILE substance, such as a solvent, from a product by EVAPORATION in a vacuum.

VALENCY

The combining power of an ATOM, ION or RADICAL.

VAPOUR

As usually employed, this term refers to a gas under such conditions that a small increase of pressure or decrease of temperature will cause it to condense, as water vapour condenses at the dew point.

VAPOUR PIPE

The pipe leading from the STILL HEAD to the condenser of a still.

VEGETABLE OIL

A nonVOLATILE oil, consisting largely of ESTERS of higher ALCOHOLS and higher CARBOXYLIC ACIDS, from a vegetable source such as sweet almonds, jojoba seeds or wheat germ. Most purified vegetable oils are faintly odorous from traces of volatiles they contain.

VIBRATIONAL THEORY

A theory of odour detection, recently (1996) advanced by Luca Turin, which suggests that odorous molecules stimulate odour-sensitive sites on the OLFACTORY HAIRS by their vibrations. This theory is subject to confirmation by further research as an alternative to the SITE-FITTING THEORY of Amoore.

VISCOSITY

The internal friction experienced by a liquid which opposes its tendency to flow freely.

'VITAL FORCE'

The hypothetical force which was held to exist only in living matter and which was believed to be necessary for the SYNTHESIS of ORGANIC COMPOUNDS. The idea of a 'vital force' was overthrown in 1845 by the German chemist Hermann Kolbe, who performed a total synthesis of acetic acid from its ELEMENTS.

VOLATILE

Descriptive of substances which evaporate when exposed to the air. Used also as a generic name for low boiling-point constituents of a natural source of aroma or flavour.

VOLATILITY

The speed or rate at which a substance evaporates. In perfumery, the concept of volatility leads to the classification of aromatic materials as TOP, middle or BASIC NOTES.

WATER DISTILLATION

A slow process of DISTILLATION in which aromatic plant material is kept in contact with boiling water for the purpose of volatilizing its ESSENTIAL OIL for subsequent CONDENSATION and collection. Only essential oils which resist THERMAL DECOMPO-SITION and the HYDROLYSIS of their constituents, such as Clove Bud Oil, can be produced successfully by water distillation.

WAVELENGTH

The distance between two successive crests or two successive troughs of a train of TRANSVERSE WAVES, or between two successive points of maximum compression or of maximum rarefaction in a train of LONGITUDINAL WAVES.

'WORM'

The coiled part of the VAPOUR PIPE of a STILL which is immersed in the cold water of the CONDENSER.

X-RAY DIFFRACTION

The scattering of X-rays by the ATOMS or IONS of a crystalline solid to form a pattern of luminous spots on a screen, from which the arrangement of the particles (ATOMS or IONS) forming the crystal may be deduced.

YLANG-YLANG

An expression in the Tagalog language of the Philippine Islands referring to something which nods and waves in the breeze, in the manner of the flowers of the Ylang-Ylang tree.

(z-)

Abbreviation for the German word *zusammen*, meaning 'together', and referring to the *cis-* form of a pair of geometrical isomers. [*See cis-/trans* ISOMERISM and also *(E-)*.]

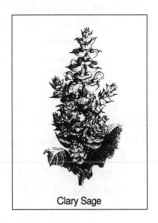

Clary Sage

Appendix

Books recommended for the further study of perfumery

Anonis, Danute Pajaujis. *Flower Oils and Floral Compounds in Perfumery.* Perfumer & Flavorist: Carol Stream, Illinois: 1993.

Calkin, Robert R., and J. Stephan Jellinek. Perfumery, Practice and Principles. John Wiley: New York, 1994.

Curtis, Tony, and David G. Williams. *Introduction to Perfumery.* Ellis Horwood: London, 1994.

Müller, P.M., and D. Lamparsky, eds. *Perfumes: Art, Science and Technology.* Elsevier Science: London, 1991.

Publications on essential oil safety

Tisserand, Robert, and Tony Balacs. *Essential Oil Safety: A Guide for Health Care Professionals.* Churchill Livingstone: Edinburgh, 1995.

Watt, Martin. *Plant Aromatics: A Data and Reference Manual — see p. 215.*

Courses in perfumery and cosmetic science

Plymouth Business School, University of Plymouth, Drake Circus, Plymouth
Devon PL4 8AA

        B.A. Hons degree in the Business of Perfumery
        Diploma and certificate courses in perfumery by distance learning
        Short courses on the Business of Perfumery

The London Institute, School of Fashion Promotion, London College of Fashion
20 John Princes Street, London W1M 0BJ

        Cert. H.E. in Cosmetic Science

Society of Cosmetic Scientists
   G.T. House, 24-26 Rothesay Road, Luton, Bedfordshire LU1 1QX
      Diploma in Cosmetic Science—in collaboration with the London Institute
      School of Fashion Promotion (*see above*). Facilities for distance learning are
      available.

Suppliers of aromatherapy oils

Eve Taylor (London) Limited
   9 Papyrus Road, Werrington Business Park, Werrington,
   Peterborough PE4 5BH
   [telephone: 01733-321101 and fax: 01733-321633]

Suppliers of molecular models

Molymod® 003 is particularly recommended. Details are available from:

Spiring Enterprises Limited
   Beke Hall, Billingshurst, West Sussex RH14 9HS

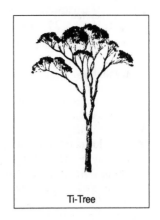

Ti-Tree

Index